Gerontology

Gerontology

Changes, Challenges, and Solutions

Volume 1: Social and Life Course Issues

Madonna Harrington Meyer and
Elizabeth A. Daniele, Editors

PRAEGER™

An Imprint of ABC-CLIO, LLC
Santa Barbara, California • Denver, Colorado

Library of Congress Cataloging-in-Publication Data

Names: Harrington Meyer, Madonna, 1959– , editor. | Daniele, Elizabeth A., editor
Title: Gerontology : changes, challenges, and solutions / Madonna Harrington Meyer, Elizabeth A. Daniele, editors.
Description: Santa Barbara, California : Praeger, 2016. | Includes bibliographical references and index.
Identifiers: LCCN 2015039168 | ISBN 9781440834264 (set) | ISBN: 978-1-4408-4491-1 (vol. 1) | ISBN: 978-1-4408-4492-8 (vol. 2) | ISBN: 978-1-4408-3427-1 (set : ebook)
Subjects: | MESH: Aging. | Geriatrics. | Aged.
Classification: LCC RC952.55 | NLM WT 100 | DDC 618.97—dc23
LC record available at http://lccn.loc.gov/2015039168

ISBN: 978-1-4408-3426-4 (set)
978-1-4408-4491-1 (vol 1)
978-1-4408-4492-8 (vol 2)
EISBN: 978-1-4408-3427-1

20 19 18 17 16 1 2 3 4 5

This book is also available on the World Wide Web as an eBook.
Visit www.abc-clio.com for details.

Praeger
An Imprint of ABC-CLIO, LLC

ABC-CLIO, LLC
130 Cremona Drive, P.O. Box 1911
Santa Barbara, California 93116-1911

This book is printed on acid-free paper ∞

Manufactured in the United States of America

To my family,
my greatest joy
M.H.M.

To my family,
my first teachers and greatest support
E.A.D.

Contents

Introduction

Madonna Harrington Meyer

Volume 1: Social and Life Course Issues

Like most other nations, the population of the United States is aging and, in the process, reshaping demographic, social, economic, and health trends. Currently there are about 40 million people, aged 65 and older, comprising 13 percent of the U.S. population. By 2030 there will be over 70 million, comprising 20 percent of the U.S. population (Ortman, Velkoff, & Hogan 2014; Aging Stats 2012). Even then, however, the United States will not catch up to many other aging nations. In 2015, for example, 26 percent of Japan's population was aged 65 or older. Thus the United States is aging, but in moderation compared with many other nations. Nonetheless, the share of the U.S. population that is aged 65 or older is growing steadily and will continue to do so for the foreseeable future. What will the impact be? Given our changing demographics and a wide variety of other sociodemographic trends, many challenges and opportunities lay ahead.

Aging of the U.S. population is linked largely to the aging of the baby boomers. As the largest generation in U.S. history, they have played an enormous role in shaping U.S. traditions, programs, and policies. Born in the victorious post–World War II era between 1946 and 1964, boomers peaked at nearly 79 million in 1999 (Fry 2015). In the earlier years, communities scrambled to accommodate the windfall of babies. Like many American schoolchildren during the 1960s, I spent my childhood in overcrowded classrooms located in annexes in school parking lots. Now baby boomers are entering old age, and communities are scrambling to accommodate the windfall of older Americans. The oldest among them are now aged 69, and the youngest are now aged 51. These growing legions of older Americans are becoming grandparents, working, volunteering, planning retirements, traveling, and, increasingly, skyping and using social media. But some are also becoming ill, less mobile, and disabled; even dying. By 2050, the boomer population will dwindle to less than 17 million. In their wake, the millennials, born between 1981 and 1997, will become the largest remaining generation (Fry 2015). In the decades to come, millennials are likely to play an enormous role in reshaping our aging society.

Understanding the impact of current old-age policies—and building new traditions, programs, or policies for the future—requires that we take the diversity of older Americans into account. At least 25 percent of people aged 65 and older have moderate to severe physical limitations, are widowed or divorced, have not completed high school, or are poor or near poor (Ortman, Velkoff, & Hogan 2014; Aging Stats 2012). Put differently, however, about 75 percent have good or excellent health, few if any physical limitations, are married, have completed high school, or report income substantially above the poverty line (Ortman, Velkoff, & Hogan 2014; Aging Stats 2012). The first group is not likely to have sufficiently good income and health to pursue comfortable lifestyles and leisure pursuits, while the second and much larger group most certainly will. Taken together these groups provide many challenges and opportunities that will reshape all aspects of American life.

The impact of an aging population depends on the impact of a multitude of other sociodemographic trends in the United States. The United States has undergone substantial transitions in recent decades, including the retreat from marriage, the rise of single parenting, increases in the proportion of working and in hours of work, rising education rates, increasing use of technology, growing inequality, retrenching welfare programs, declining savings, rising life expectancies, increasing disability rates, increasing race and ethnic diversity, increasing globalization, and increasing reliance on family members for care (see Harrington Meyer 2014). How these trends impact older people and their families, and how that impact varies by gender, race, class, and other key sociodemographic variables, is the subject of this two-volume set. Written by a mix of long-standing and emerging leaders in a broad array of disciplines, ***Gerontology: Changes, Challenges, and Solutions*** provides undergraduates, graduate students, scholars, professionals, and policy makers with an overview of the changing old-age landscape, as well as the key challenges and solutions in the field of aging.

Volume 1 focuses on socioeconomic disparities across the life course, linked to gender, race, ethnicity, immigration status, marital status, and other sociodemographic variables. These chapters demonstrate how millions reach old age having enjoyed a lifetime of cumulative advantages, including well-off parents, good schools, high-paying jobs, and multitudes of opportunities to develop a substantial nest egg for old age (Aging Stats 2012; Ferraro, Shippee, & Schafer 2009). They also demonstrate how millions reach old have having faced a lifetime of cumulative disadvantages, including poor or single parents, inadequate education, sporadic or lower-paying jobs, and fewer opportunities to accumulate a nest egg to protect themselves during old age (Aging Stats 2012; Ferraro, Shippee, & Schafer 2009). The authors analyze these disparities and examine how our traditions, programs, and policies both minimize and maximize inequality in old age.

Diversity among older Americans is evident in a comparison of the situations of Sarah and Jamica, both of whom I interviewed for my book, *Grandmothers at Work: Juggling Families and Jobs* (Harrington Meyer 2014). Sarah is a 67-year-old married, white, mother of two and grandmother of four. She and her husband both have PhDs, a household income in excess of $200,000 a year, private pensions, and substantial assets. When I asked Sarah about their economic situation she reported that they had a lot more resources than most their age, a lot more than they need, and had no worries about money during their old age. They are both in excellent health and live very active lifestyles. She told me that she travels, swims, plays tennis, golfs, bikes, hikes, and walks regularly. Now that she is retiring she is focusing on her favorite hobby, watercolor painting. At the time of the interview they were busy planning trips that would allow her to paint throughout Europe.

By contrast, Jamica is a 48-year-old divorced, black mother of four and grandmother of three. She went to college on and off but was never able to complete her nursing degree. She completed a mortuary science degree but was never able to put it to use. She held a variety of mostly part-time jobs and then, 25 years ago, began cleaning houses. She appreciated the flexible work hours, which allowed her to care for her young children, and, more recently, her young grandchildren. But the income is low and there are no benefits such as paid vacation, paid sick days, health insurance, or private pensions. Her household income is less than $40,000 a year. When asked about her economic situation she reported that she has less than she needs, a lot less than most her age, and as a result, she is worried about having enough money for her old age. "I have no money put away for my retirement. I cannot stop cleaning, I would not have income." Her car recently broke, so she has been walking to her cleaning jobs. At the time of the interview, she had just been to the doctor for the first time in eight years. "And I am behind on the dentist. I am more worried about getting physicals for the kids and the grandkids. I make choices. I do not have dental insurance. So do I let my 16-year-old son lose a tooth, or do I lose a tooth." While she loves to read, knit, and crochet, it has been six years since she has been able to find the time and money to travel to the southern United States to see her extended family.

Given the degree of inequality among the aged, and the sweeping sociodemographic changes that are underway, this is a unique moment in history. We are poised to make decisions that will impact not only those who are older today, but those who will be older in the years ahead. Old-age programs and policies can be strengthened or weakened. Inequalities among the aged can be fueled or quelled. To fully understand the dynamics of gerontology, experts from numerous disciplines should concentrate their attention on the causes, meanings, and implications of these sweeping changes. The chapters in this volume assess the life-course changes, challenges, and solutions that face our aging nation.

Overview of Chapters

The United States is an aging nation, but we are nowhere near the leaders. In Chapter 1, Janet Wilmoth locates U.S. sociodemographic patterns within worldwide patterns. She shows how some countries, mainly with greater economic and health parity than the United States, are already older than we ever expect to become, while other nations, mainly those plagued by economic, military, and health crises, may not age much at all. She concludes by reviewing the impacts of aging nations for families, health and health care, and economic productivity.

Why do some older people fare so much better than others? Over recent decades a wide variety of theories have emerged to explore the relationship between social factors and well-being in later life. In Chapter 2, Vern Bengtson and Marguerite DeLiema review and critique theories concerned with social stratification and the life course, social-psychological models of well-being, and interpretive or social constructionist perspectives on aging. They also discuss recent interdisciplinary perspectives on successful aging and the rise of micro- and midlevel theories. They conclude with a call for all scholars to pay greater attention to theories of aging.

If you are lucky enough to live long enough, you will most surely face age discrimination. You may have already practiced it, perhaps by avoiding a particular cash register because either the clerk, or the next customer, seemed too old. In Chapter 3, Meika Loe, Ariel Sherry, and Evan Chartier examine how ageism, a system of inequality that generally privileges the young at the expense of the old, is embedded in patterns of behavior and serves as a social organizing principle. The authors lay out the common definitions and stereotypes associated with ageism, the key social theories that help us to understand the causes of ageism, and the social and personal impacts of ageism. They conclude with strategies for countering ageism.

The U.S. old-age welfare state provides income and health security for the vast majority of older Americans, mainly through Social Security, Supplemental Security Income, Medicare, and Medicaid programs. These programs effectively pull millions above the poverty line each year. But access to, and the impact of, old-age programs varies by gender, race, ethnicity, age, SES, and marital status. In Chapter 4, Debra Street and Sarah Desai provide a brief history of each program; review eligibility, benefit, and funding mechanisms; and assess current policy issues, many of which are hotly contested. They conclude by discussing future directions for old-age policies in the context of changing demographic and political climates.

With age, demographic groups grow increasingly unequal in terms of virtually all socioeconomic measures. Across the life course, growing disparities in education, employment, income, wealth, health, and well-being are linked to key sociodemographic variables, particularly gender, race, and ethnicity. These variables shape well-being through virtually every life-course event from birth until death. In Chapter 5, Jan Mutchler and Ceara Somerville review the literature on inequalities linked to gender, race, and ethnicity, focusing on key examples including economic security, health and health-care access, and long-term care and care work. They conclude by evaluating solutions to these persistent challenges.

Poverty rates among the elderly are among the lowest they have ever been in U.S. history. But pockets of poverty persist. Roughly 40 percent of older black or Hispanic single women fall below the poverty line (Aging Stats 2012). In Chapter 6, Andrea Willson and Nicole Etherington use a life-course perspective to explore why some have so much, and some so little, in their old-age nest egg. They then focus on the relationship between socioeconomic status and health across the life course. They conclude with a discussion of the changing dynamics of income, poverty, wealth, and inequality in later life and challenges to its study.

Older people are remaining in the workforce longer than they have in decades. But employment rates vary by age, gender, race, ethnicity, and nativity. When workers decide to retire, retirement is increasingly a process rather than event. Instead of retiring on a specific date, many workers convert to part-time work, become consultants, or enter entirely new encore careers. In Chapter 7, Jeanette Zoeckler and Michael Silverstein characterize the demographics of the workforce. They evaluate the links between employment and health and well-being, consider key accommodations for older workers, and explore the incentives, and disincentives, of accommodation for employers. Finally they describe the factors that shape retirement decisions and retirement satisfaction.

One group of older persons that many scholars and policy makers tend to overlook are aging veterans. Over the next few decades, older veterans will largely consist of those who served in Vietnam. In Chapter 8, Andrew London employs a cumulative inequality approach to explore the lifelong impact of military service by age, gender, race, and ethnicity. He describes the Vietnam-era veteran population; reviews the life-course literature on Vietnam-era military service and socioeconomic, marriage/family, and health outcomes; and analyzes the 2009 American Community Survey data that compares Vietnam-era nonveterans, veterans with no service-connected disability, and veterans with service-connected disability on a range of life-course outcomes in late midlife. He concludes by discussing the implications, challenges, and directions for future research.

Immigration to the United States is steadily increasing. In Chapter 9, Ynesse Abdul-Malak and Rebecca Wang review the reasons why people migrate and the impact over the life course. Though historically most immigrants arrive during working-age years, in recent decades we have seen a substantial growth of immigrants arriving in later life. Using key theoretical perspectives, they analyze immigrants' socioeconomic circumstances and health outcomes, revealing substantial economic and health disparities between various groups of immigrants. They conclude by analyzing the capacity of U.S. social programs to alleviate those disparities.

As in many other nations, marriage has been on the decline in the United States for decades. Many are married for only short periods or skip marriage altogether. Living arrangements have become decidedly more complex. In Chapter 10, Judith Treas and Tanya Sanabria analyze family and household formation across the life course and reveal a wide variety of pathways. They analyze how partnerships have been redefined by cohabitation and same-sex marriage—and demonstrate how institutional living arrangements such as prisons and nursing homes have reshaped our understanding of living arrangements. They pay careful attention to how gender, socioeconomic status, race, and ethnicity shape living arrangements and the impacts on well-being for individuals and families.

Grandparenting is a particularly important role in middle and older ages for many, but certainly not all. By age 50, one-half of Americans are grandparents. While some have little regular contact with their grandchildren, many provide tremendous amounts of care and financial support. A small percent become custodial grandparents, raising their grandchildren in the absence of parents. In Chapter 11, Bert Hayslip and Heidemarie Blumenthal take a life span approach to exploring the grandparent-grandchild dyad. They examine how sociohistorical and cultural changes, combined with socioeconomic disparities, shape the experience for all generations. They look carefully at how grandparents pitch in during hard times, including divorce, sickness, disability, or death. They conclude with directions for future research that will take into account the dynamic nature of the grandparent-grandchild dyad.

As the number and proportion of older people change, so does their political clout. But not always in the ways you might expect. In Chapter 12,

Robert Hudson reveals how, after several decades of growing slowly and accompanied by little controversy, aging policies have more recently expanded dramatically and have yielded more highly charged politics. Will older voters—or younger voters—support old-age programs? He takes us on a historical journey ranging from the New Deal to the present, analyzing changes in political standing, presence in Washington, D.C., and constraints on old-age policies. He describes periods of expansion, retrenchment, and conflict, and concludes with a discussion of what may be in store for the future.

The chapters in this volume reveal changing trends, and enormous variation, in what it means to be an aging person in an aging country. They help us to understand why some face so many more challenges with so many fewer resources in the later years and what we, as a society, may, or may not, decide to do about those disparities.

References

Aging Stats. (2012). Older Americans 2012. Washington, DC: Federal Interagency Forum on Aging-Related Statistics. http://www.agingstats.gov/Main_Site/Data/2012

Ferraro, K. F., Shippee, T. P., & Schafer, M. H. (2009). Cumulative inequality theory for research on aging and the life course. In V. L. Bengtson, D. Gans, N. M. Putney, & M. Silverstein (Eds.), *Handbook of theories of aging* (2nd ed., pp. 413–433). Springer: New York.

Fry, Richard. (2015). This year Millennials will overtake Baby Boomers. January 16, 2015. PEW Research Center. http://www.pewresearch.org/fact-tank/2015/01/16/this-year-millennials-will-overtake-baby-boomers/

Harrington Meyer, Madonna. (2014). *Grandmothers at work: Juggling families and jobs*. New York: NYU Press.

Ortman, J. M., Velkoff, Victoria A., & Hogan, Howard. (2014). An aging nation: The older population in the U.S. U.S. Census Bureau. https://www.census.gov/prod/2014pubs/p25–1140.pdf

CHAPTER ONE

Demographic Perspectives on Global Population Aging

Janet M. Wilmoth

Demographers are trained to be attentive to age given fertility, mortality, and migration among human populations are inherently age-based. However, the demography of aging did not emerge as a distinct subfield until the second half of the twentieth century, when low fertility and mortality rates were creating dramatic shifts in the age structure of developed countries (Wilmoth and Simpson 2013). Demographers studying aging are concerned with documenting changes in age structures and understanding cohort flow, identifying trends in mortality, morbidity, and disability, making connections between cellular/physiological processes and demographic processes, explaining the geographic distribution and migration of older adults, exploring living arrangements, care provision and retirement trends, and considering the economic and policy implications of population aging (Siegel 1980; Hardy and Skirbekk 2012; Schoeni and Ofstedal 2010; Uhlenberg 2009).

Much of what is known about population aging is based on national-level data collected by periodic censuses, vital statistics registries, and cross-sectional surveys, all of which provide information about individuals at one point in time. Consequently, our empirical understanding of variation in the aging across countries is primarily descriptive. But over the past 25 years there has been a concerted effort among social scientists to develop comparable, high-quality, nationally representative longitudinal surveys that track individuals as they age. These surveys, which were initially deployed in developed countries like the United States, Germany, and Sweden, have now been launched in over 30 countries and more are under development. Consequently, our understanding of population aging is becoming more nuanced over time. This chapter provides an overview of what we know about aging from a demographic perspective, including variation in the rate of population aging, the factors contributing to the growth of the older adult population, the characteristics of the older adult population, the implications of shifting age structures for families, health and health care, and economic productivity, and ongoing advancements in survey research that inform our understanding of population aging. The focus is on highlighting global trends, with an emphasis on regional variation. Select country-specific examples are provided to demonstrate variation in population aging.

Global Population Aging

The rate of growth in the number and proportion of adults aged 60 and older has increased steadily across all regions of the world over the past 75 years. As shown in Figure 1.1, the total number of people aged 60 and older increased from 130 million in 1950 to more than 809 million in 2012 and is projected to be over 2 trillion by 2050 (Rowland 2009; United Nations 2012).[1] Currently Asia and Europe have the largest number of people aged 60 and older, but Asia will experience more growth in the number of older adults over the next 45 years than other regions.

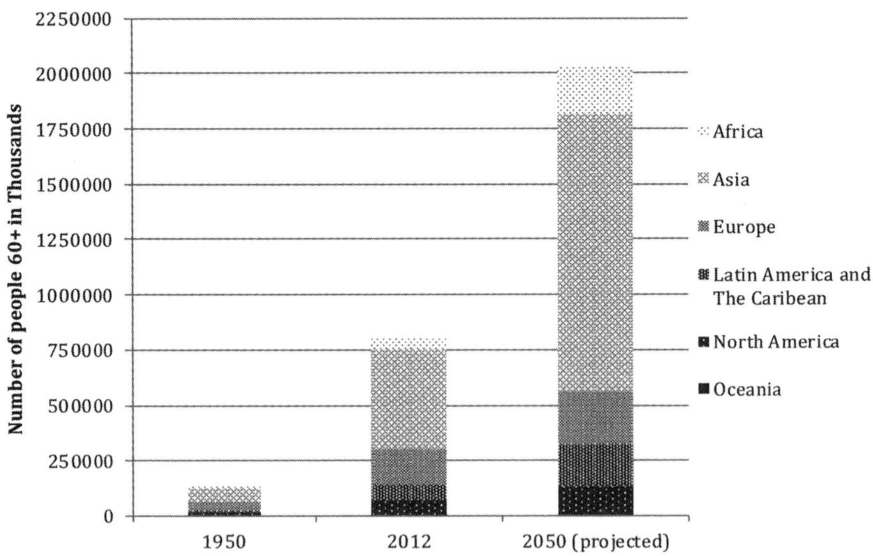

Figure 1.1 Population aged 60 years and over, total and by region, 1950, 2012, and 2050. (Data from Rowland [2009] and United Nations [2012])

Most countries within Africa have relatively small older adult populations, although many are growing at a rapid rate. Nigeria has the largest number of older adults, with nearly 9 million in 2012 and nearly 29 million expected in 2050. Egypt and Ethiopia also have relatively large older adult populations, with 7 million and 4 million respectively in 2012 and nearly 25 million and 17 million respectively expected in 2050.

The number of older adults in Latin American and Caribbean countries is relatively low but expected to grow rapidly over the next 45 years. This growth is exemplified most dramatically by Brazil, which had over 21 million older adults in 2012 but is expected to have nearly 65 million in 2050. Mexico also has a relatively large older adult population that is expected to grow from 11 million in 2012 to 37 million in 2050.

Within Asia, China and India have the largest share of older adults because both countries have the largest populations in the region. China and India currently have over 180 million and 100 million older adults, which is expected to increase to over 439 and 323 million in 2050, respectively. Japan also has a large number of older adults, almost 40 million in 2012, but that population is only expected to increase to 45 million by 2050. Rates of growth among the older adult population is also substantial in Bangladesh, which is expected to increase from 10 million in 2012 to 43 million in 2050, and in Indonesia, which is expected to increase from 20 million to nearly 75 million.

The size of the older adult population is relatively small in the countries of Oceania given many are island nations. Australia has the largest older adult population in the region, with 4 million in 2012 and a projected increase to 9 million in 2050. Within North America, the United States has 60 million older adults, which is expected to increase to 107 million by 2025. The older adult population in Canada is considerably smaller given the size of that country's population. Canada has 7 million older adults, which is expected to increase to over 13 million by 2050.

Several European countries with relatively large total populations also have high numbers of older adults. But the rate of growth over the next 45 years among older adults will be slower in European countries than Asian countries. For example, the Russian Federation has the largest number of older adults in Europe—26 million in 2012 and 39 million in 2050, followed by Germany—21 million in 2012 and 28 million in 2050, and Italy—16 million in 2012 and 22 million in 2050.

Although it is important to consider the number of older adults in a given country, the proportion of the population that is aged 60 and older is another relevant indicator of population aging. As shown in Figure 1.2, the percentage of older adults varies substantially across regions but has been systematically increasing over time for all regions.

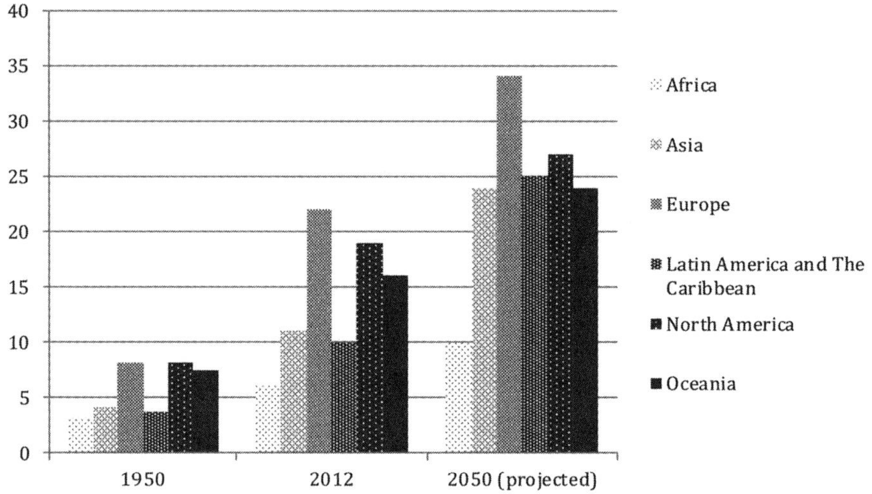

Figure 1.2 Percentage of the total population aged 60 years and over by region, 1950, 2012, and 2050. (Data from Rowland [2009] and United Nations [2012])

The region with the smallest percentage of older adults is Africa: approximately 3, 6, and 10 percent in 1950, 2012, and 2050, respectively. However, these percentages for the region mask substantial growth in the proportion of older adults in some countries. For example, 12 percent of the population was aged 60 and older in Mauritius and Reunion in 2012, and the percentage is expected to climb to 29 percent and 26 percent, respectively, by 2050. Tunisia is similar with 7 percent of the population being aged 60 and older in 2012 and an expected increase to 26 percent by 2050. Although Nigeria has a large number of older adults, their portion of the population is relatively low—5 percent in 2012 and 7 percent in 2050. The percentages in Ethiopia are similar—5 percent in 2012 and 12 percent in 2050. But Egypt is expected to have more of an increase—from 8 percent in 2012 to 20 percent in 2050.

The percentage of older adults in the Latin American and Caribbean region was slightly below 4 percent in 1950 but has been increasing more rapidly to 10 percent in 2012 and 25 percent in 2050. The countries with the highest proportions of older adults in that region are Martinique, Uruguay, Cuba, Guadeloupe, and Puerto Rico with 21, 19, 18, 18, and 18 percent of their respective populations aged 60 and older in 2012. Each of these countries is expected to have more than one-fourth to one-third of their population aged 60 and older by 2050. Brazil and Mexico, both of which are expecting large increases in the number of older adults, are also expecting dramatic increases in the percentage of the population aged 60 and older. The older adult portion was 11 percent of Brazil's population in 2012 but will be 29 percent by 2050. Similarly, the older adult population was 10 percent of Mexico's population in 2012 but will be 26 percent by 2050.

The Asian region has experienced a similar pattern of growth in the proportion of older adults in the population. Only 4 percent of the population in Asia was aged 60 and older in 1950 but that grew to 11 percent in 2012 and is expected to be 24 percent in 2050. This region is characterized by substantial differences across countries. The country with the highest proportion of older adults is Japan, with 32 percent of the population being aged 60 and older in 2012, which is expected to be 41 percent by 2050. In contrast, only 4 percent of the population in Afghanistan was aged 60 and older in 2012, and that is expected to increase to only 7 percent by 2050. Comparable percentages for Iraq are 5 percent in 2012 and 10 percent in 2050. There are numerous countries in the region that currently have a relatively low percentage of older adults but are expected to experience substantial increases in that percentage over the next 45 years. For example, among the Asian countries expecting large numerical increases in the older adult population—China, India, Bangladesh, and Indonesia—the percentages will increase from 13, 8, 7 and 9 percent in 2012 to 24, 19, 22, and 25 percent in 2050, respectively.

The countries in Oceania have a slightly larger percentage of older adults than Asia: over 7 percent in 1950, which increased to 16 percent in 2012 and 24 percent in 2050. However, there is substantial variation across this region also. The countries with the highest proportion of older adults in the region are Australia and New Zealand, which had 20 percent and 19 percent, respectively, in 2012, and both are expected to increase to 29 percent by 2050. Some island nations in the region will experience substantial change in the percentage of the population aged 60 and older, such as French Polynesia in which it will increase from 10 percent to 27 percent. Other island nations will continue to have a relatively low percentage of older adults, such as Papua New Guinea in which it will increase from 5 percent to 11 percent.

North America is similar to Oceania: 8.2 percent of the population was older adults in 1950, which increased to 19 percent in 2012 and is expected to increase to 27 percent in 2025. In North America, the United States has a slightly lower percentage of older adults compared to Canada—19 percent versus 21 percent in 2012 and 27 percent versus 31 percent expected in 2050.

Europe is similar to North America in the uniformity of the population that is aged 60 and older. Europe's population aged 60 and older which was 8.2 percent in 1950, increased to 22 percent in 2012, and is expected to be 24 percent in 2050. Almost all the countries in this region currently have one-fifth to one-fourth of their populations aged 60 and older, and all of them will be near or above one-third by 2050. Albania, has the smallest proportion of older adults in the region; the percentage of the population age 60 and older was 14 percent in 2012 and is expected to increase to 34 percent by 2050. The countries with the largest numbers of older adults—Russia, Germany, and Italy—are currently at 17, 27, and 27 percent, respectively, and are projected to be at 31 percent, 37 percent, and 38 percent, respectively, by 2050.

Why Do Populations Age?

The process of population aging in the developed countries of western Europe was initially described by the Demographic Transition Theory, which states that fertility and mortality rates change predictably in response to economic development (Teitelbaum 1975). According to this theory, countries move through several distinct phases (see Figure 1.3).

During the pretransition phase, fertility rates are high and stable while mortality rates are high but fluctuating and life expectancy at birth is low. Consequently, the pyramid-shaped age structure of the population is young

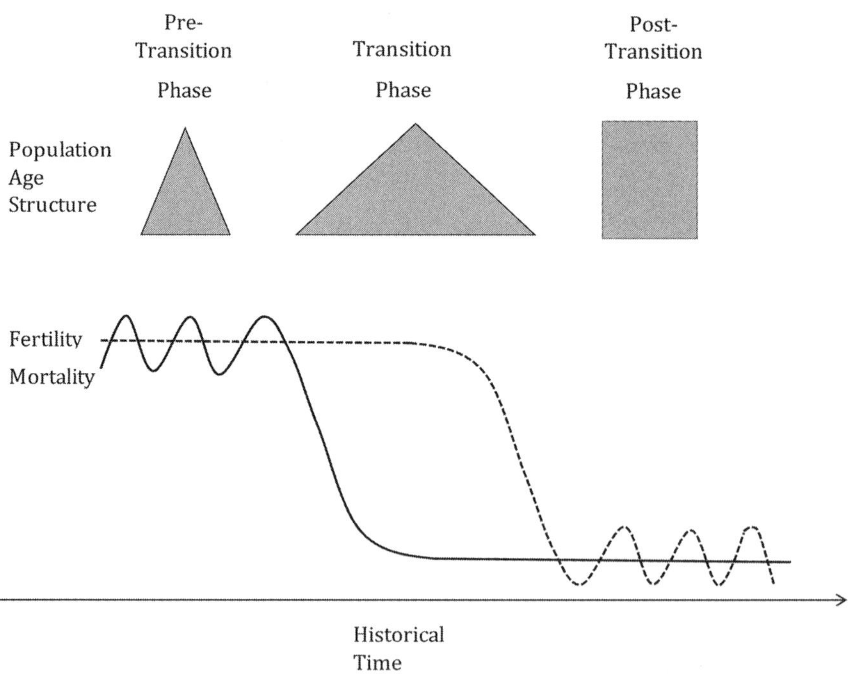

Figure 1.3 Stages of the demographic transition.

and relatively stable, as the number of births replenishes the population that has died at relatively young ages. During this stage the percentage of older adults in the population is very low. In the early parts of the transition stage, mortality rates begin to decline, particularly mortality due to infectious disease among infants, children, and childbearing-aged women, in response to improved sanitation. Life expectancy at birth begins to increase. Drops in fertility rates typically lag behind improvements in mortality, resulting in population growth. The age structure of the population becomes younger as more children survive to reproductive ages. Later during the transition stage, fertility rates continue to decline and eventually reach replacement levels of 2.1 children per woman. Mortality rates also continue to decline but at a slower rate. The population continues to grow, and the age structure remains relatively young. The population does not begin to age dramatically until the posttransition stage, when fertility rates remain at or below replacement level and mortality rates, due to man-made and degenerative diseases, decline. Life expectancy at birth and at age 65 continues to increase. The age structure of the population becomes more rectangle shaped, as each successive cohort essentially replaces itself, and the proportion of the population that survives into advanced ages increases. The original formulations of this theory predicted that the percentage of older adults in the population would peak at 20 percent during the posttransition phase, although many countries have exceeded, or are projected to exceed, this expectation.

This general pattern of demographic change occurred slowly in most developed countries as the industrial revolution spurred economic development and improvements in the standard of living. Consequently, developed countries have experienced a gradual increase in the proportion of the older adult population during the latter part of the twentieth century. For example, the percentage of the population aged 65 and older doubled from 7 percent to 14 percent in France over a 115-year period, from 1865 to 1980, and in the United States over a 69-year period, from 1944 to 2013 (Kinsella and He 2009). However, the classic demographic transition model does not adequately describe the experience of developed countries, many of which experienced more closely timed declines in fertility and mortality that occurred over a shorter period of time. As a result, developing countries are experiencing population aging at a much faster rate than developed countries. For example, the doubling of the percentage of the population aged 65 and older from 7 percent to 14 percent is expected to take 21 years, from 2011 to 2032, in Brazil and 26 years, from 2000 to 2026, in China (Kinsella and He 2009).

Furthermore, fertility and mortality rates have not reached equilibrium as expected; fertility declines have outpaced mortality declines. Consequently, some nations—particularly in Europe—have very low, and in some cases negative, annual population growth rates (Population Reference Bureau 2014). This contributes to the aging of the population because, as cohorts fail to fully replace themselves through fertility, the age structure shifts more toward older ages and the median age of the population increases substantially. The median age of the global population is currently 29.2 (United Nations 2013a), with the highest median ages being in Japan, 46, and European countries such as Germany, 46, and Italy, 45 (United States Central Intelligence Agency 2015). Therefore, while Demographic Transition Theory provides a general framework for understanding how fertility and mortality change with economic development, it does not adequately account for the unprecedented levels of worldwide population aging during the twenty-first century.

Characteristics of the Older Adult Population

Not only is the global population growing older, but the older adult population itself is also aging as mortality rates in later life continue to improve and more people survive to advanced ages. Only 7 percent of the population aged 60 and older was aged 80 or older in 1950, but by 2013 it had increased to 14 percent, which represents over 120 million people (United Nations 2013a; 2013c). The five countries with the largest percentage of the older adult population aged 80 or older in 2012 were France, 24 percent, Italy, 23 percent, Spain, 23 percent, Belgium, 22 percent, and Japan, 22 percent, whereas the countries with the largest number of adults aged 80 or older were China, 23 million, the United States, 12 million, India, 10 million, Japan, 9 million, and Germany, 4 million (United Nations 2012).

Due to gender differences in late-life mortality, which produce longer life expectancies at age 60 for women in every country, the ratio of men to women in later life is unbalanced. In 2012, worldwide there were 84 men per 100 women aged 60 and older (United Nations 2012). Countries with the most unbalanced later-life sex ratios below 60 men per 100 women are primarily in Eastern and Northern Europe, such as Belarus, Ukraine, Russian Federation, Estonia, Latvia, and Lithuania, which reflects the legacy of World War II on mortality among cohorts born in the early twentieth century. But older men outnumber older women in some countries in Africa, such as Western Sahara, Cote d'Ivorie, and Gambia, in South-Central Asia, such as Bhutan, Iran, Maldives, and Pakistan, and in Western Asia, such as Bahrain, Jordon, Kuwait, Oman, Qatar, Saudi Arabia, and the United Arab Emirates, where maternal mortality rates and gender-based migration patterns likely contribute to later-life sex imbalances.

Although it is challenging to make cross-national comparisons across a wide range of sociodemographic characteristics due to a lack of comparable data, measures of marital status, living arrangements, and labor-force participation tend to be consistently measured across surveys. Figure 1.4 presents those characteristics for the population aged 60 and over across regions separately for men and women.[2]

In every country, older men are more likely to be married than older women (United Nations 2012). Approximately four-fifths of older men are married, although the proportion is higher in Africa, 82 percent, and Asia, 82 percent, than Europe, 77 percent, North America, 75 percent, Latin America and the Caribbean, 74 percent, and Oceania, 73 percent. The variation across countries in the percentage of older men who are married is substantial, with a range of 95 percent in Senegal to a low of 46 percent in French Guiana. Only 50 percent of older women are married, with the highest percentages being in Asia, 51 percent, Africa, 50 percent, and Oceania, 50 percent, and the lowest percentages being North America, 48 percent, Europe, 45 percent, and Latin America and the Caribbean, 42 percent. The percentage of older women who are married is highest in Nepal, 71 percent and lowest in Chad, 16 percent. It is noteworthy that many countries with relatively high percentages of married older men have relatively low percentages of married older women.

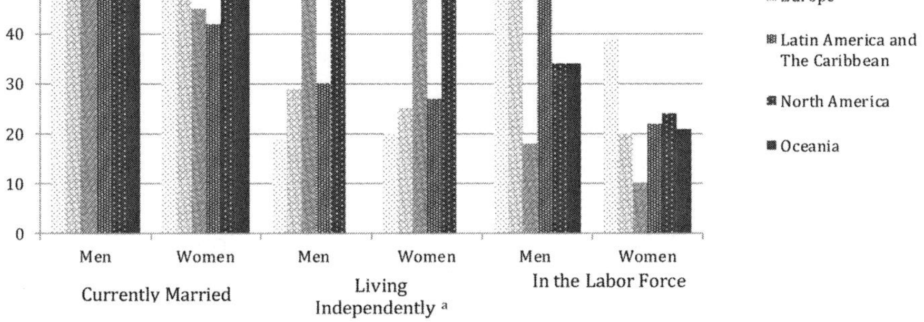

[a] Includes living alone or with spouse only. Data from Oceania are not available.

Figure 1.4 Select sociodemographic characteristics of the population aged 60 and older by region. (Data from United Nations [2012])

For example, in the United Arab Emirates 93 percent of older men are married compared to 31 percent of older women and the comparable percentages in Bangladesh are 91 percent and 28 percent, respectively. Also, the difference in marriage rates between older men and women within a given country is rarely less than 20 percent. These percentages are closest in Iceland, where 68 percent of older men are married and 52 percent of older women are married.

Independent living among older adults, which includes living with a spouse only or alone, is closely related to economic development. In developed countries older adults often have access to more economic resources that enable independent living. In addition, older adults in these countries tend to have fewer children with whom they can live given lower fertility rates and migration patterns that draw younger adults into urban areas within their own country and abroad. Given this, the highest rates of independent living among older adults are in regions with the most developed countries, in particular North America and Europe, where approximately three-fourths live with a spouse only or alone (United Nations 2012). Within these two regions, the countries with the highest rates of independent living among older adults are Denmark, Sweden, and Belgium, where over 95 percent of older men and women live with a spouse only or alone. In contrast, the lowest rates of independent living are in Africa, which are approximately one-fifth for men and women, Asia, which are approximately one-quarter for men and women, and Latin America and the Caribbean, which are less than one-third for men and women. Within these regions, the countries with the lowest rates of independent living among older adults are Senegal, Sierra Leone, Bahrain, and Bangladesh, where less than 10 percent of older men and women live with a spouse only or alone. It is important to note that, given the previously discussed gender differences in marriage, older men living independently are more likely to be living with a spouse only whereas older women living independently are more likely to be living alone.

Globally, older men are more likely to be in the labor force than older women (United Nations 2012). Rates of labor-force participation are high among older men living in Africa, 60 percent, Latin America and the Caribbean, 49 percent, and Asia, 48 percent, moderate among men living in North America and Oceania, 34 percent, and low in Europe, 18 percent. But these regions' rates mask substantial country variation. For example, within Africa, 95 percent of older men in Malawi are in the labor force compared to 11 percent in Reunion, and within Europe, the older male labor-force participation rate is highest in Iceland, 47 percent, and lowest in France, 8 percent. Rates of labor-force participation among older women are relatively high in Africa, 39 percent, moderate in Asia, Latin

America and the Caribbean, North America, and Oceania, approximately 20 percent, and low in Europe, 10 percent. Similar to the older male rates, there is substantial variation among the older female rates within regions. For example, within Africa older female labor-force participation is 89 percent in Malawi and 2 percent in Algeria, and within Europe it is 33 percent in Iceland and 3 percent in Malta. These differences across countries are due to variation in economic conditions, statutory retirement ages, historical labor-force participation rates among working-aged adults, and cultural norms regarding employment among women and older adults.

Implications of Population Aging

The demographic characteristics of the older adult population discussed in the previous section set the stage for considering the implications of population aging for families, health and health care, and economic productivity. The following discussion highlights some of the relevant demographic issues in each of these areas.

Families. The aging of the population has been accompanied by substantial shifts in family structure that have altered older adults' informal support networks. As life expectancies have improved, four- and five-generation families have become more common which has increased the number of elders within a family who might need care. At the same time, lower fertility rates have reduced the size of younger generations, including the pool of potential adult child caregivers. But these changes in family structure have not necessarily reduced the level of support given to older adults from family members (Knodel et al., 1992; Tomassini and Wolf 2000). Families continue to meet older adults' needs by coordinating care across members in a given generation and relying on skip-generation care arrangements in which, for example, grandchildren provide care to grandparents. In addition, improvements in life expectancy mean that more spouses and siblings are available to provide support to older adults in need of assistance (Redfoot and Pandya 2002; Tomassini et al., 2004; Miner and Uhlenberg 2004).

Despite migration patterns that tend to encourage the movement of young adults away from their family of origin, most older adults in developed countries have family members in relatively close proximity and interact with them on a regular basis, which provides a potential network from which support can be obtained. In the United States approximately three-fourths of older adults live within an hour of their children (Silverstein 1995) and the majority of U.S. older adults see at least one of their children at least once a week (Crimmins and Ingegneri 1990). Over half of U.S. older adults live within 25 miles of at least one sibling, and they are most likely to receive support from these proximate siblings when spouses and children are not available (Miner and Uhlenberg 2004). A study of 10 European countries indicated that 85 percent of parents have a child within 25 kilometers, and 90 percent are in contact with a child at least once a week, although proximity and contact rates tend to be lower among northern Europeans than southern Europeans (Hank 2007). As previously discussed, rates of coresidence between older adults and family members are higher in developing countries than developed countries, which suggests support networks are readily accessible. Research suggests that older adults in developing countries who live independently have access to proximate children and other relatives who provide support (Knodel and Ofstedal 2003). However, rural elders in developing countries are at risk of having unmet care needs given that younger generations may have migrated to urban areas for employment and formal supports are often not available.

Access to potential caregivers is undermined by childlessness, which has been increasing across cohorts in many countries. Approximately 6 percent of women aged 40–44 are childless worldwide, with childlessness rates being particularly high in Austria, 23 percent, the United Kingdom, 20 percent, Finland, 20 percent, Bahrain, 20 percent, and Canada, 19 percent (United Nations 2013b). In addition, the rate of childlessness is increasing across recent cohorts in some countries (Dykstra 2009). For example, in Germany less than 10 percent of women born in the mid-1930s were childless compared to over 25 percent of women born in the late 1950s, and comparable rates across cohorts over the same time period in the United States were approximately 11 percent and 19 percent (United Nations 2003). Childless older adults are more likely to live alone or in an institution and have lower levels of overall social contact (Koropeckyj-Cox and Vaughn 2007; Grundy and Read 2012). This suggests childless older adults are not able to compensate for the lack of child caregivers by expanding their social networks and therefore are at risk of needing formal care services.

Health and Health Care. As previously mentioned, the aging of the population is associated with improvements in life expectancy. Global life expectancy at birth is currently 70 years and is expected to increase to nearly 76 years by 2050. Those who survive to age 65 can expect to live 16 years currently and 18 years by 2050 (United Nations 2013a). There has been debate whether longer life is associated with a compression of morbidity (Fries 1982), in which added years are lived in good health and disability-free, or an expansion of morbidity, in which added years are lived in poor health with disability (Gruenberg 1977; Olshansky et al., 1991). Recently, there has been growing evidence for dynamic equilibrium

(Manton 1982) in which the prevalence of chronic diseases increases, but the rate of chronic disease progression slows such that a larger portion of the population experiences low levels of disability for a longer period of their lives (Laditka and Laditka 2009).

Given that chronic conditions often lead to disablement that requires personal assistance with instrumental and physical activities of daily living, countries worldwide need to prepare for the long-term care needs of their aging populations. Difficult choices about the appropriate balance of support provided by families, the public sector, and the private sector will have to be made that may require some combination of expanding support to family caregivers, developing additional community-based programs, and increasing access to assisted living and skilled nursing care facilities. Long-term care provision will be particularly essential to the growing number of older adults with dementia. The global number of people with dementia is projected to increase from nearly 36 million in 2010 to more than 115 million in 2050, with more rapid increases in low- and middle-income countries than high-income countries (Alzheimer's Disease International 2010).

Chronic conditions and other noncommunicable diseases are the main cause of death among older adults; globally among adults aged 60 and older, 85 percent die from a noncommunicable disease, 11 percent die from communicable diseases, and 4 percent die from injuries (United Nations 2013c). Thus, as the population ages, more attention has to be paid to preventing, delaying, and slowing the progression of noncommunicable diseases. Health-care providers also have to be increasingly prepared to meet the end-of-life needs of older adults. As populations age, the distribution of deaths shifts to older ages such that the majority of deaths occur among adults aged 60 and older. For example, globally 27 percent of deaths were among adults aged 60 and older in 1950–1955, but by 2005–2010 it was 60 percent, with regional percentages of 82 percent for North America, 81 percent for Europe, 73 percent in Oceania, 64 percent in Asia, 61 percent in Latin America and the Caribbean, and 27 percent in Africa (United Nations 2013c).

Given that medical costs associated with the treatment of noncommunicable diseases and end-of-life care are high, increases in the proportion of the older adult population in need of these services raises concerns about rising health-care expenditures. Health-care expenditures are higher among older adults. For example, in the United States per capita spending on health care in 2010 was $8,370 for ages 45–64, $15,857 for ages 65–84, and $34,783 for ages 85 and older (Centers for Medicare and Medicaid Services 2014). However, the United States is an outlier in health-care spending, and overall in high-income Organization for Economic Cooperation and Development (OECD) countries there is little correlation between

GDP spent on health care and the percentage of the population that is aged 65 and older. Crystal and Siegel (2009, p. 628) concluded that ". . . the crisis of 'sustainability' of health benefits for the elderly has more do to with the internationally idiosyncratic and remarkably inefficient structure of U.S. health-care financing and delivery systems than with the coming aging of the population." Thus, population aging does not necessarily translate into unmanageable health-care costs.

Economic Productivity. Most discussions about the economic implications of population aging are situated in a discussion of old-age dependency ratios and old-age support ratios. Both these ratios measure the relative size of the older adult population that is potentially in need of support to the working-aged population that generates tax revenue that finances old-age programs and serves as a pool of potential care workers. The old-age dependency ratio, which represents the number of adults aged 65 and older per 100 working-aged adults between the ages of 15 to 64, is expected to increase from 12 in 2013 to almost 25 in 2050. Over that same time period the old-age support ratio, which is number of working-aged adults per older person, will decrease from approximately 8 to 4 (United Nations 2013a). As shown in Figure 1.5, every region is expected to experience declines in the old-age support ratio, but by 2050 the absolute level will be lowest in Europe, which will only have two working-aged adults for every older adult.

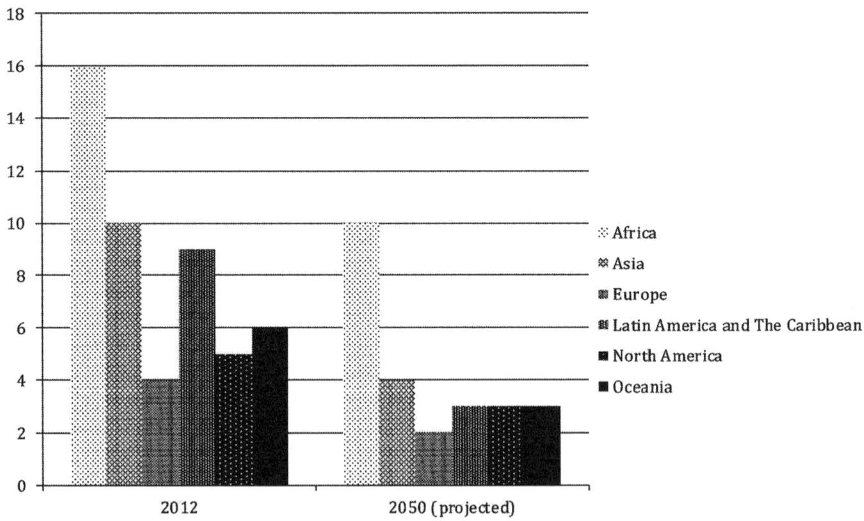

[a] The old-age support ratio represents the number of adults ages 15 to 64 per adult ages 65 and older.

Figure 1.5 Old-age support ratio by region, 2013 and 2050 (a) (United Nations [2012])

Although there is widespread concern that global population aging will lower economic growth due to expected increases in public debt, labor shortages, and lower rates of saving and investment (England 2002; Hateley and Tan 2003), these fears may be unfounded. The specific mechanisms through which population aging affects economic growth are rarely explicated (Mullan 2000) and there is no historical evidence that population aging slowed economic growth in developed nations (Easterlin 1991; Mullan 2000). Further, a United Nations report concluded that "worries that ageing populations and ageing workforces will lead to acute declines in economic growth appear unfounded" (United Nations 2007, p. 84). In addition, a National Research Council panel concluded there is "ample reason to believe that nations will be able to cope with current and projected demographic changes provided policy makers have access to information about the emerging economic and social forces that will shape future society well-being" (National Research Council 2001, p.17).

Improving Our Understanding of Population Aging through Survey Research

Planning for population aging requires high-quality, population representative data. While almost all nations collect demographic data through periodic censuses, which provides basic information about the size and characteristics of the older adult population, there is substantial variation across countries in the availability of national registries of vital statistics or detailed survey data based on representative samples of older adults. For more than 25 years, many developed countries have initiated a series of increasingly sophisticated longitudinal data collections that have yielded substantial insight into the aging process. Most notable among these is the Health and Retirement Study and its associated family of "sister studies," which are listed in Table 1.1.

These studies contain relatively comparable longitudinal measures of demographic characteristics, health conditions and physical functioning, cognition, health-care utilization, employment and retirement, income and wealth, family structure, and intergenerational exchanges from middle-aged and older adults in various developed and developing countries. Increasingly, researchers are interested in harmonizing these HRS "sister studies," as exemplified by the "Gateway to Global Aging Data" that is available at https://g2aging.org/, and evaluating the reproducibility of results based on various samples of older adults, such as the work being done with the "Integrative Analysis of Longitudinal Studies on Aging" that is explained in more detail at http://www.ialsa.org/. Collectively, these efforts are laying a foundation that will substantially advance our

Table 1.1 International "Sister Studies" of the Health and Retirement Study

Data Set Name	Study Waves	Sample Ages	Notes
Health and Retirement Study(HRS)	1992, 1993, 1994, 1995, 1996, 1998, 2000, 2002, 2004, 2006, 2008, 2010, 2012	50 and older	United States
The Brazilian Longitudinal Study of Aging (ELSI-BRASIL)			Under development as a HRS sister study. Data was collected from respondents aged 35–37 in 2008–2010 and 2012–2013 in the "Brazilian Longitudinal Study of Adult Health."
Canadian Longitudinal Study of Aging			Under development as a HRS sister study. Data collection from respondents aged 45 and older began in 2010.
Costa Rican Longevity and Healthy Aging Study – Pre-1945 cohort – 1945–1955 cohort	2005, 2007, 2009 2010, 2012	60 and older 55 and older	
The China Health Aging and Retirement Longitudinal Study (CHARLS)	2011, 2013	45 and older	
English Longitudinal Study of Ageing (ELSA)	2002, 2004, 2006, 2008, 2010, 2012	50 and older	

Data Set Name	Study Waves	Sample Ages	Notes
Health and Aging in Africa: Longitudinal Studies in Three INDEPTH Communities (HAALSI)			Under development as a HRS sister study. Data collection from respondents aged 40 and older living in South Africa was initiated in 2014.
Indonesia Family Life Survey (IFLS)	1993	26 and older	The study was redesigned in 2007 to be similar to the HRS.
The Irish Longitudinal Study on Ageing (TILDA)	2010, 2012	50 and older	
Japanese Study of Aging and Retirement (JSTAR)	2007, 2009, 2011	50 and older	
Korean Longitudinal Study on Ageing	2006, 2008, 2010, 2012	45 and older	
Longitudinal Aging Study in India (LASI)			Under development as a HRS sister study. Pilot data for respondents 45 and older is available
Mexican Health and Aging Study (MHAS)	2001, 2003, 2012, 2015	50 and older	
New Zealand Health and Aging Research Team	2010, 2012	50 and older	
Northern Ireland Cohort for the Longitudinal Study of Ageing (NICOLA)			Under development as a HRS sister study. Initial data was collected from respondents aged 50 and over in 2013.

(continued)

Table 1.1 *(continued)*

Data Set Name	Study Waves	Sample Ages	Notes
The Scottish Longitudinal Survey of Ageing (THSLS)			Under development as a HRS sister study. Plans to sample respondents aged 50 and older are underway.
Study on Global Ageing and Adult Health (SAGE)	2011	50 and older	Countries include: China, Ghana, India, Mexico, Russia, and South Africa
Survey of Health, Aging and Retirement in Europe (SHARE)	2004, 2006, 2008, 2010, 2012	50 and older	Countries include: Austria, Belgium, the Czech Republic, Estonia, Denmark, France, Germany, Greece, Hungary, Ireland, Israel, Italy, the Netherlands, Poland, Portugal, Slovenia, Spain, Sweden, and Switzerland. Country participation and field time vary across waves.

For additional details go to the HRS International Sister Studies webpage located at: http://hrsonline.isr.umich.edu/index.php?p=sisters

understanding of aging across different cultural contexts and policy environments, which will enable us to effectively meet the challenges of global population aging.

However, this is inherently difficult work, given the problems associated with standardizing survey instruments across different languages and cultural contexts. This type of large-scale research requires significant sustained investment in social science research activities, including survey development, construction, and implementation; subject recruitment, retention, and compensation; data collection, storage, and analysis; and dissemination of results. Sufficient infrastructure, including computing and accounting systems, and human resources, including well-trained scientists and staff, are also essential. But supporting these initiatives is crucial to developing high-quality data that can track trends and provide insights that will assist policy makers plan for the growing older adult population.

Discussion

This chapter has documented the unprecedented aging of the global population and its implications for families, health and health care, and economic productivity. The timing and pace of population aging have varied substantially across countries, which makes it an immediate pressing issue in the developed countries of Europe, North America, Oceania, and Asia and a longer-term issue in developing countries in Africa, Latin America and the Caribbean, and Asia. The social and economic impact of changing age structure on specific countries in these regions will depend on a range of factors.

The first and foremost factor is the overall health of the population. Lowering chronic disease prevalence, delaying the onset and slowing the progression of disability, and providing access to high-quality health care throughout the life course are likely to foster improvements in the health of older adults. However, in many developed and developing countries, the health of future cohorts of older adults is likely to be undermined by rising rates of obesity among young and middle-aged adults (Wilmoth and Simpson 2013). At the same time, substantial differences across countries in health behaviors such as smoking, substance use, and exercise will also shape the health of older adult populations. Tracking changes in population health at all ages will provide insight into future demand among older adults for health care and long-term care.

A second factor to consider is evolving family forms. Rising rates of divorce and remarriage in developed countries are creating complex family arrangements that are calling into question the nature of family obligations (Connidis 2015). It remains to be seen whether adult children whose parents were never married or are divorced provide the same level of support to each of their aging parents as those whose parents' marriages remain intact or dissolved through the death of one partner. Similarly, the conditions under which stepchildren are willing to provide instrumental and personal assistance to aging stepparents are not fully understood. At the same time, increasing acceptance of cohabitation and same-sex unions in many countries is legitimizing relationships in ways that could expand and strengthen older adults' informal support systems. Obtaining a better understanding of changes in family structure and personal relationships is essential for accurately estimating the supply of informal caregivers available to older adults and the potential demand for formal long-term care services.

A third factor is public policy. In planning for the societal changes that will accompany population aging, it is essential that policy makers take into account structural lag, which occurs when the operation of social institutions lags behind the circumstances experienced by individuals (Riley and Riley 1994). In this situation, public policies that were designed during an earlier historical time have to be updated to ensure they are effectively meeting the needs of citizens and serving national interests (Wilmoth 2014). For example, improvements in later-life health and mortality mean that older adults are spending a longer portion of their lives as retirees who are not in the labor force. The average number of years men spend in retirement in OECD countries is almost 19, with much higher averages in some European countries such as Spain, 21, Italy, 22, Austria, 23, and France, 24 (Organization for Economic Cooperation and Development 2009). Increasing statutory retirement ages and providing older adults with incentives to stay in the labor force would alleviate some of the pressures generated by declining old-age support ratios and provide older adults with an opportunity to continue engaging in work roles. Such changes in policy would help nations proactively address the challenges generated by population aging.

However, there is no one-size-fits-all strategy for addressing population aging; policies that arose in one country may or may not be effective in another country. Governments will have to develop strategies for addressing population aging that will meet the unique needs of their citizens. In doing so, existing variation among the older adult population in a given country will need to be recognized. As the other chapters in this edited volume explore in more detail, socially constructed categories such as gender, race, ethnicity, and class shape inequalities that accumulate across the life course and produce heterogeneity in the older adult population. Understanding the sources of later-life heterogeneity can serve as a foundation for formulating effective policies that not only address the issues associated with population aging but also benefit all segments of the population regardless of age.

Notes

1. All numbers and percentages reported in this section for 1950 are from Rowland (2009). All numbers and percentages for 2012 and 2050 are based on

United Nations (2012). Please see these sources for additional information about countries not discussed here.

2. All numbers reported in this section are from United Nations (2012). Please see this source for additional information about countries not discussed here.

References

Alzheimer's Disease International. (2010). *World Alzheimer Report, 2010.* Accessed 6/1/2015 http://www.alz.co.uk/research/files/WorldAlzheimerReport2010.pdf.

Centers for Medicare and Medicaid Services. (2014). *National Health Expenditure Data—Age and Gender.* Accessed 6/1/2015 http://www.cms.gov/Research-Statistics-Data-and-Systems/Statistics-Trends-and-Reports/NationalHealthExpendData/Downloads/2010GenderandAgeTables.pdf

Connidis, I. (2015). Commitment and change: Constants of family ties over time. Presented at the Aging Families/Changing Families International Conference, Syracuse University, June 3–6.

Crimmins, E. M., & Ingegneri, D. G. (1990). Interaction and living arrangements of older parents and their children. *Research on Aging,* 12, 3–35.

Crystal, S., & Siegel, M. J. (2009). Population aging and health care policy in cross-national perspective. In P. Uhlenberg (Ed.), *International handbook of population aging* (pp. 608–630). New York: SpringerScience+Business Media.

Dykstra, P. A. (2009). Childless old age. In P. Uhlenberg (Ed.), *International handbook of population aging* (pp. 671–690). New York: SpringerScience+Business Media.

Easterlin, R. (1991). The economic impact of prospective population changes in advanced industrial countries. *Journal of Gerontology: Social Sciences,* 46, S299–S309.

England, R. S. (2002). *The macroeconomic impact of global aging: A new era of economic frailty?* Washington, DC: Center for Strategic and International Studies Press.

Fries, J. (1982). The compression of morbidity. *The Milbank Memorial Fund Quarterly,* 61, 397–419.

Gruenberg, E. M. (1977). The failures of success. *Milbank Memorial Fund Quarterly,* 55, 3–24.

Grundy, E., & Read, S. (2012). Social contacts and receipt of health among older people in England: Are there benefits of having more children? *Journals of Gerontology, Series B: Psychological and Social Sciences,* 67, 742–754.

Hank, K. (2007). Proximity and contact between older parents and their children: A European comparison. *Journal of Marriage and Family,* 69, 157–173.

Hardy, M., & Skirbekk, V. (2012). Research opportunities in the demography of aging. In L. J. Waite (Ed.), *Perspectives on the future of the sociology of aging* (pp. 32–59). Washington, DC: National Academies Press.

Hateley, L., & Tan, G. (2003). *The graying of Asia: Causes and consequences of rapid aging in Asia.* New York: Eastern Universities Press.

Kinsella K., & He, W. (2009). *An aging world: 2008.* Washington, DC: National Institute on Aging and U.S. Census Bureau.

Knodel, J., Chayovan, N., & Siriboon, S. (1992). The impact of fertility decline on family support for the elderly: An illustration from Thailand. *Population Development Review,* 18, 79–103.

Knodel, J. E., & Ofstedal, M. B. (2003). Gender and aging in the developing world: Where are the men? *Population and Development Review,* 29(4), 677–698.

Koropeckyj-Cox, T., & Vaughn, R. A. C. (2007). Characteristics of older childless persons and parents: Cross-national comparisons. *Journal of Family Issues,* 28, 1362–1414.

Laditka, S. B., & Laditka, J. N. (2009). Active life expectancy: A central measure of population health. In P. Uhlenberg (Ed.) *International handbook of population aging* (pp. 543–565). New York: SpringerScience+Business Media.

Manton, K. G. (1982). Changing concepts of morbidity and mortality in the elderly population. *Milbank Memorial Fund Quarterly,* 60, 183–191.

Miner, S., & Uhlengberg, P. (2004). Intergenerational proximity and the social role of sibling neighbours after midlife. *Family Relations,* 46, 145–153.

Mullan, P. (2000). *The imaginary time bomb: Why an ageing population is not a social problem.* New York: I. B. Tauris.

National Research Council. (2001). *Preparing for an aging world: The case for cross-national research.* Washington, DC: National Academy Press.

Olshansky, S. J., Rudberg, M. A., Carnes, B. A., Cassel, B. A., & Brady, J. A. (1991). Trading off longer life for worsening health: The expansion of morbidity hypothesis. *Journal of Aging and Health,* 3, 194–216.

Organization for Economic Cooperation and Development. (2009). *OECD society at a glance.* Accessed 6/1/2015 http://public.tableausoftware.com/views/Retirement/LFEA

Population Reference Bureau. (2014). *2014 world population data sheet.* Accessed 5/29/2015 http://www.prb.org/pdf14/2014-world-population-data-sheet_eng.pdf

Redfoot, D. L., & Pandya, S. M. (2002). *Before the boom: Trends in long-term supportive service for older Americans with disabilities.* Washington, DC: The AAPR Public Policy Institute.

Riley, M. W., & Riley, J. W., Jr. (1994). Structural lag: Past and future. In M. W. Riley, R. L. Kahn, & A. Foner (Eds.), *Age and structural lag* (pp. 15–26). New York: John Wiley and Sons, Inc.

Rowland, D. T. (2009). Global population aging: History and prospects. In P. Uhlenberg (Ed.), *International handbook of population aging* (pp. 37–65). New York: SpringerScience+Business Media.

Schoeni, R. F., & Ofstedal, M. B. (2010). Key themes in research on the demography of aging. *Demography,* 47, 5–15.

Siegel, J. (1980). On the demography of aging. *Demography,* 17, 345–364.

Silverstein, M. (1995). Stability and change in temporal distance between the elderly and their children. *Demography,* 32, 29–45.

Teitelbaum, M. S. (1975). Relevance of demographic transition theory for developing countries. *Science,* 188(4187), 420–425.

Tomassini, C., Glaser, K., Wolf, D. A., Broese van Broenou, M. I., & Grundy, E. (2004). Living arrangements among older people: An overview of trends in Europe and the USA. *Population Trends*, 115, 24–34.

Tomassini, C., & Wolf, D. A. (2000). Shrinking kin networks in Italy due to sustained low fertility. *European Journal of Population Studies*, 16, 353–372.

Uhlenberg, P. (Ed.) (2009). *International handbook of population aging*. New York: SpringerScience.

United Nations (2003). Partnership and reproductive behavior in low-fertility countries. Accessed 6/2/2015 http://www.un.org/esa/population/publications/reprobehavior/partrepro.pdf

United Nations (2012). Population aging and development, 2012 wallchart. Accessed 5/29/2015 http://www.un.org/esa/population/publications/2012WorldPopAgeingDev_Chart/2012PopAgeingandDev_WallChart.pdf

United Nations (2013a). Profiles of aging. Accessed 5/29/2015 http://esa.un.org/unpd/popdev/AgingProfiles2013/default.aspx

United Nations (2013b). World Fertility Report 2012. Accessed 6/1/2015 http://www.un.org/en/development/desa/population/publications/dataset/fertility/wfr2012/MainFrame.html

United Nations (2013c). World population ageing 2013. Accessed 5/29/2015 http://www.un.org/en/development/desa/population/publications/pdf/ageing/WorldPopulationAgeing2013.pdf

United States Central Intelligence Agency. (2015). *The world factbook: Median age*. Accessed 5/29/2014 https://www.cia.gov/library/publications/the-world-factbook/fields/2177.html

Wilmoth, J. M. (2014). The implications of structural lag for old age policy. In R. Hudson (Ed.), *The new politics of old age policy* (3rd ed., pp. 20–38). Baltimore: Johns Hopkins Press.

Wilmoth, J. M., & Simpson, N. M. (2013). Demographic perspectives on aging. In J. M. Wilmoth & K. F. Ferraro (Eds.), *Gerontology: Perspectives and issues* (4th ed., pp. 199–222). New York: Springer Pub.

CHAPTER TWO

Theories of Aging and Social Gerontology: Explaining How Social Factors Influence Well-Being in Later Life

Vern L. Bengtson and Marguerite DeLiema

In science, theories are explanations, and the purpose of theories is to provide an explanation of *why* and *how* things happen. Social gerontology as a scientific field is concerned with understanding how social factors affect older individuals' well-being at both the macrolevel of society and the microlevel of individuals and their relationships.

Social gerontology is a multidisciplinary field that was originated by sociologists, psychologists, social workers, and public policy advocates interested in aging, then expanded by demographers, economists, and scholars in the humanities. The common intent underlying their efforts has been a humanitarian goal to understand and improve the lives of older adults through research that can lead to interventions. Research efforts of social gerontologists have been directed at a wide variety of topics, such as explaining why there are disparities among older persons in well-being, and how the diversity of people's aging experience affects and is affected by their location in social structures.

In this chapter, we examine some of the major theories that have been developed to date in social gerontology. We begin by discussing what is meant by theory in social gerontology and the history of theorizing in our field. We then present some of the major theories or perspectives in social gerontology and what they try to explain about well-being later in life. We organize these along three major dimensions: theories concerned with social stratification and the life course in relation to well-being, those concerned with social-psychological models of well-being, and interpretive or social constructionist perspectives on aging and well-being. We conclude with some recent models of well-being in later life and a call for future efforts at theorizing—which is much needed in our field, and often badly neglected in our current emphasis on training of graduate students.

What Is Theory and Why Does It Matter?

While the term *theory* may be used in many ways, in science theory means the development of *explanations* to account for empirical findings (Bengtson et al., 2009). Theories of aging help to explain the *how* and *why* behind the *what* that is reported in data about age differences and age changes. The end product of a good theory in science can be a successful *intervention,* which involves changing existing conditions to improve some outcome, such as a new vaccine to prevent disease, or (hopefully) a more equitable old-age Medicare insurance policy to improve health outcomes for all sociodemographic groups (Bengtson, Burgess, & Parrott, 1997).

The systematic progression of theory-based explanation over time is the standard by which the progression and status of any field of scholarly or scientific research is judged (Brown, 1986). If empirical results are not presented within the context of explanations or theory, this limits the process of building, revising, and interpreting how and why phenomena occur. It is through the ability to explain specific empirical findings with more general theories that knowledge develops (Turner, 2005).

Theories also provide understanding, which is somewhat different from explanation (Bengtson & Settersten, 2016). We can posit a theory about the causal relationship between two variables without having insight into the mechanisms that underlie the relationships; a theory that includes mechanisms achieves a deeper level of understanding. Moreover, in social gerontology it can be said that there are two general types of theory: (1) theories of *explanation* concerning how and why something occurs—for example, cumulative advantage/disadvantage theories in aging, which explain *why* variability among older people partly reflects social inequalities, and *how* social processes generate those inequalities over time; and (2) theories of *orientation* that provide a worldview and even a set of explicit assumptions or propositions, that lead us to see and interpret aging phenomena in particular ways—for example, postmodern theory, feminist theory, critical gerontology, or the life-course perspective. While the latter are often called "theories," they are, from another perspective, more often broader "paradigms" than theories. But the frame and propositions they provide are extremely useful in developing more specific theories. In any case, both types are represented in gerontology today, and we discuss both in this chapter.

But theory, and particularly the process of theory development (which we suggest is central to the future of social gerontology), may seem irrelevant to some students and junior researchers who are readers of this chapter. Yet theory is part and parcel of every research project, recognized or not. When we put together a plan to study some problem of importance, we already have some hunch, or explanation, about possible outcomes. These reflect some implicit theory about how a set of phenomena may be related, and these expectations or hunches are indebted to previous explanations. Yet too often researchers appear to be unaware of this conceptual and theoretical inheritance and proceed without any acknowledged theory (Hendricks, Applebaum, & Kunkel, 2010). In social gerontology, particularly in public policy applications or program interventions, it is crucial to specify the theoretical assumptions of the research or program intervention before investing large sums of money and hoping for the best. If the underlying theory is missing or inadequate, it is unlikely the intervention program or public policy will achieve its objectives. And if the intervention is not backed by tested theory-based knowledge, it will be difficult to judge why it worked—or, more important, why it *didn't* work (Bengtson, Burgess, & Parrott, 1997; Settersten & Bengtson, 2016).

Concepts are the building blocks of theory. Concepts are terms, like "successful aging" or "cumulative disadvantage" or "social roles," that represent a great number of observations, or data, collected through research procedures. Concepts are linked to these empirical phenomena through operational definitions, from which hypotheses are derived and then tested through more empirical observations (data collection). The process of theory building engages researchers in developing explanations about what lies behind these data—the *why* and *how* underlying these phenomena (Turner, 2005; Wallace & Wolf, 1991). Theories are useful in predicting and hence manipulating naturalistic phenomena and environments. Thus they are important for designing programs aimed at ameliorating problems associated with aging, such as programs and services provided by the Older Americans Act, Medicare, and Adult Protective Services.

Another major approach shaping research in social gerontology has been the interpretive perspective, which historically has taken a somewhat different approach to theory (Marshall, Matthews, & McMullen, 2016). Many researchers using interpretive approaches focus on describing and understanding how social interactions proceed, as well as the subjective meanings or interpretations of age and aging phenomena. From this perspective, a "theory" is useful to the extent it provides a deeper understanding of particular social events and settings that have meaning for older persons in the context of their social worlds (Gubrium & Holstein, 1999). This reflects what Berger and Luckman (1966) called the *social construction of reality*. A major contribution of the interpretive perspective is its emphasis on agency—seeing individuals as active agents who can change the nature of their social environments, which is an important consideration for social gerontologists (Marshall, 2005).

Another perspective is critical theory, which questions scientific methods as a means for understanding the diverse manifestations of aging. Rather, the process of critical understanding of meanings, the analysis of power and domination, and the constraints imposed by social structures or forces—which, taken together, constitute *critical knowledge*—are equally as important as objective or scientific knowledge in understanding the phenomena of aging (Bengtson, Burgess, & Parrott, 1997; Moody, 2001).

Some critical theorists argue that values cannot be separated from what are termed "facts," and that all research is inherently value-laden—subject to the biases of the investigator (Marshall, 1999). Social gerontologists operating in the scientific mode would argue instead that their vigorous and peer-reviewed methods guard against such biases. We suggest that one way to address these issues is to regard each of these perspectives as providing different lenses to approach the different problems at hand. Interpretive and critical approaches to knowledge may be different in their objectives and methods, yet they also involve the identification of concepts, which are the building blocks of any theory. All these theoretical perspectives can thereby enrich understanding of the multiple facets of well-being in later life.

Early Explanations: Social Roles and Their Relation to Well-Being in Later Life

The development of gerontology, as a field of research and intervention, has owed much to its progressive development of theory (for a comprehensive review, see Bengtson, 2016). The earliest researchers in aging, such as Burgess (1923, 1960), Hall (1922), Cowdry (1939), Linton (1942), Parsons (1942), and Havighurst (1943), integrated empirical findings into theoretical insights and established the foundations of gerontology. Then, as social gerontology developed in the post–World War II period, it drew theoretical insights from the prevailing social theories of the time, such as structural functionalism and symbolic interactionism, and later Marxism and rational choice theory.

Activity Theory

What are the social factors that influence well-being in later life? What are the social requisites for successful aging? These were the research questions that formed the basis for the first major social science study of aging (Cavan et al., 1949; Havighurst & Albrecht, 1953). The answer appeared relatively straightforward: older people should maintain a high level of activity in the social roles they had in middle life, and when they lose these roles (through retirement, for example) they should replace them, as in volunteer activities. This became the activity theory of aging, an informal and implicit theory until Havighurst (1963) discussed it and Lemon, Bengtson, and Peterson (1972) formalized it.

Activity theory postulated that older individuals who are more active would be more satisfied with their lives. Underlying the theory was an assumption that social interaction was important to a positive self-development, and that an individual's self-concept is related to his or her social roles. A natural consequence of aging, unfortunately, is an involuntary reduction in roles, through events like retirement, widowhood, and the loss of friends. In order to maintain a positive sense of self, older persons must compensate for these role losses and find substitute roles. Well-being in later life, therefore, results from increased activity in newly acquired roles, such as volunteer work, hobbies, and participating in social clubs.

Activity theory provided a conceptual justification for an assumption underlying many programs and interventions for the elderly—that social activity in and of itself is beneficial and will result in greater life satisfaction. But activity theory received relatively little empirical support (Lemon, Bengtson, & Peterson, 1972), and there were many criticisms (Maddox, 1965). First, the theory assumed that all older persons need and desire high levels of social activity, although some old people may prefer to be couch potatoes. Second, the theory overlooked variations in the meaning of particular activities in the lives of older people. For example, baby-sitting grandchildren may improve self-esteem and sense of self-worth for some people but be viewed as a chore and burden to others.

Nevertheless, the ideas underlying activity theory were attractive in the 1960s, in part because they reinforced American cultural values of independence and autonomy. Moreover, they can be readily discerned in recent successful aging models that have become increasingly visible today, as we will discuss later. Not unlike activity theory, the successful aging model has been criticized for its excessive individualism, its discounting of social/economic inequality, and its "one size fits all" stereotyping (Schmeeckle & Bengtson, 1999).

Disengagement Theory

While activity theory maintained that high role involvement was the explanation (and prescription) for successful aging, disengagement theory provided a much different view. Here, older persons who follow a gradual retrenchment to more diminished and focused levels of activities are likely to have higher well-being. Disengagement theory (Cumming & Henry, 1961) was the first explicitly social-psychological theory of aging. It was based on an impressive multidisciplinary project of data collected from the Kansas City Studies of Adulthood and Aging. The data demonstrated gradual but progressive declines by age in social interaction, psychological involvement, and physiological functions of aging individuals. The theory explained these decreases as inevitable processes, which would occur intrinsically within older people; they would occur across all cultures, time periods, and communities, as part of developmental disengagement. The theory postulated that aging individuals and social structures mutually disengage as death approaches, an adaptation that could be seen as beneficial for the individual and society because it allows younger generations to replace older adults in positions of increasing power and importance (Cumming & Henry, 1961).

Disengagement was a truly general theory of aging, explaining many aging processes under one general set of mechanisms that fit together. Moreover, as a theory it was elegant, multidisciplinary, parsimonious, and intuitively provocative (Achenbaum & Bengtson, 1994). However, its ambitious propositions were roundly criticized (Hochschild, 1975). The theory had attempted to explain both macro- and microlevel changes with one grand theory, but when tested against other data, its validity and generalizability claims were not supported. While many older people did appear to be disengaging or withdrawing from their social connections and activities while maintaining high life satisfaction, many did not, particularly in other social settings (Bengtson, 1969).

One outcome of the criticism of disengagement theory was to curtail further attempts to develop a general theory of aging. However, disengagement theory had a significant effect in social gerontology by prompting development of alternative theories of aging, in particular, activity theory, and, much later, socioemotional selectivity theory (Carstensen, 1992), described later in this chapter.

Modernization Theory

A few years after the theoretical controversy sparked by disengagement versus activity theory, another grand theory emerged. Cowgill and Holmes

(1972) presented a theory based on ideas that had been first articulated by the pioneer of American sociology of aging, Ernest Burgess, in the 1920s (Burgess, 1960). Modernization theory proposed that the status and well-being of the elderly is inversely related to the level of industrialization in a society, and that this explains why the aged are less valued in, say, North America than in traditionally agrarian Asian societies (Cowgill, 1974; Cowgill & Holmes, 1972). It attempted to explain variations in age status both historically and across societies. While the elderly held high status in preindustrial societies as a result of their control of scarce resources and their knowledge of tradition, they have lower status in modern industrialized societies. Four elements of industrialization are related to the reduced status of older people: economic technology, urbanization, mass education, and health technology (Cowgill, 1974).

This was an attractive theory, and it was often cited as a critique of the position of the elderly in American society. Yet, like many general theories, it could not be documented empirically except at somewhat superficial levels (Laslett, 1976). Historical research examining the loss of authority of elders (Fisher, 1977), the timing and sequencing of the proportion of aged (Laslett, 1985), and the appearance of retirement (Quadagno, 1982) did not support the theory. Large-scale comparative research on the effects of modernity suggested that the aged were actually better off in more modernized contexts (Bengtson et al., 1975). Still, though modernization theory is no longer used as a general explanation of the status of the aged, it has been applied in more narrowly defined settings, for example, Aboderin's (2004) qualitative study of the intergenerational relations and the status of elders under conditions of poverty in urban Ghana in the late 1990s.

Continuity Theory

At the individual level, Atchley's (1989) continuity theory proposed that despite some disruptions of established roles and behavior patterns across the life span, individuals are inclined to maintain the same habits, personalities, and lifestyles they developed in earlier years. If necessary, individuals actively make adaptations that allow them to gain a sense of continuity between the past and the present. The theory posited that it is this sense of continuity across the life span that contributes to well-being in later life.

Continuity theory's implicit reference to trajectories and their constitutive roles, identities, values, and behaviors across life stages finds parallels in aspects of the life-course perspective described later on. However, assumptions contained in our perceptions of the meaning of time—our own constructions or culture-bounded views—may call into question the usefulness of continuity theory. Kenyon, Ruth, and Madder (1999) questioned whether continuity theory is about aging *per se*, or whether in some cases it reflects a cohort, cultural, or period effect based on an unexamined belief in a linear view of time.

In support of continuity theory, research by Agahi, Ahacic, and Parker (2006) reported that average levels of leisure participation were mostly stable from midlife into older age, yet there were significant *intra*individual differences in participation over time and variation across activity types. For example, participation in religious activity remained relatively constant over a 34-year period for those who engaged in religious activity in midlife, but restaurant visits varied considerably. There were individuals who rarely ate at restaurants in midlife who then dined out frequently in later life (perhaps their wives got tired of cooking!). The researchers contend that these changes may reflect historical trends in the growing popularity of dining out instead of age-related effects. In a review of the literature on retirement satisfaction, researchers found that continuity theory can accommodate longitudinal patterns in retirement adjustment, helping to explain *inter*individual differences in well-being; however, the theory does not adequately explain *intra*individual fluctuations in life satisfaction over time (Wang, Henkens, & van Solinge, 2011).

Social Competence/Breakdown Model

How do problems of aging occur for individuals, and how can gerontological interventions be constructed to help them? Social competence/breakdown theory (Kuypers & Bengtson, 1973) represented an attempt to explore both normal and problematic aspects of aging by linking micro- and macrosocial dimensions. This model started from an interpretive theoretical perspective, looking at meanings of age and aging in a culture where ageism is rampant.

The social breakdown model sought to explain the negative consequences that follow an age-related crisis and pose a threat to well-being. The precipitating event is often an age-related crisis in health, a job loss to a younger worker, or the death of a spouse. These role losses can activate the older person's internalized beliefs that he is frail and incompetent, which are further reinforced by a culture that devalues the contributions of older people. Internalized ageism manifests outward, leading to further atrophy of the older person's previous competency skills and his self-confidence. Once the older person recharacterizes himself as sick, inadequate, or incompetent, he becomes more vulnerable still, resulting in further negative social and psychological well-being.

This process can be reversed, and competence promoted, by intervening before the downward spiral begins. Interventions may include providing improved environmental supports, such as senior transportation, modified housing, or job retraining, while facilitating expression of personal strength. It is this aspect of the social breakdown/competence model that made it appealing as an explanatory theory for social workers. However, it has seldom been tested in empirical studies.

Social Stratification, the Life Course, and Well-Being

The theories described above were innovative and useful in calling attention to the newly developing field of social gerontology. But they tended to focus on individuals and their social roles, and how these related to well-being in later life. The next stage of theory development would expand this to integrate the social structure with the life course (Bengtson, 2016). New theoretical perspectives emerged. Prominent among them were the age stratification model, the life-course perspective, and the cumulative advantage/disadvantage model. This theoretical work reflected an effort to synthesize the distinct micro- and macrolevel approaches of earlier theorizing (Hendricks, 1992).

The Age Stratification Perspective

Both the age stratification and the life-course perspectives began in gerontological theory with the insights of Leonard Cain (1964). He drew from sociologists (such as Mannheim and Eisenstadt) on the importance of generations, and anthropologists (such as Van Gnepp and Malinowski) for the concept of age grading and age statuses in preliterate societies, to build a persuasive case that age, and aging, were important phenomena in American society.

A few years later Matilda Riley developed what she at that time called the age stratification model, which became one of the most important traditions of macrolevel theorizing in social gerontology (Riley, Johnston, & Foner, 1972). This model sought to bring together and explain: (1) cohort flow or the movement of different age cohorts across time in order to identify similarities and differences between them; (2) the interdependence of age cohorts and social structures; and (3) the asynchrony between structural and individual change over time. It developed concepts such as age cohorts, age roles, age-graded social structures, age segregation/integration, and structural lag. Structural lag occurs when social structures cannot keep pace with the changes in population dynamics and individual lives. A useful example of structural lag (Riley, Kahn, & Foner, 1994) is the discordance between the increasing needs of elderly parents for caregiving support, the concurrent reductions in state resources to provide long-term care services, and the resultant increased demands placed on families to provide parent care, even as adult children are less able to do so because of employment demands. Using this theoretical perspective, Riley and Loscocco (1994) argued that a more age-integrated society brought about by policy changes can compensate for structural lag and improve the lives of older adults. Restructuring the social institutions of work, education, and the family, through such policies as extended time off for education or caregiving, can bring social structures in balance with individuals' lives.

The Life-Course Perspective

This perspective is perhaps the most widely cited theoretical framework in social gerontology today. It is based on the premise that to understand the present circumstances of elderly people, we must take into account the social and psychological forces operating throughout the earlier course of their lives (George, 1996). This represents a convergence of thinking in sociology and psychology about processes at both macro- and microsocial levels of analysis and how they apply to populations and individuals over time. It is a multidisciplinary perspective, drawing concepts and methods from sociology, psychology, biology, anthropology and history.

Researchers using the life-course perspective were attempting to explain: (1) the dynamic, contextual, and processual nature of aging; (2) age-related transitions and life trajectories; (3) how aging is related to and shaped by social contexts, cultural meanings, and social-structural location; and (4) how time, period, and cohort shape the aging process for individuals as well as for social groups (Bengtson & Allen, 1993; Elder, 1992; Elder & Johnson, 2002).

Several basic assumptions were part of the life-course perspective (Elder & Johnson, 2002; Settersten & Godwelski, 2016). The first is that *development and aging are lifelong processes*—relationships, events, and processes of earlier life stages have consequences for later-life relationships, processes, and outcomes. The second principle concerns the *interdependence of lives over time,* especially in the family, where individuals are linked across generations by bonds of kinship and processes of intergenerational transmission. For example, economic declines can have reverberating effects on the interconnected life paths of family members. The third principle concerns *agency* in human development—the idea that individuals make choices within the constraints of social structures and historical conditions. The fourth principle is the impact of *history and place*. Research designs should nest individual lives and family processes within social and historical contexts. A fifth principle emphasizes *historical time*, or the importance of transitions and their timing relative to structural and historical contexts. There can be a "best fit" in the timing of individual development and family life stages as they converge with structural and historically created opportunities.

An example is the epidemiologic transition theory, which expanded the life-course perspective to a population scale using an anthropological perspective (Omran, 1971, 2005). The theory examines how demographic, economic, and sociological factors interact with health and disease over time to alter the structure and composition of populations. In Western societies, degenerative diseases replaced infectious diseases as the drivers of mortality. This created an epidemiological transition from high mortality and high fertility to low mortality and low fertility, and an increasing divide between males and females in longevity. Longer, healthier lives were accompanied by changes in work roles, family structure—more generations alive at one time—overall economic productivity, and an overall improvement in living standards for older adults. While not a social gerontology theory, the epidemiological transition theory is a useful macrolevel explanation for how modernization affects population health, life expectancy, and social roles, which then affects the overall well-being of older societies (Gaziano, 2010).

Cumulative Advantage/Disadvantage Theory

The cumulative disadvantage/advantage theory applied a life-course approach to the analysis of stratification among the aged. The theory sought to explain how inequality is produced across the life course and maintained in old age (O'Rand, 2016). As applied to older people, those already advantaged (across a range of domains, such as health or wealth) will accumulate more benefits, while those who are disadvantaged early will accumulate more loss (O'Rand, 1996).

In the 1970s and 1980s, two themes emerged in social gerontology that the cumulative advantage/disadvantage perspective was uniquely positioned to examine: the heterogeneity or diversity of older persons, and poverty and inequality among the aged (Dannefer, 2003). A central concept was intracohort heterogeneity. Structural or institutional arrangements operate to stratify cohorts as they allocate differential opportunities for the accumulation of value and reward. Inequality is seen as the product of institutional arrangement as well as aggregated individual actions over time. People who begin in a position of social advantage generally are better positioned to acquire additional resources than those who begin life at the bottom of the hierarchy (Quadagno & Reid, 1999). This also explains the differences within cohorts along significant life-course trajectories in terms of health, family, work, income, and wealth.

The cumulative inequality theory suggested by Ferraro, Shippee, and Schafer (2009) uses an interdisciplinary lens to integrate the life-course perspective with the cumulative advantage/disadvantage perspective. Originally based on the Matthew effect in science (Merton, 1968), cumulative inequality is premised on five axioms. The first is that social systems, not individual behaviors, generate inequality, and that these social systems set a course for demographic and developmental processes. Second, disadvantage increases exposure to risk, while advantage increases exposure to opportunity. Those who begin in poverty are more likely to experience food insecurity, joblessness, and negative life events like divorce, bankruptcy, and poor heath; whereas those born into wealth are more likely to have access to good nutrition, education, and eventually greater economic security in retirement. Inequality can accumulate over generations, so that the family one is born into affects the availability of both physiologic and social resources throughout his or her life; and prenatal conditions—the mother's diet, lifestyle choices, and her exposure to environmental pathogens—affect developmental trajectories. The third principle is that accumulation of risk, available resources, and human agency all influence a person's ultimate life-course trajectory.

Fourth, subjective feelings about where people stand relative to others are more important in shaping their life-course trajectory than their actual position in the social hierarchy. In other words, believing that one is doing better than one's peers increases self-efficacy, and self-efficacy may improve physiological well-being. In this way, the cumulative inequality theory diverged from cumulative advantage/disadvantage theory by borrowing concepts from social constructionism. Fifth, individuals who have accumulated the most disadvantages will have the greatest health problems in older age, leading to higher mortality rates. The strengths of the cumulative inequality theory are its interdisciplinary focus and its ability to explain the heterogeneity of older cohorts, thus making it very popular among health disparity researchers.

Social-Psychological Models of Well-Being in Later Life

Other perspectives in social gerontology take a more narrow approach to explaining well-being in later life. These theories focus less on how broad social forces influence well-being—like how cultural, economic, and political contexts produce social stratification—to instead focus on the individual and the individual's relationships with others. These mid-level theories include the social exchange theory applied to aging (Dowd, 1975), selective optimization with compensation (Baltes & Baltes, 1990), and the socioemotional selectivity theory (Carstensen, 1992). They explain adaptive changes in emotion regulation and decision making with age, in addition to exploring the costs and benefits of social relationships over the life course.

Social Exchange Theory: A Rational Choice Perspective

Social exchange theory has been useful in analyses focusing on intergenerational social support and transfers. Developed and extended by Dowd (1975), this theory of aging drew from sociological formulations by Homans (1961) and Blau (1964) and work in economics that assumes a rational choice model of decision making and behavior. Applied to aging, this perspective attempted to account for exchange behavior between individuals of different ages as a result of the shift in roles, skills, and resources that accompany advancing age (Hendricks, 1995). A central assumption was that the various actors (such as parent and child or elder and youth) bring resources to the interaction or exchange. Resources can be nonmaterial, such as social support and companionship, and will most likely be unequal. For example, in caregiving relationships a dependent older person requires increasing levels of support over time but can provide fewer resources in return for care. A second assumption of social exchange theory was that the actors will continue to engage in the exchange only as long as the personal benefits are greater than the personal costs, and that there are no better alternatives. This theoretical approach also assumed that exchanges are governed by norms of reciprocity: when we give something, we trust that something of equal value will be given in return.

A contribution of social exchange theory is its ability to explain exchanges of contact and social support as well as how these exchanges are influenced by emotional, social, or financial support (Silverstein et al., 2002). However, simplistic formulations of social exchange theory may ignore the fact that many interactions are not driven solely by rationality or an economic calculation on the part of each actor, but rather by irrational motivations such as altruism, affection, or a sense of familial obligation.

Another issue is that in contrast to social constructionist theories, the quality and the meaning of the exchange are ignored in rational choice-type theories. Yet Merz et al. (2009) note that relationship quality moderates the association between providing intergenerational support to parents and the well-being of adult children, such that in high-quality relationships, the challenges of providing intergenerational support are perceived as less burdensome. In a separate study, Merz and Consedine (2009) found that receiving *emotional* support from family members was related to greater well-being, whereas receiving *instrumental* support was either negatively or not associated with well-being. These associations depended on whether the older person's attachment style was open and emotionally secure. Thus, the quality of the relationship and the type of resources provided—emotional versus instrumental—were important in determining whether there were barriers or facilitators to intergenerational exchange.

The social exchange theory was premised on the assumption of an imbalance in the relative power of the parties to the exchange and has been used as an explanation for caregiver stress leading to elder abuse and neglect (Dong, Simon, & Gorbien, 2007; Walker & Allen, 1999). The idea is that as an elder becomes more and more impaired, his or her increasing dependency becomes stressful to a caregiver who responds by physically and/or emotionally harming the older person in order to rebalance the distribution of power. While this paradigm was attractive to researchers for its simplicity, other researchers have found that it is more often the abuser who is dependent on the elder for financial and emotional support rather than the other way around (Jackson & Hafemeister, 2013; Pillemer & Finkelhor, 1989).

Selective Optimization with Compensation Theory

This psychologically oriented theory explained how individuals cope with age-related losses to manage adaptive (successful) development in later life (Baltes & Baltes, 1990). The theory identified three fundamental mechanisms or strategies: selection, optimization, and compensation. The central focus of this model of psychological and behavioral adaptation was on maximizing gains—optimization—and minimizing losses—selection and compensation—as one ages.

Selection refers to the increasing restriction of an individual's life to fewer domains of functioning because of age-related losses in the range of adaptive potential. Optimization reflects the idea that people engage in behaviors that augment or enrich their general reserves and maximize their chosen life courses. Like selection, compensation results from restriction of the range of adaptive potential and becomes operative when specific behavioral capacities are lost or are reduced below a standard required for adequate functioning. This lifelong process of selective optimization with compensation enables people to age successfully (Schroots, 1996).

These concepts have been tested empirically, particularly in the areas of work-related demands and coping with chronic disease. For example,

Young, Baltes, and Pratt (2007) found that selective optimization with compensation strategies were effective for people whose time and energy resources were constrained by having young dependents, receiving little support at work, and being older. And in a qualitative study, researchers found that resource allocation strategies are used by adults adapting to physiological constraints due to chronic health conditions (Rozario, Kidahashi, & DeRienzis, 2011).

Socioemotional Selectivity Theory

This has become one of the most highly used theories across a wide range of individually focused social gerontological studies. In constructing this theory, Carstensen (1992) combined insights from developmental psychology—particularly the selective optimization with compensation model developed by Baltes and Baltes (1990)—with social exchange theory to explain why the social exchange and interaction networks of older persons are reduced over time, a phenomenon disengagement theory tried to explain. According to the socioemotional selectivity theory, constricting the range of social partners is a lifelong adaptation performed to maximize emotional and social gains and minimize emotional risks. While social interactions benefit the individual by providing opportunities to acquire new information, get assistance, identify and select mates, and maintain one's self-concept, new social interactions also require effort and can pose a risk to one's self-concept. Through mechanisms of socioemotional selectivity, individuals reduce interactions with people in their peripheral social network while increasing emotional closeness with significant others, such as adult children and siblings.

The theory has been empirically tested in both young and old populations. Studies showed that future time perspective is more important than age in determining whether socioemotional selectivity will occur (Carstensen, 2006; Fung, Carstensen, & Lutz, 1998). When individuals perceive there is less time left in life, they selectively devote more effort to emotion regulation and bonding with close friends and family than to investing in future relationships and rewards. For example, Carstensen and Fredrickson (1998) found that HIV-positive men with limited time left to live behaved more like older adults in their interest in interacting with various social partners.

Carstensen's (1992) socioemotional selectivity theory, which is a lifespan theory of motivation, provided a concise development-behavioral explanation for selective interactions in old age. The theory explained age-related declines in the level of contact with distal social partners in exchange for more meaningful interactions with significant others. Such chosen interactions reflect the levels of reward these exchanges of emotional support provide for older persons. An extension of this theory—the positivity effect, or older adults' selective memory for positive stimuli over negative stimuli—has been supported by results from neuroimaging studies on anticipation, exposure, and encoding of emotional stimuli (Samanez-Larkin & Carstensen, 2011).

Interpretive Perspectives on Well-Being in Later Life

Additional theories emerged in another period of theorizing in social gerontology, including the political economy of aging perspective (Estes et al., 1984), which drew from Marxist thinking and conflict theory in sociology, as well as development of socially constructed and ideological theories. The growing presence in the field of social constructivist theories, critical perspectives, political economy of aging perspectives, feminist theories of aging, and postmodernist perspectives reflects this trend.

Social Constructionist and Interpretive Theories

When social constructionist theories emerged several decades ago, they became the most frequently cited perspectives in social gerontology. Social constructionist theories drew from a long tradition of microlevel analysis in the social sciences: symbolic interactionism (Mead, 1934), phenomenology (Berger & Luckmann, 1966), and ethnomethodology (Garfinkel, 1967). They are often associated with the postmodern era in qualitative research (Andrews, 2012). Using hermeneutic or interpretive methods, social constructionism focused on individual agency and social behavior within larger structures of society and particularly on the subjective meanings of age and the aging experience.

Key concepts of social constructionist and interpretive theories of aging included social meaning, social realities, social relations, attitudes toward aging and the aged, and life events (Marshall et al., 2016). Researchers working in the social constructivist tradition emphasized their interest in understanding, if not explaining, individual processes of aging as influenced by social definitions and social structures. Examples include Gubrium's (1993) study of the subjective meanings of quality of care and quality of life for residents of nursing homes, and how each resident constructs meanings from her or his own experiences. There are critiques: the microlevel focus of social constructionist theories obscures macrolevel effects such as cohort, historical, and age stratification influences. Also, meanings emerge from analyses of life narratives, and thus cannot be measured by predefined measurement scales, such as those used by most survey researchers. This perspective may also minimize the effects of social structure or the role of power.

A more recent application of social constructionism is Gilleard and Higgs's (2010) conceptualization of the "fourth age," which was a response to Bernice Neugarten's (1974) initial conceptualization of the third age as a postretirement/predisability life stage. According to Neugarten, third agers—55 through 75-year-olds—are generally healthy, affluent, politically active, and free from the responsibilities of child care and work. Peter Laslett (1987) popularized this concept by arguing that modernization is what facilitated the lifestyles and behaviors of adults in the third age. Because of better health and financial security, older people could productively engage with society in a way that previous generations could not.

Gilleard and Higgs (2010) applied a social constructionist perspective to these concepts. According to their revised perspective, generational identity is socially constructed. They argued that shifting work identities, consumerism, and community structures lead to a fracturing between the young-old and oldest-old cohorts. While third agers are socially positioned to participate in public discourse due to better health and financial resources, fourth agers are characterized by increasing frailty, cognitive decline, and institutionalization. According to this reconceptualization of Neugarten's original framework, the divide between the third and fourth ages and the marginalization of the oldest-old is driven by the anti-aging movement, youth-oriented culture, consumerism, and society's general reluctance to accept the aging process.

Critical Gerontology

Critical gerontology was less a formal theory than a framework for understanding the status of the aged within the broader social context (Quadagno & Reid, 1999). Critical perspectives are reflected in several theoretical trends in contemporary social gerontology, including the political economy of aging theory, feminist theories, theories of diversity, and humanistic gerontology. Coming primarily out of the Frankfort school of critical theory (Horkheimer & Adorno, 1944; Habermas, 1971), and poststructuralism (Foucault, 1977), these perspectives shared a common focus on criticizing "the process of power" (Baars, 1991) as well as traditional positivistic approaches to knowledge. The strength of critical theory was its focus on how class structure and the distribution of resources affect opportunities for social interaction and human capital, yet it ignored individual agency as a factor that shapes the lives of older people (Victor, 2013).

Critical gerontology developed two distinct patterns, one that focused on humanistic dimensions of aging, and one that emphasized structural components. Moody (1993) postulated four goals of the humanistic strand of critical theory: (1) to theorize subjective and interpretive dimensions of aging; (2) to focus on praxis (involvement in practical change) instead of technical advancement; (3) to link academics and practitioners through praxis; and (4) to produce "emancipatory knowledge." A second strand emphasized that critical gerontology should create positive models of aging focusing on the strengths and diversity of age, in addition to critiquing positivist knowledge (Bengtson, Burgess, & Parrott, 1997). To reach the goals of critical gerontology, researchers focused on the key concepts of power, social action, and social meanings in examining the social aspects of age and aging. For example, Wild, Wiles, and Allen (2013) used critical gerontology as a lens to question whether *resiliency* is an acceptable benchmark to assess how well people cope with the challenges of older age. They argue that most resilience research fails to explore the role that social inequality and community structure play in limiting or enabling access to resilience resources.

Political Economy of Aging

This perspective, which drew originally from Marxism (Marx, 1967/1867), conflict theory (Simmel, 1904/1966), and critical theory (Habermas, 1971), has used the interaction of economic and political forces to explain how social resources are allocated, and how variations in the treatment and status of the elderly can be understood by examining public policies, economic trends, and social-structural factors (Estes, 2001; Quadagno & Reed, 1999). A political economy perspective applied to aging maintains that socioeconomic and political constraints shape the experience of aging, resulting in the loss of power, autonomy, and influence of older persons. Life experiences are seen as being patterned not only by age, but also by class, gender, race, and ethnicity (Phillipson, 2009). These structural factors, often institutionalized or reinforced by economic and public policies, constrain opportunities, choices, and experiences of later life.

The political economy of aging perspective has been used to critique positive gerontology's focus on civic engagement as a beneficial and necessary role for retired older adults (Martinson & Minkler, 2006). The authors argued that the civic engagement movement devalues older adults for whom engagement is either not desired or impossible because of conditions of poverty or disability. They claimed that the movement is driven by the politics of retrenchment in American political and economic life. Policy makers turn to retired older adults to fill service gaps in their communities, with volunteer work replacing paid work and government-funded social programs designed to serve a community's needs.

The political economy of aging theory would argue that social programs created for older adults benefit capitalist interests and the existing social order more than the elderly themselves (Quadagno & Reid, 1999). Because those in power decide what programs are needed and differentially allocate services across socioeconomic and demographic groups, programs reinforce social stratification and reproduce existing class divisions rather than empower those who are oppressed. Thus, a major focus of the political economy of aging perspective is how ageism is constructed through social practices and policies, and how it harms the well-being of older people.

Feminist Gerontology

Feminist theories of aging, or feminist gerontology, was a form of critical gerontology that gave priority to gender as an organizing principle for social life across the life span that significantly alters the experience of aging in inequitable ways (Calasanti, 1999; McMullin, 1995). Feminist theories regarded current theories and models of aging as insufficient because they failed to address differences in power and privilege in gender relations, the experience of women in the context of aging, civic engagement, and caregiving demands, and issues of race, ethnicity, and class (Blieszner, 1993; Calasanti, 1999; Netting, 2011; Ray, 1996).

Feminist gerontology recognized that gender is socially constructed and has different meanings throughout the life course (Hooyman & Gonyea, 1995). Gender roles for older women are shaped by cultural expectations and historical, political, and economic forces. At the macrolevel of analyses, feminist theories of aging combined with political economy and critical perspectives to examine differential access to key material, health, and caring resources, which substantially alter the experience of aging for women compared to men (Arber & Ginn, 1991; Calasanti & Slevin, 2006). For example, feminist researchers sought to explain the comparatively high rates of poverty among older women and to propose changes in the ideologies and institutions that perpetuate it.

From a feminist perspective, family caregiving can be understood as an experience of obligation, structured by the gender-based division of domestic labor and the devaluing of unpaid work (Stroller, 1993). At the microlevel, feminist perspectives held that gender should be examined in the context of social meanings, reflecting the influence of the social constructivist approach. Like critical gerontology, feminist theories are oriented toward social justice. Proponents advocate for structural change in the institutions of work, retirement, and caregiving to produce greater equity between the sexes (Hooyman et al., 2002).

Social constructionism and critical perspectives have gained prominence in social gerontological theorizing, mirroring theoretical developments in sociology and in the humanities. Social gerontologists often combine insights from these perspectives to guide their research and interpret findings. At the same time, these theoretical perspectives pose a challenge to the scientific assumptions that have traditionally guided much gerontological research.

The Rise of Successful Aging Models and Positive Gerontology

Following the often savage criticisms of disengagement theory (Maddox, 1965; Hochschild, 1975), some social gerontologists simply moved away from explaining how things *are* for older adults, to how things *should be* to improve well-being—hence the popularity of successful and productive aging theories. These theories prescribed ways to maximize and improve the aging experience (Havighurst, 1963; Johnson & Mutchler, 2014; Rowe & Kahn, 1998). Unlike critical gerontology perspectives, frameworks for successful, productive, and positive aging focused less attention on macrolevel political and institutional forces that affect social roles for the aged. Rather, they viewed individuals as active agents in society, directly shaping their aging trajectories through personal lifestyle choices. Positive gerontology emphasized the multiple ways older people contribute to their own health, to their families and communities, and to society (Johnson & Mutchler, 2014).

Successful Aging

The concept of "successful aging" has become perhaps the most popular and frequently cited concept in the history of gerontology (Rowe & Coscoe, 2016). The successful aging perspective is rooted in Havighurst's (1963) activity theory and also Baltes and Baltes's (1990) model of selective optimization with compensation. Rowe and Kahn's (1998) frequently cited recipe for successful aging involves a combination of low probability of disease and disease-related disability, high cognitive and physical functional capacity, and active engagement with life. Modifiable factors that can improve well-being include healthy eating, exercise, and increased social engagement.

Although successful aging has dominated the literature, there are many other positive aspects of aging that have been subjects of theory development—and, importantly, may be less value-laden or politically volatile, more precise, easier to operationalize, and theoretically fecund. These include theories of "optimal" aging, coping, and resilience (Aldwin & Igarashi,

2016), spirituality (Coleman, Schroeder-Butterfill, & Spreadbury, 2015), and wisdom (Ardelt & Oh, 2016).

Productive Aging and Civic Engagement

Productive aging advocated that older adults participate in paid and unpaid work that benefits society (Butler, 1989). Civic engagement refers not only to unpaid volunteer work, but also to work in organizations that pursue activities that benefit the public (Kaskie et al., 2008). The concepts emerged following the 1961 White House Conference on aging, where it was stated that older adults had a "right to be useful" and an "obligation" to participate in meaningful social roles through civic participation, work, and leisure (U.S. Senate Special Committee on Aging, 1961).

According to Bass and Caro's (2001) productive aging framework, social institutions and cultural values that devalue older adults' contributions to society restrict their engagement and exclude them from many positive roles. Activity choices can be improved through organizational and public policies to increase the quality and quantity of civic engagement for older adults. Like Bass and Caro's (2001) framework, many models of productive aging focused on ways that older people can give back to society and the ways policies can promote those roles.

Generativity

The theory of generativity is another successful aging perspective for improving well-being in later life. It was based on Erik Erikson's (1950) lifespan theory of personality development. According to Erikson, generativity is a later stage of adult development that involves nurturing, teaching, leading, and promoting the next generation (McAdams, Saint Aubin, & Logan, 1993). Generativity can be cultivated through volunteering, community activism, religious participation, and work and leisure pursuits. Although not construed as an innate biological drive, generative actions are motivated by a combination of cultural demand and personal desire to build a legacy by promoting younger generations.

The value of generative actions is determined by the aging person's subjective belief in the goodness of humankind and a conscious concern for the well-being of future cohorts (McAdams & Saint Aubin, 1992). In this way the theory borrowed from social constructionism and interpretive theoretical perspectives. The *generativity script*, as described by McAdams (1988), represented individuals' inner accounts of how generative actions fit into their larger life stories, contemporary society, and the social world. As such, the generativity script contributes to one's personal identity, providing a sense of intergenerational unity and life purpose (McAdams & Saint Aubin, 1992). Generativity, like other productive aging frameworks, emphasized social engagement in later life but with a special focus on engaging with younger generations, leading to improved physical and mental well-being.

Recent Efforts at Unified Models of Well-Being in Later Life

Theory development in social gerontology has shifted over time from attempts at grand explanations of the social position of the aged toward discipline-specific micro- and midlevel theories. Midlevel theories are useful in building a bridge between observable social problems and midrange conceptualization (Hendricks, Applebaum, & Kunkel, 2010). Often labeled *models* or *frameworks*, these theories apply existing theoretical concepts to current problems facing older adults, or they apply new concepts to explain specific age-related phenomena, such as elder abuse and intergenerational roles and relationships. Examples of micro- and midlevel theories that have received attention include Andersen's (1995) behavioral health utilization model, the Roy adaptation model applied to caregiver stress (Roy, 1991; Tsai, 2003), and environmental gerontology perspectives that examine the relationship between older persons and their sociospatial surroundings (Wahl & Weisman, 2003).

A trend in gerontology has been to bridge theories across disciplines related to aging—psychology, biology, sociology, and public policy. Bass's (2009) integrative model of social gerontology, for example, examined the cumulative and interacting forces of historical events, economic conditions, power structures, and political environments on an aging individual. These broad sociopolitical conditions shape family and cultural norms around religion, tradition, and role expectations. These contexts also affect a person's access to social and economic resources—health care, housing, jobs, and social relationships.

Bass's (2009) integrative model depicted the life course as proceeding along a dynamic, fluid path. Physiological and psychological conditions interact with the environment to direct individual development and affect well-being in old age. As with the cumulative inequality theory (Ferraro, Shippee, & Schafer, 2009), Bass's (2009) comprehensive life-course model helps explain the heterogeneity among older people in well-being, but its layered, multifaceted dimensions are hard to test using empirical data.

A more recent interdisciplinary perspective is the spectrum model of aging (Martin & Gillen, 2013). It is perhaps the most recent attempt to create a unified lifespan model of aging and human development. Grounded in the positivist perspective, it was conceived as an individual-specific framework that bridged objective and subjective influences on human development and well-being over the life course: genetics, sociodemographic circumstances, childhood events, and lifestyle choices. The spectrum model used a game theory approach (Marshall, 1973) and evidence-based research from many disciplines to plot strategies for improving the aging experience. Similar to Rowe and Kahn's (1998) successful aging framework, it posited that individuals can modify their subjective aging position through behavior modification, pharmacological interventions, social support, health promotion, and other strategies that improve well-being. Each person must choose from a range of options based on the economic, political, and social resources available. A modification in one domain can create new opportunities in other domains, so individuals face limitless possibilities for progressing through a developmental trajectory. The framework allowed individuals to construct their own meanings of successful aging and what they must do to achieve it. Thus, it provides more interpretive approaches to defining successful aging than previous successful aging models (Havighurst, 1963; Rowe & Kahn, 1998).

Opportunities for Future Theory Development in Social Gerontology

Social gerontology is ripe with opportunities to incorporate new concepts into theoretical models that explain well-being in later life. For example, with better tools for collecting physiological data from thousands of participants in longitudinal studies, gerontologists and epidemiologists are now examining the lifelong interplay between genes and the environment, *epigenetics*, and how these interactions affect later-life outcomes. Epigenetics concerns how environmental exposure and lifestyle choices affect the expression of genes, particularly those involved in aging and disease. While little is known about how social support and social structures affect gene expression and ultimately influence well-being, theory development in this area can help guide researchers in designing studies to examine these interactions, leading to targeted interventions.

Another opportune area for theory development is elder mistreatment. This is an expanding interdisciplinary area of research in gerontology that has major implications for well-being in later life. In the early 1980s, caregiver stress and burden was the predominant explanation for elder abuse (Steinmetz, 1978). This perspective was rooted in the social exchange theory (Dowd, 1975) and proposed that as people age they rely more on others who are ill prepared to meet the demands caregiving requires. To rebalance the distribution of power in the relationship, caregivers respond by harming the elder or failing to meet the elder's needs.

Empirical evidence has largely discredited the caregiver stress and burden theory as the sole cause of elder mistreatment (Suitor & Pillemer, 1988; Bristowe & Collins, 1989). Studies in the later 1980s found that caregivers who abused older adults did not necessarily care for more impaired or dependent elders than nonabusing caregivers (Bristowe & Collins, 1989; Pillemer, 1985; Suitor & Pillemer, 1988), and in many cases abusers are not caregivers at all. Despite these findings, researchers still rely on this theory to explain conflict and violence in caregiving relationships.

Other researchers have developed broader theoretical explanations for elder abuse, such as the ecological perspective. This focused on the contextual risk factors that give rise to abuse, such as living with dependent younger relatives with mental health or substance abuse issues (Schiamberg & Gans, 2008). Jackson and Hafemeister (2013) argue that although symptoms and risk factors vary by type of mistreatment, such as neglect versus physical abuse, interventions must be guided by a comprehensive theory. An inclusive theory of elder abuse should explain the underlying phenomenon and take into account the characteristics of both the older victim and the abuser, because successful interventions will likely involve both individuals.

Discussion

Emerging scholars in gerontology should prioritize theory in their area of specialization, as well as try to connect theories across disciplines. In the past, gerontology was characterized as data rich and theory poor (Birren & Bengtson, 1988), although this is slowly changing (Alley et al., 2010; Hendricks, Applebaum, & Kunkel, 2010). Still, applied researchers generally conduct studies that are problem-driven rather than theory-driven. They would argue that their goal is to improve the lives of older adults through research, rather than to generate knowledge for the sake of advancing science. Yet no applied research is devoid of theory. Even descriptive researchers are operating under implicit assumptions about how the world works and how to effect social and political change to enhance the well-being of older adults. Their efforts could be more effective in creating a cumulative knowledge base if they would pay more explicit attention to the theory underlying their findings.

To build a better roadmap for addressing social problems through research, future gerontologists should make their assumptions about cause and effect more explicit using a theoretical framework. Perhaps focusing on midlevel theory development is a promising enterprise for emerging scholars. Midlevel theories do not try to explain everything, but can act as scaffolding to help researchers make sense of their observations and synthesize knowledge across disciplines.

References

Aboderin, I. (2004). Decline in material family support for older people in urban Ghana, Africa: Understanding processes and causes of change. *Journal of Gerontology: Social Sciences, 59B*, S128–S137.

Achenbaum, W. A., & Bengtson, V. L. (1994). Re-engaging the disengagement theory of aging: On the history and assessment of theory development in gerontology. *The Gerontologist, 34*, 756–763.

Agahi, N., Ahacic, K., & Parker, M. G. (2006). Continuity of leisure participation from middle age to old age. *The Journals of Gerontology, Series B: Psychological Sciences and Social Sciences, 61*(6), S340–S346.

Aldwin, C. M., & Igarashi, H. J. (in press). Coping, optimal aging, and resilience in a sociocultural context. In V. L. Bengtson & R. J. Settersten, Jr. (Eds.), *Handbook of theories of aging* (Ch. 25). New York: Springer.

Alley, D. E., Putney, N. M., Rice, M., & Bengtson, V. L. (2010). The increasing use of theory in social gerontology: 1990–2004. *Journal of Gerontology: Social Sciences, 65B*, 583–590.

Andersen, R. M. (1995). Revisiting the behavioral model and access to medical care: Does it matter? *Journal of Health and Social Behavior, 36*, 1–10.

Andrews, T. (2012). What is social constructionism? *Grounded Theory Review, 11*(1), 39–46.

Arber, S., & Ginn, J. (1991). *Gender and later life: A sociological analysis of constraints*. Newbury Park, CA: Sage.

Ardelt, M. A., & Oh, H. D. (2016). Theories of wisdom and aging. In V. L. Bengtson & R. J. Settersten, Jr. (Eds.), *Handbook of theories of aging* (Ch. 29). New York: Springer.

Atchley, R. C. (1989). A continuity theory of normal aging. *The Gerontologist, 29*, 183–190.

Baars, J. (1991). The challenge of critical theory: The problem of social construction. *The Journal of Aging Studies, 5*, 219–243.

Baltes, P. B., & Baltes, M. M. (1990). Psychological perspectives on successful aging. The model of selective optimization with compensation. In P. B. Baltes & M. M. Baltes (Eds.), *Successful aging: Perspectives from the behavioral science* (pp. 1–34). New York: Cambridge University Press.

Bass, S. A. (2009). Toward an integrative theory of social gerontology. In V. L. Bengtson, D. Gans, N. M. Putney, & M. Silverstein (Eds.), *Handbook of theories of aging* (2nd ed., pp. 347–374). New York: Springer.

Bass, S. A., & Caro, F. G. (2001). Productive aging: A conceptual framework. In N. Morrow-Howell, J. Hinterlong, & M. Sherraden (Eds.), *Productive aging: Concepts and challenges* (pp. 37–78). Baltimore, MD: Johns Hopkins University Press.

Bengtson, V. L. (1969). Cultural and occupational differences in level of present role activity in retirement. In R. J. Havighurst, J. M. A. Munnichs, B. L. Neugarten, & H. Thomas (Eds.), *Adjustment to retirement: A cross-national study* (pp. 33–53). Assen, The Netherlands: Van Gorkum.

Bengtson, V. L. (in press). The social forces of later life: Early theory development in the sociology of aging. In V. L. Bengtson & R. J. Settersten Jr. (Eds.), *Handbook of theories of aging* (Ch. 5, pp. 101–123). New York: Springer.

Bengtson, V.L., & Allen, K.R. (1993). The life course perspective applied to families over time. In P.G. Boss, W.J. Doherty, R. LaRossa, W.R. Schumm, & S.K. Steinmetz (Eds.), *Sourcebook of family theories and methods: A contextual approach* (pp. 469–504). New York: Plenum Press.

Bengtson, V. L., & Settersten, R. J., Jr. Theories of aging: Developments within and across disciplinary boundaries. In V. L. Bengtson & R. J. Settersten Jr. (Eds.). *Handbook of theories of aging* (3rd ed., pp. 1–17). New York: Springer.

Bengtson, V.L., Burgess, E.O., & Parrott, T.M. (1997). Theory, explanation, and a third generation of theoretical development in social gerontology. *Journal of Gerontology, 52B*, S72–S88.

Bengtson, V.L., Dowd, J.J., Smith, D.H., & Inkeles, A. (1975). Modernization, modernity, and perceptions of aging: A cross-cultural study. *Journal of Gerontology, 30*(6), 688–695.

Bengtson, V.L., Gans, D., Putney, N.M., & Silverstein, M. (2009). Theories about age and aging. In V.L. Bengtson, D. Gans, N.M. Putney, & M. Silverstein (Eds.), *Handbook of theories of aging* (2nd ed., pp. 3–23). New York: Springer.

Bengtson, V.L., Rice, C.J., & Johnson, M.L. (1999). Are theories of aging important? Models and explanations in gerontology at the turn of the century. In V.L. Bengtson & K.W. Schaie (Eds.), *Handbook of theories of aging* (pp. 3–20). New York: Springer.

Berger, P.L., & Luckmann, T. (1966). *The social construction of reality*. New York: Doubleday.

Birren J., & Bengtson, V. (1988). Preface. *Emergent theories of aging* (pp. ix–x). New York: Springer.

Blau, P. M. (1964). *Exchange and power in social life*. New York: Wiley.

Blieszner, R. (1993). A socialist–feminist perspective on widowhood. *Journal of Aging Studies, 7*, 171–182.

Bristowe, E., & Collins, J.B. (1988). Family mediated abuse of noninstitutionalized frail elderly men and women living in British Columbia. *Journal of Elder Abuse & Neglect, 1*(1), 45–64.

Brown, H. (1986). *The wisdom of science*. New York: Random House.

Burgess, E.W. (1923). The Study of the delinquent as a person. *American Journal of Sociology, 28*(6), 657–680.

Burgess, E.W. (Ed.). (1960). *Aging in western societies*. Chicago, IL: University of Chicago Press.

Butler, R.N. (1989). Dispelling ageism: The cross-cutting intervention. *Annals of the American Academy of Political and Social Science, 503*, 138–147.

Cain, L.D., Jr. (1964). Life course and social structure. In R.E.L. Faris (Ed.), *Handbook of modern sociology* (pp. 272–309). Chicago, IL: Rand McNally.

Calasanti, T.M. (1999). Feminism and gerontology: Not just for women. *Hallym International Journal of Aging, 1*, 44–55.

Calasanti, T. M., & Slevin, K. F. (2006). *Age matters: Realigning feminist thinking*. New York: Taylor & Francis.

Carstensen, L. L. (1992). Social and emotional patterns in adulthood: Support for socioemotional selectivity theory. *Psychology and Aging, 7*, 331–338.

Carstensen, L. L. (2006). The influence of a sense of time on human development. *Science, 312*(5782), 1913–1915.

Carstensen, L. L., & Fredrickson, B. L. (1998). Influence of HIV status and age on cognitive representations of others. *Health Psychology, 17*(6), 494–503.

Cavan, R. S., Burgess, E. W., Havighurst, R. J., & Goldhamer, H. (1949). *Personal adjustment in old age*. Chicago, IL: Science Research Associates.

Coleman, P. G., Schroeder-Butterfill, E. S., & Spreadbury, J. H (2016). Religion, spirituality and aging. In V. L. Bengtson & R. J. Settersten Jr. (Eds.), *Handbook of theories of aging* (Ch. 29). New York: Springer.

Cowdry, E. V. (1939). *Problems of aging*. Baltimore, MD: Williams and Wilkins.

Cowgill, D. A. (1974). Aging and modernization. A revision of the theory. In J. F. Gubrium (Ed.), *Late life* (pp. 126–146). Springfield, IL: Charles C. Thomas.

Cowgill, D. A., & Holmes, L. D. (1972). *Aging and modernization*. New York: AppletonCentury-Crofts.

Cumming, E., & Henry, W. (1961). *Growing old: The process of disengagement*. New York: Basic Books.

Dannefer, D. (2003). Cumulative advantage/disadvantage and the life course: Cross-fertilizing age and social science theory. *Journal of Gerontology: Social Sciences, 58B*, S327–S337.

Dong, X., Simon, M. A., & Gorbien, M. (2007). Elder abuse and neglect in an urban Chinese population. *Journal of Elder Abuse & Neglect, 19*(3–4), 79–96.

Dowd, J. J. (1975). Aging as exchange: A preface to theory. *Journal of Gerontology, 30*, 584–594.

Elder, G. H., Jr. (1992). Models of the life course. *Contemporary Sociology: A Journal of Reviews, 21*, 632–635.

Elder, G. H., Jr., & Johnson, M. K. (2002). The life course and aging: Challenges, lessons, and new directions. In R. A. Settersten Jr. (Ed.), *Invitation to the life course: Toward new understandings of later life* (pp. 49–81). Amityville, NY: Baywood.

Erikson, E. (1950). In M. J. E. Senn (Ed.), *Symposium on the healthy personality* (pp. 91–146). Oxford, England: Josiah Macy, Jr. Foundation.

Estes, C. L. (2001). Political economy of aging: A theoretical framework. In C. L. Estes et al. (Eds.), *Social policy and aging: A critical perspective*. Thousand Oaks, CA: Sage.

Estes, C. L., Gerard, L. E., Jones, J. S., & Swan, J. H. (1984). *Political economy, health, and aging*. Boston, MA: Little, Brown.

Ferraro, K. F., Shippee, T. P., & Schafer, M. H. (2009). Cumulative inequality theory for research on aging and the life course. In V. L. Bengtson, D. Gans, N. M. Putney, & M. Silverstein (Eds.), *Handbook of theories of aging* (2nd ed., pp. 413–433). New York: Springer.

Fisher, D. H. (1977). *Growing old in America*. New York: Oxford University.

Foucault, M. (1977). *Discipline and punish: The birth of a prison* (A. Sheridan, Trans.). New York: Vintage/Random House.

Fung, H. H., Carstensen, L. L., & Lutz, A. M. (1999). Influence of time on social preferences: Implications for life-span development. *Psychology and Aging, 14*(4), 595–604.

Garfinkel, H. (1967). *Studies in ethnomethodology*. Englewood Cliffs, NJ: Prentice Hall.

Gaziano, J. M. (2010). Fifth phase of the epidemiologic transition: The age of obesity and inactivity. *Journal of the American Medical Association, 303*(3), 275–276.

George, L. K. (1996). Missing links: The case for a social psychology of the life course. *The Gerontologist, 36*, 248–255.

Gilleard, C., & Higgs, P. (2010). Theorizing the fourth age: Aging without agency. *Aging and Mental Health, 14*, 121–128.

Gubrium, J. F. (1993). *Speaking of life: Horizons of meaning for nursing home residents*. New York: Aldine de Gruyter.

Gubrium, J. F., & Holstein, J. A. (1999). Constructionist perspectives on aging. In V. L. Bengtson & K. W. Schaie (Eds.), *Handbook of theories of aging* (pp. 287–305). New York: Springer.

Habermas, J. (1971). *Knowledge and human interests* (J. J. Shapiro, Trans.). Boston, MA: Beacon Press.

Hall, G. S. (1922). *Senescence*. New York: Appleton.

Havighurst, R. J. (1943). *Human development and education*. New York: Longman.

Havighurst, R. J. (1963). Successful dying. In R. Williams, C. Tibbits, & W. Donahue (Eds.), *Processes of aging*. New York: Atherton.

Havighurst, R. J., & Albrecht, R. (1953). *Older people*. New York: Longmans, Green.

Hendricks, J. (1992). Generations and the generation of theory in social gerontology. *International Journal of Aging and Human Development, 35*, 31–47.

Hendricks, J. (1995). Exchange theory in aging. In G. Maddox (Ed.), *The encyclopedia of aging* (2nd ed.). New York: Springer.

Hendricks, J., Applebaum, R., & Kunkel, S. (2010). A world apart? Bridging the gap between theory and applied social gerontology. *The Gerontologist, 50*(3), 284–293.

Hochschild, A. R. (1975). Disengagement theory: A critique and a proposal. *American Sociological Review, 40*, 553–569.

Hooyman, N. R., & Gonyea, J. (1995). *Feminist perspectives on family care: Policies for gender justice*. Thousand Oaks, CA: Sage.

Hooyman, N. R., Browne C. V., Ray, R., & Richardson, V. (2002). Feminist gerontology and the life course. *Gerontology & Geriatrics Education, 22*(4), 3–26.

Homans, G. C. (1961). *Social behavior: Its elementary forms*. New York: Harcourt Brace Jovanovich.

Horkheimer, M., & Adorno, T. W. (1944). The cultural industry: Enlightenment as mass deception. In M. Horkheimer & T. W. Adorno (Eds.). *Dialectic of enlightenment* (J. Cumming, Trans.). New York: Continuum Publishing.

Jackson, S. L., & Hafemeister, T. L. (2013). *Understanding elder abuse: New directions for developing theories of elder abuse occurring in domestic settings*. Research in Brief, National Institute of Justice. No. NCJ 241731.

Johnson, K.J., & Mutchler, J.E. (2014). The emergence of a positive gerontology: From disengagement to social involvement. *The Gerontologist, 54*(1), 93–100.

Kaskie, B., Imhof, S., Cavanaugh, J., & Culp, K. (2008). Civic engagement as a retirement role for aging Americans. *The Gerontologist, 48*(3), 368–377.

Kenyon, G.M., Ruth, J., & Mader, W. (1999). Elements of a narrative gerontology. In V.L. Bengtson & K.W. Schaie (Eds.), *Handbook of theories of aging* (pp. 40–58). New York: Springer.

Kuypers, J.A., & Bengtson, V.L. (1973). Social breakdown and competence: A model of normal aging. *Human Development, 16*, 181–201.

Laslett, P. (1976). Societal development and aging. In R. Binstock & E. Shanas (Eds.), *Handbook of aging and the social sciences* (pp. 87–116). New York: Van Nostrand Reinhold.

Laslett, P. (1985). Societal development and aging. In R. Binstock & E. Shanas (Eds.), *Handbook of aging and the social sciences* (2nd ed., pp. 199–230). New York: Van Nostrand Reinhold.

Laslett, P. (1987). The emergence of the third age. *Ageing & Society, 7*, 113–160.

Lemon, B.W., Bengtson, V.L., & Peterson, J.A. (1972). An exploration of the activity theory of aging. *Journal of Gerontology, 27*, 511–523.

Linton, R. (1942). Age and sex categories. *American Sociological Review, 7*, 589–603.

Maddox, G.L. (1965). Fact and artifact: Evidence bearing on disengagement theory from the Duke Geriatrics Project. *Human Development, 8*(2–3), 117–130.

Marshall, V.W. (1973). Game-analyzable dilemmas in a retirement village: A case study. *The International Journal of Aging and Human Development, 4*(4), 285–291.

Marshall, V.W. (1999). Analyzing social theories of aging. In V.L. Bengtson & K.W. Schaie (Eds.), *Handbook of theories of aging* (pp. 434–455). New York: Springer.

Marshall, V.W. (2005). Agency, events, and structure at the end of the life course. *Advances in life course research, 10*, 57–91.

Marshall, V. W., Matthews, A. M., & McMullin, J. A. (2016). The interpretive perspective on aging. In V. L. Bengtson & R. J. Settersten Jr. (Eds.), *Handbook of theories of aging* (Ch. 20). New York: Springer.

Martin, D.J., & Gillen, L.L. (2014). Revisiting gerontology's scrapbook: From Metchnikoff to the spectrum model of aging. *The Gerontologist, 54*(1), 51–58.

Martinson, M., & Minkler, M. (2006). Civic engagement and older adults: A critical perspective. *The Gerontologist, 46*(3), 318–324.

Marx, K. (1967[1867–1895]). *Capital: A critique of political economy*. New York: International Publishers.

McAdams, D.P. (1988). *Power, intimacy, and the life story: Personological inquiries into identity*. Hey York: Guilford Press.

McAdams, D.P., & de Saint Aubin, E.D. (1992). A theory of generativity and its assessment through self-report, behavioral acts, and narrative themes in autobiography. *Journal of personality and social psychology, 62*(6), 1003–1015.

McAdams, D.P., de Saint Aubin, E.D., & Logan, R.L. (1993). Generativity among young, midlife, and older adults. *Psychology and Aging, 8*(2), 221–230.

McMullin, J. (1995). Theorizing age and gender relations. In S. Arber & J. Ginn (Eds.), *Connecting gender and aging: A sociological approach*. Philadelphia, PA: Open University Press.

Mead, G.H. (1934). *Mind, self, and society*. Chicago, IL: University of Chicago Press.

Merton, R.K. (1968). The Matthew effect in science. II: Cumulative advantage and the symbolism of intellectual property. *Isis, 79*, 606–623.

Merz, E.M., & Consedine, N.S. (2009). The association of family support and wellbeing in later life depends on adult attachment style. *Attachment & Human Development, 11*(2), 203–221.

Merz, E., Consedine, N.S., Schulze, H.J., & Schuengel, C. (2009). Wellbeing of adult children and ageing parents: Associations with intergenerational support and relationship quality. *Ageing and Society, 29*(05), 783–802.

Moody, H.R. (1993). Overview: What is critical gerontology and why is it important? In T.R. Cole, W.A. Achenbaum, P.L. Jakobi, & R. Kastenbaum (Eds.), *Voices and visions: Toward a critical gerontology*. New York: Springer.

Moody, H.R. (2001). The humanities and aging: A millennial perspective. *The Gerontologist, 41*, 411–415.

Netting, F.E. (2011). Bridging critical feminist gerontology and social work to interrogate the narrative on civic engagement. *Affilia, 26*(3), 239–249.

Neugarten, B. (1974). Age groups in American society and the rise of the young–old. *The Annals of the American Academy of Political and Social Science, 415*(1), 187–198.

Omran, A.R. (1971). The epidemiologic transition: A theory of the epidemiology of population change. *The Milbank Memorial Fund Quarterly, 49*(4), 509–538.

Omran, A.R. (2005). The epidemiologic transition: A theory of the epidemiology of population change. *Milbank Quarterly, 83*(4), 731–757.

O'Rand, A M. (1996). The precious and the precocious: Understanding cumulative disadvantage and cumulative advantage over the life course. *The Gerontologist, 36*, 230–238.

O'Rand, A. M. (2016). Long, broad and deep: New research directions in aging and inequality. In V. L. Bengtson & R. J. Settersten Jr. (Eds.), *Handbook of theories of aging* (Ch. 19). New York: Springer.

Parsons, T. (1942). Age and sex in the social structure of the United States. *American Sociological Review, 7*, 604–616.

Pillemer, K. (1985). The dangers of dependency: New findings on domestic violence against the elderly. *Social Problems, 33*(2), 146–158.

Pillemer, K., & Finkelhor, D. (1989). Causes of elder abuse: Caregiver stress versus problem relatives. *American Journal of Orthopsychiatry, 59*(2), 179–187.

Phillipson, C. (2009). Social welfare, aging, and globalization in a post-industrial society. In J. Hendricks & J. Powell (Eds.), *The welfare state in post-industrial society* (pp. 57–70). New York: Springer.

Quadagno, J. (1982). *Aging in early industrial society: Work, family and social policy in nineteenth century England*. New York: Academic Press.

Quadagno, J., & Reid, J. (1999). The political economy perspective in aging. In V.L. Bengtson & K.W. Schaie (Eds.), *Handbook of theories of aging* (pp. 344–358). New York: Springer.

Ray, R. E. (1996). A postmodern perspective on feminist gerontology. *The Gerontologist, 36*, 674–680.
Riley, M. W., Johnson, M., & Foner, A. (1972). *Aging and society. Vol III: A sociology of age stratification*. New York: Russell Sage Foundation.
Riley, M. W., Kahn, R. L., & Foner, E. (1994). *Age and structural lag: Society's failure to provide meaningful opportunities in work, family and leisure*. New York: John Wiley.
Riley, M. W., & Loscocco, K. A. (1994). The changing structure of work opportunities: Toward an age-integrated society. In R. P. Abeles, H. C. Gift, & M. G. Ory (Eds.), *Aging and quality of life*. New York: Springer.
Rowe, J. D., & Kahn, R. L. (1998). *Successful aging*. New York: Pantheon Books.
Rowe, J. W., & Cosco, T. D. (2016). Successful aging. In V. L. Bengtson & R. J. Settersten Jr. (Eds.), *Handbook of theories of aging* (Ch. 27). New York: Springer.
Roy, C. (1991). *The Roy adaptation model: The definitive statement*. Norwalk, CT: McGraw-Hill/Appleton & Lange.
Rozario, P. A., Kidahashi, M., & DeRienzis, D. R. (2011). Selection, optimization, and compensation: Strategies to maintain, maximize, and generate resources in later life in the face of chronic illnesses. *Journal of Gerontological Social Work, 54*(2), 224–239.
Samanez-Larkin, G. R., & Carstensen, L. L. (2011). Socioemotional functioning and the aging brain. In J. Decety & J. T. Cacioppo (Eds.), *The Handbook of social neuroscience* (pp. 507–521). New York: Oxford University Press.
Schiamberg, L. B., & Gans, D. (2008). An ecological framework for contextual risk factors in elder abuse by adult children. *Journal of Elder Abuse & Neglect, 11*(1), 79–103.
Schmeeckle, M., & Bengtson, V. L. (1999). Successful aging. Conclusions from a longitudinal study: Cross national perspectives. *Contemporary Gerontology, 5*, 87–90.
Schroots, J. F. (1996). Theoretical developments in the psychology of aging. *The Gerontologist, 36*, 742–748.
Settersten, R. J., Jr., & Bengtson, V. L. (2016). Prospects for future theory development in aging. In V. L. Bengtson & R. J. Settersten Jr. (Eds.), *Handbook of theories of aging* (Ch. 35). New York: Springer.
Settersten, R. J., Jr., & Godlewski, R. A. (2016). Concepts and theories of age and ageing. In V. L. Bengtson & R. J. Settersten Jr. (Eds.), *Handbook of theories of aging* (Ch. 2). New York: Springer.
Silverstein, M., Conroy, S. J., Wang, H., Giarrusso, R., & Bengtson, V. L. (2002). Reciprocity in parent–child relations over the adult life course. *Journal of Gerontology: Social Sciences, 57B*, S3–S13.
Simmel, G. (1904/1966). *Conflict* (K. H. Wolff, Trans.). Glencoe, CL: Free Press.
Steinmetz, S. K. (1978). Battered parents. *Society, 15*(5), 54–55.
Stroller, E. P. (1993). Gender and the organization of lay health care: A socialist–feminist perspective. *Journal of Aging Studies, 7*, 151–170.
Suitor, J. J., & Pillemer, K. (1988). Explaining intergenerational conflict when adult children and elderly parents live together. *Journal of Marriage and the Family, 50*(4), 1037–1047.

Tsai, P.F. (2003). A middle-range theory of caregiver stress. *Nursing Science Quarterly, 16*(2), 137–145.

Turner, J.H. (2005). Is a scientific theory of the family desirable? In V.L. Bengtson, A.C. Acock, K.R. Allen, P. Dilworth-Anderson, & D.M. Klein (Eds.), *Sourcebook of family theory & research* (pp. 26–29). Thousand Oaks, CA: Sage.

U.S. Senate Special Committee on Aging. (1961). *The 1961 White House Conference on aging: Basic statement and recommendations.*

Victor, C. (2013). Social gerontology: Older people and everybody else. In K. Komp & M. Aartsen. (Eds.), *Old age in Europe* (pp. 45–58). Amsterdam: Springer Netherlands.

Wahl, H. W., & Weisman, G. D. (2003). Environmental gerontology at the beginning of the new millennium: Reflections on its historical, empirical, and theoretical development. *The Gerontologist, 43*(5), 616–627.

Walker, A.J., & Allen, K.R. (1999). Relationships between caregiving daughters and their elderly mothers. *The Gerontologist, 31*(3), 389–396.

Wallace, R.A., & Wolf, A. (1991). *Contemporary sociological theory: Continuing the classical tradition* (3rd ed.). Englewood Cliffs, NJ: Prentice Hall.

Wang, M., Henkens, K., & van Solinge, H. (2011). Retirement adjustment: A review of theoretical and empirical advancements. *American Psychologist, 66*(3), 204–213.

Wild, K., Wiles, J.L., & Allen, R.E. (2013). Resilience: Thoughts on the value of the concept for critical gerontology. *Ageing and Society, 33*(1), 137–158.

Young, L.M., Baltes, B.B., & Pratt, A.K. (2007). Using selection, optimization, and compensation to reduce job/family stressors: Effective when it matters. *Journal of Business and Psychology, 21*, 511–539.

CHAPTER THREE

Ageism: Stereotypes, Causes, Effects, and Countermovements

Meika Loe, Ariel Sherry, and Evan Chartier

Do you remember that awful feeling in the pit of your stomach when you turned 40? Bet you'd like to feel that again! Happy 50th!

—Hallmark birthday card

Ageism, or the systematic stereotyping of and discrimination against people because they are old, manifests across overlapping individual, interpersonal, and institutional or societal axes (Wilkinson & Ferraro, 2004). As seen above, ageist birthday cards perpetuate prejudicial attitudes toward elders on an individual level. Young people can also experience age-based individual discrimination when they are considered incompetent at work simply due to their age. These individual manifestations of ageism may include affective, cognitive, and behavioral components (Cuddy & Fiske, 2004).

Unlike other kinds of oppression, with the exception, perhaps, of oppression based on disability, every individual will experience ageism in his or her lifetime. The dichotomy between those privileged and those marginalized by ageism is not as clear as it is with other identities, because who is perceived as old is subjective, there is no obviously defined group of victims, making this a complicated form of discrimination (Kite & Wagner, 2004). Ageism is also more commonplace and socially acceptable than other forms of oppression; most members of American society hold ageist beliefs and/or implicit prejudices such as disproportionately valuing youth

(Levy & Banaji, 2004). Implicit attitude tests have demonstrated that the old exhibit internalized ageism by revealing negative attitudes toward elders, which demonstrates that most people do not age out of ageism (Levy & Banaji, 2004). The widespread nature of ageism makes it less surprising that elders internalize these negative views, such as rejecting the label old or perpetuating the idea of a senior moment (Levy & Banaji, 2004).

We are troubled by the extent to which ageism has pervaded contemporary American society. We therefore write this chapter with an eye toward social change. We hope that Robert Butler's prediction will come true: that the baby boomer generation, in collaboration with other generations, will be successful in eradicating ageism. To that end, we dedicate the final section of this chapter to countering ageism.

We approach this chapter from a social justice perspective that prioritizes agency and self-determination. And yet, our own agency as authors of this chapter is constrained when we consider how language is age-based and politically charged. In order to maintain some level of consistent language use, we support the efforts of sociologists of aging Toni Calasanti and Kathleen Slevin (2001), who make a strong case for using the adjective "old" to reclaim its positive connotations, to naturalize and neutralize it. However, we are aware that attempts to counter ageism can themselves be perceived as ageist. When Meika Loe surveyed several hundred people aged 55 to 95, asking which words they prefer to use to describe their age group, most noted dislike for common terms that highlight age like "elderly," "old," or "senior citizen." When pressed, the majority was most comfortable with "mature adult" or "elder." Similarly, a recent Pew Research Report revealed that 75 percent of Americans associate the term "old" with those who are aged 85 and older, and those who are no longer independent (Taylor, 2009). "Elder" was more warmly received, as it tends to connote respect and refer to a broad age spectrum. Thus, while we have chosen to employ the terms "old" and "elder" as the best of problematic terms to counter ageism, we cannot avoid how charged *age-based language* is in an age-stratified society.

In this chapter, we examine ageism from multiple perspectives to account for the often diffuse and pervasive ways that people of all ages experience *age-based discrimination*. We employ an *age-relations approach* that examines structural ageism by exposing ageism as a system of inequality that generally privileges the young at the expense of the old (Calasanti, 2003). We show how, similar to racism and sexism, ageism is embedded in patterns of behavior and serves as a social organizing principle (Dressel, Mickler, & Yen, 1997). We also use an *intersectional feminist lens* to intentionally uncover how experiences with ageism can differ in frequency and intensity across members of various classes, professions, genders, sexualities, ethnicities, and geographic communities (Bergling,

2004; Cruikshank, 2009; Gullette, 2004). Such a multitiered approach explicitly identifies how ageist policies, institutional practices, and attitudes pervade our individual psyches, social interactions, and biomedical practices. Thus, this chapter analyzes not only *macrolevel age-based stratification*, but also *microlevel ageism* including that which may be internalized by the old themselves (Joyce & Loe, 2010). Accordingly, we have divided our chapter into four subsections. The first section lays out common definitions and stereotypes associated with ageism as well as social theories attempting to understand the causes of ageism; the second explores effects of structural ageism; the third takes an intersectional approach in understanding ageism; and the final section is dedicated to countering ageism.

Ageism: Definitions, Stereotypes, and Social Causes

Ageism Defined

Pulitzer prize winning geriatrician Robert Butler coined the term *ageism* in 1969 to refer to the "systematic stereotyping of and discrimination against people because they are old, just as racism and sexism accomplish this with skin color and gender" (p. 243). Such judgments were based on a "deep-seated uneasiness on the part of the young and the middle aged—a personal revulsion to and distaste for growing old, disease, disability, and fear of powerlessness, uselessness and death" (Butler, 1969, p. 243). Butler (1975) felt that such learned revulsion led younger generations to "subtly cease to identify with their elders as human beings" (p. 12).

In 1980, Butler expanded his definition of ageism for use in social science by developing three distinguishable but interrelated concepts: *prejudicial attitudes, discriminatory practices*, and *institutional practices and policies that perpetuate stereotypes and undermine dignity*. All three social aspects of ageism are interrelated and mutually reinforcing.

Although Butler's work was well known in academic circles, founder of the Gray Panthers Maggie Kuhn is credited with popularizing the term *ageism* in America. Kuhn founded the Gray Panthers organization in 1970, in response to her forced retirement at the age of 65 (Wilkinson & Ferraro, 2004). Among their many initiatives and achievements, the Gray Panthers established a U.S. national media watch task force designed to track ageist stereotyping.

Ageist Stereotypes

Cuddy and Fiske (2004) argue that individuals can have multiple, often contradictory views of older persons. Even elders themselves often internalize contradictory ageist notions called self-ageism. *Self-ageism*, or "a learned set of beliefs and practices that prevent us from functioning in an optimal way in relation to aging, our own bodies, and people more than ten years older than we are," is one form of internalized oppression (Gullette, 2011, p. 34). Self-ageism encourages elders into one of a limited number of culturally acceptable roles, such as the grandmotherly and family-oriented older woman, distinguished elder statesman and respected conservative gentleman, or the isolated and inactive senior citizen (Cuddy & Fiske, 2004). Hess's classic work on stereotypes and stereotype threat revealed a deep-seated prejudice in American culture that may prime older adults to enact self-ageism through slowed walking and displaying worse memory, thereby making ageism a self-fulfilling prophecy (Hess, 2006; Whitbourne & Sneed, 2004).

Word association studies indicate that Americans tend to associate old people who are white and middle class with words such as "incompetent" and "warm." However, these associations change dramatically when asked about elders with different racial, gender, and class identities (Cuddy & Fiske, 2004). The *stereotypes* associated with our culturally acceptable roles for elders intersect with race, class, and gender-based oppressions to especially marginalize people of color, low income, and transgender individuals who are often unable to embody one of society's acceptable elder roles. Other common stereotypes of elders include being diseased, lonely and depressed, physically and cognitively impaired, unattractive, unproductive, and asexual (Joyce & Mamo, 2006; Whitbourne & Sneed, 2004; Wilkinson & Ferraro, 2004).

Ageist stereotypes are perpetuated through our language use, mass media, and academic scholarship. Media outlets, such as television and greeting card companies, often underrepresent the elderly, cast them in peripheral or negatively depicted roles, and rely on ageist notions as the punch line for jokes (Palmore, 1999; Pasupathi & Löckenhoff, 2004; Wilkinson & Ferraro, 2004). The societal taboo of asking someone his or her age points to the implicit assumption that it is something to be ashamed of (Palmore, 1999). In scholarship, ageism occurs when elders are lumped together in one group, without acknowledging variation or generational differences.

Social scientists have built upon Butler's work to link ageism with both social oppression and privilege. Positive ageism exists both in the form of discrimination in favor of old people, such as Medicare, as well as *positive stereotypes* (Wilkinson & Ferraro, 2004). Palmore (1999) notes eight positive attributes associated with elders: kindness, wisdom, political power, eternal youth, dependability, happiness, freedom, and affluence.

Causes of Ageism

Two primary theoretical perspectives have emerged in the debate over what processes cause ageism: terror management theory and social identity theory. *Terror management theory* (Becker, 1973) suggests that ageism stems from death denial, or fears about our own mortality. Scholars in this tradition propose that older adults remind the young of their inevitable death. The recognition of one's mortality threatens one's worldview, and the individual responds by physically and psychologically distancing themselves from elders (Greenberg, Schimel, & Mertens, 2004). Such distancing creates a social barrier that inhibits individuals from meeting older adults who may defy their ageist stereotypes. As a result, perceptions of elders are more greatly influenced by one's own family members or mass media outlets, which are already imbued with ageist messages.

Social identity theory, described by Kite and Wagner (2004), has also been used to explain how ageism is taught and reinforced through interactions. This theory posits that in order to feel good about oneself, one must feel good about the group to which one belongs by feeling superior to other groups. Therefore, a young person may negatively stereotype elders to increase his or her self-esteem. As the United States undergoes massive demographic changes as the population ages significantly over the next several decades, social identity theory may become an even more important perspective to explore.

Ageism: Social, Economic, and Health Effects

Ageism shapes social, economic, and health outcomes. This section reviews social science research on the effects of ageism in relationships, in the workplace, and in terms of health behaviors and outcomes.

Ageism in Relationships

Within the context of relationships, ageism can significantly influence the way individuals interact with older adults. At one level, it shapes communication. Due to the stereotype that elders are incompetent, many speak to elders using what has been termed *elder speak*. Elder speak is much like baby talk, characterized by simple words and explanations and basic topics of conversation (Cuddy & Fiske, 2004; Pasupathi & Löckenhoff, 2004). Not only does ageism alter the way others speak to elders, but it also influences the way people respond to what elders say. One contributor to the high rates of elder abuse is the fact that many people do not believe older adults when they "complain" about being mistreated (Pasupathi & Löckenhoff, 2004). Ageism may also fuel elder abuse because of the individuals' conceptions of elders as helpless and repulsive, therefore not worth respecting (Palmore, 1999). Nursing homes put elders at particular risk because the power dynamic between the employees and the residents leave elders in powerless and low-status roles (Palmore, 1999).

Additionally, many people prefer to distance themselves physically from elders. This practice takes many forms, including putting seniors in nursing homes and avoiding senior centers. Although it is illegal for real estate agents to discriminate by age, such a law indicates ageist tendencies in finding housing for elders (Palmore, 1999). *Physical distancing* is also seen in experimental contexts, such as in a study by Isaacs and Bearison (1986), in which children distanced themselves more from an elder partner (75-year-old) than a younger one (35-year-old), showing just how early such discrimination begins. Such isolation puts the old at higher risk for mental and physical illness, and even suicide (Palmore, 1999). Even more interesting, sometimes it is the old who distance themselves from the young to avoid becoming targets of ageist remarks and discrimination (MacDonald & Rich, 1983; Palmore, 1999).

For older women in particular, ageist stereotypes increase the risk of invasion of privacy and threats to safety. Within families, sometimes it is not isolation but the opposite that causes problems. Gerontologist Margaret Cruikshank (2009) explains that many families make the generalized assumption that older women require little physical and psychological space. This is in part connected with the stereotyping of all older women as grandmothers whose purpose it is to serve younger generations.

Ageism at Work

Yet another physical distancing technique involves keeping elders out of the workplace. Employers point to many common stereotypes of senior workers as rationale for *workplace discrimination*. One such stereotype is that older workers are no longer fit to continue their jobs due to physical and mental decline or age-related inability to adapt to changing technology (McCann & Giles, 2004). This stereotype is further linked with the assumption that performance and productivity decline among older workers and that senior employees are less creative than their younger counterparts (Cuddy & Fiske, 2004; McCann & Giles, 2004). Such a bias is reflected in work evaluations, where many employers rate older workers as worse than their younger counterparts, despite studies that show there are no differences in the two groups' work outputs (McCann & Giles, 2004). Even when employers are presented with identical resumes, save for the age of the applicant, they reveal a preference for the younger worker (Bendick, Jackson, & Romero, 1993). Older workers are also often charged as being close-minded and unwilling to change (Cuddy & Fiske, 2004).

These ageist views can severely impact the careers and quality of life for older workers. Those who still have a job might experience ageism on a daily basis in their work environment in the form of jokes and hostile humor, patronizing speech, and discrimination in training (McCann & Giles, 2004). Ageism is closely tied with discrimination against older adults during hiring and forcing senior workers into retirement (Greenberg, Schimel, & Mertens, 2004; Palmore, 1999). At times, such hiring discrimination is made on a judgment as basic as someone "looks too old" (Gullette, 2011, p. 119). This can make it extremely hard for older workers to find jobs and can also have a tremendous negative impact on their economic well-being. Even those in midlife can have significant difficulty securing certain jobs (e.g., those that depend on rapidly changing technology), and such "displacement among workers in their fifties and sixties often results in lower wages or lasting unemployment" (Gullette, 2011, p. 153). In addition to their negative views of older workers, employers are also motivated to reject older workers because they can pay younger workers much less and save by not having to pay pension or retirement packages (Palmore, 1999).

The U.S. government has played a notable role in protecting older workers. The Social Security Act, enacted in 1935, was the first major national policy in this realm. This act served to institutionalize retirement, presenting 65 as the proper age for retirement (McCann & Giles, 2004). Three decades later, the Age Discrimination in Employment Act (ADEA) of 1967 was created in an attempt to "protect individuals older than age 40 from employment discrimination based on age, as well as to promote opportunities for older workers who were capable of meeting job requirements" (McCann & Giles, 2004, p. 177). Many years later, in 2005, the Supreme Court ruled that with regard to the ADEA, victims only needed to show disparate impact instead of intentional discrimination (Cruikshank, 2009). Building on the ADEA is the Older Workers Benefit Protection Act of 1990 (the Older Workers Act), which was put in place with the goal to ensure that older workers receive benefits outlined in a waiver that is given "knowingly and voluntarily" (Gregory, 2001; McCann & Giles, 2004).

Despite the government's efforts to protect the rights of older workers, there are still many cases in the United States where individuals are victims of hiring discrimination or ageist comments in the workplace (McCann & Giles, 2004; Wilkinson & Ferraro, 2004). Gregory (2001) argues that the ADEA falls short in eliminating ageist stereotypes in the workplace and notes that it can be extremely challenging for older workers to prove discrimination in hiring. Similarly, because many other decisions within the workplace are subjective, such as promotions and transfers, it is hard to prove discriminatory intent (Gregory, 2001). Because it is so difficult to prove workplace age discrimination in court, many fear accusing their employers because of the retaliation that might ensue in the case of a non-conviction (Gregory, 2001). The shortcomings of these policies indicate a need for new or reformed laws that could better bring justice to the workplace.

Despite the negative impact ageism can have on older adults' employment and economic security, elders are also the beneficiaries of *positive economic ageism*. There are many programs that discriminate by age such that elders save money, such as certain tax benefits (e.g., double personal exemption) and senior discounts at many stores, restaurants, and hotels (Palmore, 1999). Social security is another institutional form of positive ageism, as those who receive benefits do so because of their age, combined with marital status and work history. Additionally, there are two government programs that attempt to increase employment opportunities for just older adults. The first, Senior Community Service Employment Program for Older Americans Act, guarantees minimum-wage pay to those over 55 for part-time public service. Similarly, the Foster Grandparent Program pays low-income elders to help care for people in need, such as special needs children, orphaned infants, and those in convalescent hospitals (Palmore, 1999).

Ageism in Health Care

Discriminatory treatment of older adults extends into the medical sphere as well. Cultural critic Margaret Gullette (2011) suggests that doctors treat older patients differently, "withholding information, diagnostic services, or treatment" (p. 51). Elder speak appears extensively in this domain, as health-care practitioners are known to oversimplify the information they share with elder patients, use slower speech, and adopt a demeaning emotional tone (Cuddy & Fiske, 2004; Palmore, 1999). Furthermore, studies show that doctors communicate more clearly and respectfully and provide much better information when dealing with younger patients as opposed to older adults (Pasupathi & Löckenhoff, 2004). In nursing homes, many employees treat residents almost as if they are children, which has the effect of depleting older adults' self-esteem and promoting dependent rather than independent behavior (Pasupathi & Löckenhoff, 2004). Other health professionals too are known to treat older patients like children (Palmore, 1999). Wilkinson and Ferraro argue that ageist attitudes of doctors begin at medical school, where they are exposed to ageist language in discussions about geriatric care. Additionally, medical professionals are most familiar with older adults who are sick, making it easier to stereotype all elders as frail and to associate aging with disease (Palmore, 1999).

Not only do elders receive less information about their health but they also receive *differential treatment*. There are many instances in which older adults remain untreated for "common and treatable medical conditions"

(Levy & Banaji, 2004, p. 50). Contributing to the problem is the fact that many believe health conditions and illnesses in older adults are inherent and irreversible, simply due to natural aging, even if that is not the case (Palmore, 1999). Comparing the diagnostic differences between younger and older patients, researchers have found that older adults are less likely to be referred for psychiatric help and that doctors tend to attribute health issues to age rather than an actual medical condition (Cuddy & Fiske, 2004; Gullette, 2011; Pasupathi & Löckenhoff, 2004). For example, memory lapses are considered much more seriously in older adults and such cognitive issues in this population are considered to arise from stable causes, rather than some temporary condition (Kite & Wagner, 2004). As a result of these biased diagnoses, many elders fail to receive the treatment they need. And many elders themselves fail to recognize signs of health issues because they too attribute many symptoms to normal aging (Palmore, 1999).

In some cases, elders experience not merely lack of treatment, but outright mistreatment. *Elder abuse* in the health-care system is a serious problem. Awareness of this issue has increased as hidden videos capturing instances of elder abuse in care facilities across America have been released online. MacDonald and Rich (1983) explain how the stereotype of older women as particularly weak and vulnerable makes them easy targets for male abusers. For more on elder abuse, see Chapter 9, Volume 2 of this series.

Just as stereotypes alter the ways health practitioners interact with, diagnose, and treat older adults, stereotypes also contribute to health issues. Much research in the social sciences has found evidence of *stereotype priming*, in which simply thinking about stereotypes of the group to which one belongs can unconsciously lead individuals to behave in the ways described by those stereotypes. This phenomenon has been observed many times with older adults. Stereotype activation among older cohorts has been shown to lead to decreases in one's will to live, worse handwriting, slower walking speeds, and decreased performance on memory tasks (Levy & Banaji, 2004). Furthermore, exposure to these stereotypes has been shown to lead to heightened cardiovascular stress responses (Levy & Banaji, 2004). The effects of stereotype priming therefore makes it hard to assess whether older adults actually display signs of serious health issues or are just influenced by the stereotypes of which they are constantly bombarded.

Further fueling ageism in the medical sphere are notions that older adults are not worth the same care as younger patients. Gullette (2011) refers to this as medical care being "rationed by age" (p. 52). Because many elder patients rely on Medicare they are less attractive to hospitals because such institutions make less money in treating them (Wilkinson & Ferraro, 2004). Additionally, many people believe that since older adults will be "dying soon" anyway, they do not deserve the same treatment as the young, even if a proper analysis of their health would reflect otherwise (Pasupathi & Löckenhoff, 2004). Others argue that treating older adults is much more complex than treating the non-old, and thus reducing their health care would alleviate some of doctors' stress (Palmore, 1999). The sentiments that elders are burdens on the health-care system and unworthy of proper medical attention can produce even more health risks for older adults. Gullette (2011) suggests that making elders feel like burdens on an institutional level may lead many older adults not to seek care when it is needed, or to contemplate and maybe even attempt suicide.

Ageism and Medicine

So far we have discussed ageism in health care primarily in terms of how it directly influences the way older adults are regarded and treated. Another key way in which health care in America is linked with ageism is *medicalization*. Medicalization is the tendency to define any emotional, mental, and physical process as medical (Conrad, 2007). Medicalization affects all ages, but it has particular implications in an ageist society. In societies that position youthful bodies as the norm, the changes associated with aging are ripe for being labeled pathological. Sociologists, anthropologists, and gerontologists have carefully documented the transformation of the emotional, mental, and physical changes associated with aging into "illnesses" (Cruikshank, 2009; Estes & Binney, 1989; Gubrium, 1986; Kaufman, 1994; Lock, 1993). For example, the medical construction of Alzheimer's disease redefined memory loss as an illness category during the 1960s and 1970s (Gubrium, 1986). Since then, what had been a normal component of aging was reconfigured into a spectrum-based, "mild-to-severe" disease through the creation and delineation of medical diagnostic categories (Joyce & Loe, 2010).

Today, *anti-aging medicine* taps into the fear of aging and represents one possible extension of medicalization processes. Instead of particular mental, physical, or emotional processes being turned into a disease, now the aging process itself is understood as pathology (Joyce & Loe, 2010). In this context, even popular medicine such as Dr. Oz's "The Power to Prevent Aging," pathologizes aging and promotes restoration to youthfulness.

Embodied ageism and medicalization intersect with sexism in particular by pressuring women to achieve what Brooks (2010) calls "the ideal of a feminized agelessness." Within this ideal, women are expected to continually work to reverse, minimize, and prevent signs of aging and maintain appearances, such as perky breasts and flat stomachs, associated with a particular version of youthful femininity. With anti-aging medicine, such as expensive pharmacological therapies and surgeries, the symbols and connotations associated with a particular body can be manipulated to present different levels of aging (Calasanti & Slevin, 2001). Brooks (2010) explores how American women's attitudes about femininity and aging are shaped in the context of deciding whether to use anti-aging medicine and technology. Because American society deems women old at a younger chronological age than men, primarily due to the cultural importance of appearance and reproductive abilities to a woman's worth in society, women experience particular pressure to utilize anti-aging techniques (Calasanti & Slevin, 2001).

Ageism: An Intersectional Approach

Ageism is a socially constructed system of discrimination that intersects with other hierarchies such as gender, race, class, and sexuality. An *intersectional approach* reveals ageism as one form of discrimination within a system of overlapping oppressions such as racism, sexism, classism, and homophobia (Collins, 1990). Ageism varies from other forms of discrimination because we all must age and die, and therefore all humans experience ageism during their lives.

Although all elders may experience ageism, other forms of discrimination—namely sexism, racism, classism, and heterosexism—make the experience of ageism different across various groups (Calasanti & Slevin, 2001). For example, we all experience some of the *social stigma* against aging bodies; however, elders in minority groups who may be black, lesbian, or poor will experience more prejudice and have access to different tools for responding to ageism than a white, wealthy, and/or straight man. At the same time, *cultural variation in attitudes* about aging and old people within the United States may translate into more reverence for elders in minority groups. For example, Loe (2011) shows how old women are often keystones in African American churches. This section is dedicated to uncovering the importance and impact of these intersectional realities.

Calasanti and Slevin's (2001) book, *Gender, Social Inequalities, and Aging*, highlights the ways in which an intersectional framework is beneficial to illuminating the persistence of ageism within society and academia. Calasanti and Slevin use a *relational approach* that recognizes how diverse elders' experiences of ageism are shaped in relation to one another by intentionally focusing on nonmajority experiences. Unfortunately, academic fields in general, and gerontological research specifically, lack significant data on diverse populations; despite increasing racial and ethnic diversity amongst America's elderly population, gerontologists continue to study primarily homogeneous populations of white elders and low-income African Americans (Calasanti & Slevin, 2001). The following analyses are therefore based on a small number of studies with limited data on nonmajority groups, perhaps due in part to racial/ethnic patterns in life expectancy; however, we believe that the conclusions drawn from even restricted sample sizes have important ramifications for how we understand ageism in contemporary society.

One reality of an intersectional approach is the impossibility of analyzing a specific hierarchy or identity in isolation. We focus the following discussion around manifestations of ageism in relation to three *guiding ageist stereotypes*: the dependent elder, the ageless elder, and the asexual elder. Woven throughout each discussion is an integrated intersectional analysis that attempts to illuminate how ageism is experienced differently across races, genders, sexualities, and social classes.

An intersectional perspective is particularly important for gerontologists given the complicit role of the discipline in perpetuating ageist practices. Gerontologists have historically used a middle-aged, white, heterosexual bias in theory and research to define the old as deviant from a middle-aged norm (Calasanti & Slevin, 2001). For example, the concept of "aging successfully" promotes the idea that aging is an individual problem that elders can adapt to (Calasanti & Slevin, 2001). If aging is seen as an individual problem that can be controlled, then elders who cannot control their aging process—for medical, financial, or other reasons—are at fault and can be blamed. "Productive aging" defines a successful elder as one who maintains their ability to produce within a capitalist society, even though capitalism disadvantages the oldest-old, women, and minorities who either cannot work or perform a majority of unpaid care work (Calasanti & Slevin, 2001). An emphasis on productive aging is ageist because it contends that the old are only valuable as long as they subscribe to middle-aged norms, which transfers ageist stereotypes to those who cannot work rather than challenging such notions (Calasanti & Slevin, 2001).

The Dependent Elder

One ageist stereotype of the old is their uniform association with increased *economic dependence* on state resources. However, research shows that the economic dependence of elders varies widely amongst individuals with different racial, class, sexual orientation, and gender identities. For example, government benefits—such as Social Security and Medicare—are allocated to assist low-income elders; however, partner benefits have previously not been available to individuals in same-sex partnerships in states without marriage equality. In these states, elders in same-sex relationships may be unable to access their spouse's benefits, therefore increasing their dependence on outside resources as compared to their straight, legally married peers (Calasanti & Slevin, 2001; LGBT Movement Advancement Project and Services and Advocacy for Gay, Lesbian, Bisexual and Transgender Elders, 2010).

Gendered care work provides another example of how particular groups become especially economically dependent with age. Traditional divisions of labor, market discrimination, and unstable employment histories make it more difficult for women to receive promotions, pay, pensions, and Social Security; women are therefore more likely than men to become dependent on state resources in old age (Calasanti & Slevin, 2001). The inability to access resources and dependence on state assistance is especially problematic for many elder women of color, who are overwhelmingly represented in low-income and care work occupations (Calasanti & Slevin, 2001). Men of color are significantly more likely than whites to have a criminal record, which has a strong negative correlation with securing a job and increases the likelihood that nonwhite elders will become dependent on state resources in old age (Pager, 2003). Given society's ageist tendency to devalue elders who are seen as economically dependent on outside resources, low-income, nonwhite, LGBT, and women elders are marginalized by ageism at rates far greater than the stereotypical white, straight, and/or male individual.

Old age in the United States has become synonymous with physical dependence and illness and is therefore something to be avoided. This ageist assumption that all elders are physically dependent ignores important nuances inherent in lives of *interdependence*. Furthermore, U.S.-based elders are constructed in contrast to a mythical ideal of human adult independence, an ideal that is virtually unattainable. Assuming that elders are completely physically dependent on family members or personal care assistants strips them of the significant personal agency that the old exercise throughout their daily lives. In her book *Aging Our Way: Independent Elders, Interdependent Lives,* Meika Loe (2011) explains how the old exercise *personal agency* by advocating for themselves, networking, innovating, growing, and learning well into old age. That said, agency itself is shaped by locational factors, privilege, and oppression. By ignoring the diverse manifestations of personal agency in old age, we construct the aging process as primarily a loss of independence.

Physical dependence and poor health do not develop among the old uniformly, nor are they experienced in the same ways across individuals. These dependence and health disparities are stratified across socioeconomic and racial lines, and become especially problematic when ageist societies give independent elders more social value, while others who are needy are marginalized and ostracized. For example, social class has a significant impact on a child's exposure to different physical and psychosocial environments, which in turn influence adult health (Cohen et al., 2010). Low-income youth who enter working-class jobs with minimal health benefits become dependent, low-income elders far sooner than their more privileged peers (Calasanti & Slevin, 2001). Moreover, members of racial minority groups report age-related physical ailments far earlier than white elders, and research indicates that black elders receive inferior health care compared to white elders regardless of their income (Newman, 2003; Wallace, 1991). *Cumulative inequality theory* suggests that the lifelong accumulation of disadvantages associated with low-income occupations, inaccessible health benefits, and inferior quality medical care lead impoverished nonwhite people into physical dependence at a far greater rate than those who are more privileged, a fact that makes "successful aging" nearly impossible (Ferraro & Kelley-Moore, 2003; Ferraro & Shippee, 2009). These minority group members are therefore more likely to become physically dependent and be marginalized by a society that increasingly values productive independence.

Even elders who rely on family members or personal care assistants are not uniformly impacted by their dependence. Class privilege affords elders with financial resources the ability to purchase care work at market value, thereby maintaining separate social, familial, and dependent care work spheres. As seen in the film, *Gen Silent* (Maddux, 2010), ageism and sexuality intersect in caring for elder gays/lesbians; many elders who become dependent on personal care assistants feel they must go back in the closet to protect their health and well-being. The LGBTQ elders who are forced to hide their sexuality due to fear of reprisal or discrimination at the hands of family members or personal care assistants are unable to maintain the heterocentric middle-aged norm touted by American society, and thus fail to age successfully in their contexts of care.

The Ageless Elder

Martha B. Holstein (2006) describes how cultural messages, the media, and the academy "support the denial of change" and imply "that age should be no more than an artifact . . . we need be no different in old age than we were in middle age" (p. 313). Successful aging is defined by the ability to maintain an "ageless" level of independence and productivity into old age (Kaufman, 1994). *Agelessness* is a social ideal marketed to the healthy and wealthy in the form of anti-aging medicine. Specifically, medicalization encourages the old to become dependent on medications and expensive procedures in an attempt to stall, or even reverse, the aging process. However, the medicalization of aging does not affect all elders equally. An intersectional approach is useful to uncover how the diverse old experience medicalization differently.

Medicalization highlights the importance of economic resources. As mentioned above, the surgeries, hormone treatments, exercise regimes, and prescriptions that help some elders avoid ageist stereotypes by passing as younger adults, or aging successfully, are an exercise in class privilege (Calasanti & Slevin, 2001, p. 19–21). These expensive medical interventions differentiate aging experiences between the rich and poor, as the former are more able to afford such treatments and thus avoid the stigma associated with aging. Given the strong relationship between gender and racialized oppressions, the class privilege associated with the ability to pass as middle-aged disproportionately marginalizes low-income women of color. In addition to being a principally ageist notion, participating in a culture of medicalized aging to distance ourselves from the old is simply not an option for most marginalized populations.

The Asexual Elder

The medicalization of aging highlights the intersections between ageism and sexuality by rendering invisible sexually active elders, particularly those beyond midlife. In so doing, medicalization continues to prioritize a middle-aged or ageless heterosexual norm as the social and cultural basis against which other expressions of sexuality are judged. As people age, they tend to rely on an increasing number of medications and medical interventions that can dampen sexual desire, such as antidepressants, drugs for high blood pressure, and chemotherapy (DeLamater, 2012). The negative impact of these medical interventions and medications on a person's libido may perpetuate the commonly held ageist assumption that aging in general subsumes all sexual desire, rather than attributing at least some of the changes to various medicinal side effects (Walz, 2002). In addition, the increased prevalence of and social reliance on expensive cosmetic surgeries, hormone replacement treatments, and erectile dysfunction drugs are attempts to avoid the stigma and shame associated with sexually inactive aging bodies by medicalizing an otherwise biologically normal phenomenon (Joyce & Mamo, 2006; Loe, 2006).

Ageist assumptions that the old are inherently asexual, along with limited research on elders' sexual experiences, render the realities of elders' sexual desire and pleasure invisible. Sexual people are conceptualized as teenagers and young adults, especially young men and couples in their teens, twenties, and thirties. Even feminist scholars have paid more attention to younger women's sexual experiences and reproductive issues associated with youth (DeLamater, 2012). The stereotype that elders do not engage in sexual behaviors is contradicted by recent findings that more than half of 65 to 74-year-olds, and more than one in four 75 to 85 year-old elders, identify as sexually active (Lindau et al., 2007). Many women over the age of 85 experience sexual intimacy and pleasure (Loe, 2006). In fact, some elders report developing an increased sense of personal agency and expanded "repertoire of physical responses" as they age (Winks & Semans, 2002). The widespread assumption that the old are not engaged in sexual behaviors may hamper efforts to provide accurate sexual health education and counseling services to the elderly population (Lindau et al., 2007).

The *social and cultural invisibility* of sexual lives of diverse elders is perpetuated in academic research. Scholars and research studies tend to focus only on straight, white, young, and/or middle-aged populations; for example, there were only three articles in family gerontology published in the 1990s that dealt with LGBT elders (Allen & Walker, 2006). This is despite the fact that 1.5 million elders over the age of 65 are currently identified as lesbian, gay, or bisexual, and this population is expected to double over the next 15 years (LGBT Movement Advancement Project and Services and Advocacy for Gay, Lesbian, Bisexual, and Transgender Elders, 2010). Understanding the sexual experiences of LGBT elders is particularly difficult because the contemporary old, particularly privileged women, grew up in a culture where they were expected not to be sexual beings let alone identify as gay, lesbian, bisexual, or transgender (Calasanti & Slevin, 2001).

Countering Ageism

How can we counter ageism in the twenty-first century? Anti-ageist work can occur on *individual, relational, and societal levels*. This section reviews efforts to counter ageism ranging from policy reform, to social media campaigns, to organizational and grassroots work. Calasanti and Slevin (2001) suggest that individuals strive to be anti-ageist by uncovering and fighting ageism in its many forms.

Countering Ageism at Individual and Relational Levels

What can you do to counter ageism? Awareness is an important first step in fighting ageism. Being *self-aware* of our potentially ageist attitudes, including being mindful of our implicit ageism, is key to changing how we view and interact with elders (Golub, Filipowicz, & Langer, 2004; Palmore, 1999). When we learn to recognize negative ageist stereotypes and discrimination, perpetuated by others or ourselves, we can better call attention to these unacceptable thoughts and behaviors. Furthermore, acknowledging age-based power and privilege, or how younger individuals benefit from ageism, puts age relations in perspective.

Spreading awareness and educating others about ageism and its many forms is crucial to combatting ageism. Braithwaite (2004) as well as Golub, Filipowicz, and Langer (2004) argue the importance of teaching people to recognize that not all elders are the same and should not be grouped as such, encouraging people to recognize the unique characteristics of older adults. Barbara MacDonald and Cynthia Rich (1983) calls on us to treat elders as fully human, and thus to "look [elders] in the eye." Education, which can include anything from gerontology workshops and classes to social studies, should also include teaching diverse positive images of elders and challenging negative stereotypes by learning why many are common misconceptions (Levy & Banaji, 2004; Palmore, 1999). One way to understand the root of many ageist misconceptions is to consider other reasons that older adults might be behaving in the ways that are stereotyped. For example, Golub, Filipowicz, Langer (2004), borrowing from disability studies, suggest that elders might have difficulty getting out of a car not because of physical weakness but rather because the car is not well designed for their needs. Similarly, there may be cases in which older adults appear forgetful to younger generations, but this could be because they are indifferent to a topic and thus do not pay attention to it (Golub, Filipowicz, & Langer, 2004).

It can be equally beneficial to change the language we use, not only in terms of referring to elders, but also in how we communicate with them and how we talk about aging. Palmore (1999) calls on us to stop using *ageist language* in a way that connotes aging as positive or negative. For example, he suggests that rather than say "stay young," we say "stay healthy, alert, vigorous, active" (Palmore, 1999, p. 92). Also, as we saw at the beginning of this chapter, humor can be a vehicle to reinforce ageism. Aging itself is regularly turned into a joke in an ageist society. We can counter ageism by limiting the ageist jokes we tell and call others out when they use ageist language or humor (Palmore, 1999). We can also use humor to reject age-based stereotypes, or to cope with ageism. For example, nonagenarian Glenn, profiled in *Aging Our Way*, confronts asexual elders stereotypes by sending lewd jokes via email, and leaving a thrift-store slip on his unmade bed for his housekeeper to find (Loe, 2011). In this way, laughing about the changes that aging inevitably brings can be healthy and beneficial.

Elders themselves can play a significant role in combatting ageism. Palmore (1999) finds that elders typically respond to ageism in four main ways: They accept ageism and tend to withdraw; they try to pass as younger so as to deny association with a negative status; they attempt to avoid ageism by isolating themselves; and they form organizations that strive to counter ageist stereotypes and promote reform. Because most elders are themselves ageist (just as women can reinforce sexism), there is a call for older adults in particular to rally against this prejudice and discrimination. Recent examples of elder activism around ageism include "Yo, is this ageist?" a blog in which Ashton Applewhite draws attention to ageist issues and has followers share the ageist situations they experience every day. Additionally, the Old Women's Project is a group of older women that call attention to how they are affected by ageism and call for an end to the injustice. Another women's group, the Raging Grannies, represents older women across the country that challenge ageist stereotypes by peacefully promoting equality for all using creativity and humor. That said, their name reinforces the view of old women as grandmotherly and doesn't leave symbolic space for old women without kids or grandkids.

In addition to calling attention to commonplace forms of ageism, Gullette (2011) argues that people, in particular elders, need to learn to accept their changing bodies; changes that are age-related or not. By embracing the physical changes of aging, individuals can more confidently confront the cultural ideal of a youthful image, such as by taking on anti-aging medicine and resisting "commerce in pathological aging and decline ideology as a whole" (Gullette, 2011, p. 101). Barbara MacDonald and Cynthia Rich (1983) also call on older adults, in particular women, to reclaim their selfhood and identify as old rather than trying to pass as younger. They must accept themselves before they can expect others to recognize them as individuals, more than just another older person.

Work by elders alone will not be sufficient to counter ageism, however; combatting ageism must be an intergenerational effort. Families can play an especially important role in helping to change the way people view the old. On the one hand, how adult children interact with their aging parents can go a long way in *confronting ageist expectations*. Palmore (1999), for example, suggests that if adults are accepting of their parents forming new relationships after the death of a spouse, this can defy the image of elders as sexless and confront messages that oppose remarriage among the old. Families also have the power to influence the way children conceive of elders and of aging. Gullette (2011) contends that "the before-and-after stories about aging that each of us internalizes in childhood can be no more than one sentence deep and yet as salient as Pike's Peak" (p. 148). We have seen evidence that we internalize *ageist messages* at a young age and carry those with us throughout our lives, but so too can we hold onto anti-ageist messages, if those are the ones we learn.

One way for families to instill anti-ageist perceptions of elders is to foster connections between grandparents and grandchildren, relationships that may be impeded by geographic mobility patterns and social privilege. *Intergenerational relationships* can be beneficial in two ways. First, recognizing elders as in-group members, such as important family members, helps prevent stereotyping (Cuddy & Fiske, 2004). Additionally, numerous studies have shown that the more exposure to elders one has, the less likely one is to stereotype them later in life (Golub, Filipowicz, & Langer, 2004). Cuddy and Fiske (2004) explain that this helps because the more personal relationships one has with elders, the more likely it is to know an older adult who does not fit common stereotypes. Having a personal connection to someone who defies those stereotypes can lead one to question those stereotypes, thereby making one less likely to apply them in the future. Such findings indicate the importance of increasing the opportunities for children and young adults to interact with older adults. Some programs that foster intergenerational connections already exist, such as Generations United and the Homeshare program. There are also foster grandparent programs that provide opportunities for older adults to connect with younger generations in educational institutions (from preschool on), via tutoring programs, and through religious institutions (Braithwaite, 2004). Braithwaite (2004) suggests that interacting with older adults in these settings helps younger generations see elders in a multitude of important social roles, expanding their perception of elders. Similar programs that promote intergenerational cooperation could go a long way in confronting ageism.

Countering Ageism at the Societal Level

As we have discussed, one of the factors contributing to ageism is our *cultural valuation of youth*. Because we view youth as the ideal, by contrast we associate elders with negative images. As such, one way to counter ageism is to change society's perceptions of older adults so as to value elders. A powerful first step is to reclaim the word "old" by using it in a positive or neutral way, as suggested by Calasanti and Slevin (2001), which is what we have tried to do throughout this chapter. Similarly, rather than perpetuate negative stereotypes of the old, promoting positive images of aging can go a long way in changing the way society thinks about the aging process and elders. Gullette (2011) recommends transforming the aging narrative from a *narrative of decline* to a *narrative of progress*, emphasizing increased resilience, for example. Cheryl Laz (1998) and Bytheway (2002) likewise encourage people to be more aware of aging in our everyday lives so as to help us view it as something that is actively "done" rather than some sudden, horrible transformation that happens to us.

We should also focus on spreading positive images of elders, revealing them as they really are, as caregivers, creative forces, designers, valued workers, and more (Loe, 2011). Beyond changing the way others view elders, positive stereotypes can actually directly impact the way older adults behave. Studies show that positive age stereotypes can in fact improve memory, increase walking speed, and improve balance (Kite & Wagner, 2004; Levy & Banaji, 2004). A particularly fascinating study by Ellen Langer in 1981 revealed that having older adults live as if they were a number of years younger, with greater responsibilities and expectations of autonomy, caused significant improvement in many measures used to assess natural decline due to aging (Grierson, 2014). Such studies illuminate how powerful the mind can be in shaping our behaviors in response to our mental constructs of age. This makes it all the more important for us to alter these *social constructs of aging* and elders in a positive way.

Along with valuing elders, we need to also strive to *destigmatize death*. Given that ageism is fueled by individuals' fear of mortality, it seems that helping society better understand and cope with death could assuage that concern and in turn reduce ageism. There are a number of ways we can destigmatize death. In Europe, for example, there is a death café movement, which is spreading to America. These death cafés provide a confidential forum for individuals to get together and discuss death in a philosophical way with the help of a facilitator (Span, 2013). Classes or more informal gatherings that directly address fears about death and aging decline could also help (Greenberg, Schimel, & Mertens, 2004). Braithwaite (2004) suggests that film, drama, television, and literature may serve a role in destigmatizing death by increasing exposure to "aspects of aging that leave us feeling conflict ridden, confused, inept, or ill at ease" (p. 322). In increasing the number of discussions about death and aging, it is important to also educate people so as to how they can better prepare for these changes, such as informing them about palliative care and advanced directives. Learning about these can give them a semblance of control over what might otherwise be extremely overwhelming.

But how can we begin to foster these crucial social norms and values? One way is through the media. Rather than bombard consumers with ageist jokes, we should promote slogans that counter ageism, such as "age is a case of mind over matter, if you don't mind it doesn't matter," "age is just a number," or "age is important only for wines and cheese" (Palmore, 1999). Media can also be an efficient way to spread positive images of elders to the masses, and as our society ages, and TV-watching demographics shift, we hope that networks will be convinced of how realistic portrayals of elders as nuanced and complex can be profitable (such as in the program *Last Tango in Halifax*). TV shows, movies, and the news can help show older adults in many different social roles and better convey their positive attributes, such as their wisdom, volunteerism, political participation, and law-abiding nature (Braithwaite, 2004; Palmore, 1999). Providing society with these new *mediated images of elders* can help them widen their conceptions of older adults and break free from the limiting negative stereotypes.

Additionally, organizations can play an important role in altering how society views aging and elders. Palmore (1999) suggests that religious institutions can be especially influential in this matter, as they can draw upon religious texts and traditions that support the valuation of elders. Other organizations combat ageism by protecting the rights of the old, sponsoring research on aging, and providing resources for elders. Though not an exclusive list, the following are some of the more well-known organizations working toward these goals: Administration on Aging, AARP, American Federation for Aging Research, American Society on Aging, Gerontological Society of America, Gray Panthers, National Association for Hispanic Elderly, National Caucus on Black Aged, National Council of Senior Citizens, National Council on Aging, Inc., National Institute on Aging, National Senior Citizen's Law Center, Older Women's League.

Countering Ageism at Organizational and Institutional Levels

Because ageism occurs at the personal, social, and institutional levels, we need changes at all of these levels too. There are three *institutional domains* in which change could go a long way in reducing ageism. The first of these is The Vita Needle factory in Needham, MA, a superb example of a workplace that is inclusive of workers of all ages. Lynch (2012) reveals how many Vita Needle employees are actually older adults, who find that financially they need the opportunity to continue working after their previous careers, appreciate the flexible hours and extra income, and take joy in the social engagement and sense of meaning the job offers. Vita Needle's organizational structure seems nothing but mutually beneficial for both the employees and the company. Other companies might also find that they benefit from offering creative opportunities to keep older adults in the workforce.

Federal changes to laws such as the ADEA can also play a major role in improving the experiences of older workers. Gregory (2001) proposes a few amendments to these policies, many of which involve making it easier for older workers to prove age discrimination. In order to remedy hiring discrimination, Gregory (2001) suggests requiring employers to file reports that reveal the breakdown of applications, interviews, and hires by age. Additionally, if class action were allowed in these situations—it currently is not—then it would be easier to challenge employers and also deter them from discriminatory practices in the first place. Abolishing the mixed-motive rule, which allows employers to prove that their decisions were in part influenced by legitimate reasons, could also make it easier for older workers to win their case. Finally, in those cases in which one can prove age discrimination, Gregory (2001) argues that older workers should also be compensated for the emotional distress unemployment causes.

It is also essential that we make changes to health care. On the one hand, this entails better preparing doctors to work with older patients. Such training must begin in medical school, where educators should eliminate negative stereotypes that are often perpetuated by the way doctors talk about older adults (Wilkinson & Ferraro, 2004). Medical schools should also teach students about the many social and psychological aspects of aging and promote compassionate interaction with older patients (Braithwaite, 2004; Palmore, 1999). Tufts Medical School, for example, brings some of its students to a local senior housing facility so they can practice developing a rapport with older adults. Practices like this can go a long way in preparing future medical practitioners for communicating effectively and respectfully with elder patients.

These programs might also be useful in generating more interest in geriatric medicine, which both Palmore (1999) and Wilkinson and Ferraro (2004) argue is necessary for improving the health-care system for older adults. Incentivizing doctors to specialize in geriatrics could also help combat ageism in health care. All in all, expanding the number of health practitioners who are sensitive to the needs of older patients not only makes elders' interactions with doctors more satisfying and helpful, but it can also improve their health. Gullette (2011) theorizes that better health care for older adults early on might mean that they are less sick when they use Medicare. If better geriatric medicine practices could lead to fewer health issues and thus less reliance on Medicare, this could mitigate society's frustration that health care for elders is a financial burden.

Finally, the government can play a major role in reducing ageism by creating and enforcing policies that protect the rights of older adults. This process should include three major components. First, it should include a thorough review of existing policies to ensure that current laws and procedures do not unnecessarily discriminate by age (Braithwaite, 2004). This also entails evaluating legislation, such as the Age Discrimination in Employment Act, to ensure that it is properly enforced (Palmore, 1999). Second, the government can create new policies and procedures that reduce ageism (Braithwaite, 2004). For example, providing subsidies for home care may decrease the number of older adults pressured into moving into nursing homes by making it easier for such elders to find and afford in-home care (Palmore, 1999). The third key component is that older adults should be included in the process of reviewing, creating, and implementing policies (Braithwaite, 2004).

Conclusion

The most effective means by which to counter ageism is an integration of the many specific methods we have just discussed. It requires individuals sparking social change, and it involves institutions creating guiding rules and norms for the individuals they affect. It will be a process of both reevaluating our behavior, beliefs, and laws, and innovation—developing new legislation and new images and roles for elders. We all need to be aware of ageism because one day we might all become the targets of this discrimination and stereotypes. If you could do something now to protect your rights for the future, why wouldn't you?

References

Allen, K. R., & Walker, A. J. (2006). Aging and gender in families. In T. M. Calasanti and K. F. Slevin (Eds.), *Age matters: Realigning feminist thinking*. New York: Routledge.

Becker, E. (1973) *The denial of death*. New York: The Free Press.

Bendick, M., Jackson, C., & Romero, H. (1993). *Employment discrimination against older workers: An experimental study of hiring practices*. Washington, DC: Fair Employment Council of Greater Washington.

Bergling, T. (2004). *Reeling in the years: Gay men's perspectives on age and ageism*. New York: Harrington Park Press.

Braithwaite, V. (2004). Reducing ageism. In T. Nelson (Ed.), *Ageism: Stereotyping and prejudice against older persons* (pp. 311–337). Cambridge: MIT Press.

Brooks, A. (2010). Aesthetic anti-aging surgery and technology: Women's friend or foe? *Sociology of Health and Illness*, 32(2), 238–257.

Butler, R. (1969). Ageism: Another form of bigotry. *The Gerontologist*, 9, 243–245.

Butler, R. (1975). *Why survive? Being old in America*. New York: Harper and Row.

Butler, R. (1980). Ageism: A foreword. *Journal of Social Issues*, 36(2), 8–11.

Bytheway, B. (2002). Positioning gerontology in an ageist world. In Lars Andersson (Ed.), *Cultural gerontology* (pp. 59–76). Westport: Auburn House.

Calasanti, T. M. (2003). Theorizing age relations. In Simon Biggs, Ariela Lowenstein, and Jon Hendricks (Eds.), *The need for theory: Critical approaches to social gerontology* (pp. 199–218). New York: Baywood Press.

Calasanti, T. M., & Slevin, K. F. (2001). *Gender, social inequalities, and aging*. Walnut Creek: AltraMira Press.

Cohen, S., Janicki-Deverts, D., Chen, E., & Matthews, K.A. (2010). Childhood socioeconomic status and adult health. *Annals of the New York Academy of Sciences*, 1186, 37–55.

Collins, P.H. (1990). *Black feminist thought: Knowledge, consciousness, and the politics of empowerment.* Boston: Unwin Hyman.

Conrad, P. (2007). *The medicalization of society: On the transformation of human conditions into treatable disorders*. Baltimore, MD: Johns Hopkins University Press.

Cruikshank, M. (2009). *Learning to be old.* Plymouth: Rowman & Littlefield.

Cuddy, A.J.C., & Fiske, S.T. (2004). Doddering but dear: Process, content, and function in stereotyping of older persons. In T. Nelson (Ed.), *Ageism: Stereotyping and prejudice against older persons* (pp. 3–26). Cambridge, MA: MIT Press.

DeLamater, J. (2012). *Sex for life: From virginity to Viagra, how sexuality changes throughout our lives.* New York: NYU Press.

Dressel, P., Minkler, M., & Yen, I. (1997). Gender, race, class, and aging: Advances and opportunities. *International Journal of Health and Services*, 27(4), 579–600.

Estes, C., & Binney, E. (1989). The biomedicalization of aging: Dangers and dilemmas. *The Gerontologist*, 29(5), 587–596.

Ferraro, K.F., & Kelley-Moore, J.A. (2003). Cumulative disadvantage and health: Long-term consequences of obesity? *American Sociological Review*, 68(5), 707–729.

Ferraro, K.F., & Shippee, T.P. (2009). Aging and cumulative inequality: How does inequality get under the skin? *Gerontologist*, 49(3), 333–343.

Golub, S.A., Filipowicz, A., & Langer, E.J. (2004). Acting your age. In T. Nelson (Ed.), *Ageism: Stereotyping and prejudice against older persons* (pp. 277–294). Cambridge, MA: MIT Press.

Greenberg, J., Schimel, J., & Mertens, A. (2004). Ageism: Denying the face of the future. In T. Nelson (Ed.), *Ageism: Stereotyping and prejudice against older persons* (pp. 27–48). Cambridge, MA: MIT Press.

Gregory, R.F. (2001). *Age discrimination in the American workplace: Old at a young age*. New Brunswick, NJ: Rutgers University Press.

Grierson, B. (2014, October 22). What if age is nothing but a mind-set? *New York Times*. Retrieved from http://www.nytimes.com/

Gubrium, J. (1986). *Old timers and Alzheimer's: The descriptive organization of senility*. JAI Press.

Gullette, M.M. (2004). *Aged by culture.* Chicago: University of Chicago Press.

Gullette, M.M. (2011). *Agewise: Fighting the new ageism in America*. Chicago: University of Chicago Press.

Hess, T. H. (2006). Attitudes toward aging and their effects on behavior. In J. E. Birren & K. W. Schaie (Eds.), *Handbook of the Psychology of Aging* (pp. 379–406). Burlington, MA: Elsevier Academic.

Holstein, M. B. (2006). On being an aging woman. In T. M. Calasanti and K. F. Slevin (Eds.), *Age matters: Realigning feminist thinking.* New York: Routledge.

Isaacs, L.W., & Bearison, D.J. (1986). The development of children's prejudice against the aged. *International Journal of Aging and Human Development*, 23, 175–194.

Joyce, K., & Loe, M. (2010). A sociological approach to ageing, technology, and health. *Sociology of Health and Illness*, 32(2), 171–180.

Joyce, K., & Mamo, L. (2006). Graying the cyborg: New directions in feminist analyses of aging, science, and technology. In T. M. Calasanti and K. F. Slevin (Eds.), *Age matters: Realigning feminist thinking*. New York: Routledge.

Kaufman, S. (1994). *The ageless self: Sources of meaning in late life*. Madison: University of Wisconsin Press.

Kite, M. E., & Wagner, L. S. (2004). Attitudes toward older adults. In T. Nelson (Ed.), *Ageism: Stereotyping and prejudice against older persons* (pp. 129–161). Cambridge, MA: MIT Press.

Laz, C. (1998). Act your age. *Sociological Forum*, 13(1), 85–113.

Levy, B. R., & Banaji, M. R. (2004). Implicit ageism. In T. Nelson (Ed.), *Ageism: Stereotyping and prejudice against older persons* (pp. 49–75). Cambridge, MA: MIT Press.

LGBT Movement Advancement Project and Services and Advocacy for Gay, Lesbian, Bisexual and Transgender Elders. (2010). Improving the lives of LGBT older adults. Retrieved on November 1, 2014. Online. http://www.lgbtmap.org/file/improving-the-lives-of-lgbt-older-adults.pdf

Lindau, S. T., Schumm, L. P., Laumann, E. O., Levinson, W. L., O'Muircheataigh, C. A., & Waite, L. J. (2007). A study of sexuality and health among older adults in the United States. *The New England Journal of Medicine*, 357, 762–774.

Loe, M. (2006). *The rise of Viagra: How the little blue pill changed sex in America*. New York: New York University Press.

Loe, M. (2011). *Aging our way: Lessons for living from 85 and beyond*. New York: Oxford University Press.

Lock, M (1993). *Encounters with aging: Mythologies of menopause in Japan and North America*. Berkeley: University of California Press.

Lynch, C. (2012). *Retirement on the line: Age, work, and value in an American factory*. Ithaca, NY: Cornell University Press.

MacDonald, B., & Rich, C. (1983). *Look me in the eye: Old women, aging, and ageism*. San Francisco: Spinsters/Aunt Lute.

Maddux, S. (Producer and Director) (2010). *Gen Silent*. [Motion Picture]. United States of America: Interrobang Productions.

McCann, R., & Giles, H. (2004). Ageism in the workplace: A communication perspective. In T. Nelson (Ed.), *Ageism: Stereotyping and prejudice against older persons* (pp. 163–199). Cambridge, MA: MIT Press.

Newman, K. S. (2003). *A different shade of gray: Midlife and beyond in the inner city*. New York: The New Press.

Pager, D. (2003). The mark of a criminal record. *American Journal of Sociology*, 108(5), 937–975.

Palmore, E. (1999). *Ageism: Negative and positive*. New York: Springer Publishing Company.

Pasupathi, M., & Löckenhoff, C. (2004). Ageist behavior. In T. Nelson (Ed.), *Ageism: Stereotyping and prejudice against older persons* (pp. 201–246). Cambridge, MA: MIT Press.

Span, Paula (June 16, 2013). Tea, Two Sugars, and Death: Café Groups Ponder the End. *New York Times*.

Taylor, Paul, et al. (June 29, 2009). Growing old in America: Expectations vs. reality. *Pew Research Report*.

Wallace, S. P. (1991). The political economy of health care for elderly blacks. In M. Minkler and C. L. Estes (Eds.), *Critical perspectives on aging: The political and moral economy of growing old*. Amityville, NY: Baywood.

Walz, T. (2002). Crones, dirty old men, sexy seniors: Representations of the sexuality of older persons. *Journal of Aging and Identity*, 7(2), 99–112.

Whitbourne, S. K., & Sneed, J. R. (2004). The paradox of well-being, identity processes, and stereotype threat: Ageism and its potential relationships to the self in later life. In T. Nelson (Ed.), *Ageism: Stereotyping and prejudice against older persons* (pp. 247–273). Cambridge, MA: MIT Press.

Wilkinson, J. A., & Ferraro, K. F. (2004). Thirty years of ageism research. In T. Nelson (Ed.), *Ageism: Stereotyping and prejudice against older persons* (pp. 339–358). Cambridge, MA: MIT Press.

Winks, C., & Semans, A. (2002). *The good vibrations guide to sex*. San Francisco, CA: Cleis Press.

CHAPTER FOUR

The U.S. Old-Age Welfare State: Social Security, Supplemental Security Income, Medicare, and Medicaid

Debra Street and Sarah Desai

Uncertainty about how older age will be experienced is an inherent part of every individual life course. Individuals growing older may wonder how aging will change their relationships, whether there will be enough income and savings to live comfortably, and if they will be healthy or struggle with chronic illness, among other things. Some individuals look forward to golden years, expecting to retire in good enough health and with sufficient income to enjoy meaningful activities and relationships, leisure, and travel. Others confront an old age plagued by vulnerabilities associated with ill health, low incomes, or both, perhaps needing to work for as long as their bodies allow because they cannot afford to retire. Even individuals who begin retirement in comfortable circumstances face the prospects of serious illness, the death of a partner, or outliving savings. For some individuals and their families, the income and health needs associated with old age simply overwhelm their capacities to manage entirely on their own.

The singular uncertainties that individuals confront—the risks and rewards associated with individual lifetimes of high or low incomes, good or poor health—look very different from a societal level, where risk is shared. The contours of the aggregate experiences of millions of elderly people in a national population are easier to predict, on average, than individualized ones. During the twentieth century, affluent countries around the world intervened in the risks of low income at older ages, by institutionalizing retirement through age-related social policies. Public pension programs became the largest single social expenditure program in most countries—the bulwark of an old-age welfare state—as public pension systems pooled risk and safeguarded elderly citizens against poverty and destitution. Public pension systems made universal or nearly universal retirement possible, giving citizens the right to stop working before wearing out (Myles, 1989). While individuals were still expected to do their part to maintain health and prepare financially for retirement, two periods of U.S. legislative activity in the twentieth century relieved individuals of exclusive responsibility for safeguarding well-being in old age by creating two centerpiece federal social insurance programs to support income and health security for older Americans. The Great Depression provided the social backdrop against which Franklin Roosevelt pushed for Social Security legislation in the 1930s. Social Security was intended, in part, to help prevent extreme poverty in old age. Lyndon Johnson's Great Society policy initiatives in the 1960s were the background for Medicare legislation that, for the first time, ensured routine access to health care for elderly Americans. Entitlement to social insurance coverage that provides income and health care at retirement age is the cornerstone of the U.S. old-age welfare state.

Supplementing and extending the reach of the social insurance entitlement programs are two parallel needs-based programs. Supplemental Security Income (SSI) augments income for impoverished elders and Medicaid plays an essential role in health-care provision for the poorest older Americans. To qualify for benefits under SSI or Medicaid, individuals must be deemed eligible by demonstrating need—usually through a means test that limits coverage to individuals with extremely low incomes and very few assets. While the threshold for eligibility under these poverty-based programs is very low and the process of qualifying for benefits can be stigmatizing, each provides essential income or access to services that improve the lives of the most vulnerable elderly Americans.

Social Security, SSI, Medicare, and Medicaid have all been adapted since their enactment to meet changing social and economic circumstances, and each program fills a distinct role in promoting the health and income security of older Americans. In the early years of the old-age welfare state, reforms often focused on broadening coverage and improving benefits. More recently, reforms have focused on containing costs and ensuring the future financial viability of the programs. For current elderly Americans, entitlement to Social Security and Medicare benefits enacted in the twentieth century provide most of their retirement income and a floor of protection for most individuals' income and health arrangements, while SSI and Medicaid provide safety nets for the most vulnerable. An intrinsic characteristic of the old-age welfare state has been the challenge of balancing two sometimes competing demands. Benefits must be adequate to meet needs, and all participants—taxpayers and beneficiaries alike—must be treated equitably. Fiscal constraints and political contests make achieving the balancing act especially difficult. Yet as the U.S. baby boomers reach retirement age in the twenty-first century, between 2011 and 2029, these social programs will doubtless be adjusted to meet future needs for an increasingly diverse elderly population.

Social Security

Social Security is a self-financed—pay-as-you-go through worker and employer payroll tax contributions—federal social insurance program that provides monthly cash benefits to retired workers in the United States. In addition to older workers and their family members, Social Security also provides benefits for disabled workers and the family members of deceased workers. Eighty years ago, when Social Security was enacted, over half of elderly Americans lived in poverty, with few prospects to change that during the Great Depression. When President Franklin D. Roosevelt signed the Social Security Act of 1935 into law, one goal was to protect older Americans from a "poverty-ridden old age." Since then, the retirement and survivor components of Social Security have been reformed numerous times, lifting more and more elderly people out of extreme poverty by providing modest monthly incomes. By the late 1950s, the poverty rate among Americans 65 and older had dropped to just below 40 percent, and by 2015 it was around 10 percent, the lowest rate for any age group. In fact, despite enduring pockets of poverty and persistent levels of near-poverty in some segments of the elderly population, some argue that Social Security has been the single most effective antipoverty policy in the United States (e.g., Herd, 2009a).

Social Security is the largest social transfer program in the United States, by far, with about 97 percent of older Americans receiving monthly income as beneficiaries. Social Security is financed through payroll taxes. Covered workers and their employers each pay 6.2 percent of covered earnings up to a ceiling ($118,500 in 2015); self-employed individuals pay the full 12.4 percent of their income, up to the ceiling. Payroll taxes for Social Security are regressive, in that covered workers with the lowest incomes pay the same rate of taxes on much smaller incomes when compared to much higher earners near the income ceiling. Earners above the ceiling pay a smaller proportion of their income in payroll taxes than the lowest-paid workers since none of their income above the ceiling is subject to payroll taxes. However, Social Security also has progressive elements. It was designed from the outset to reduce inequality in old age for covered workers, with benefit formulas giving high-wage earners a smaller percentage return and low-wage earners receiving a higher rate of return of preretirement earnings in their Social Security benefits. A high-wage earner can expect to receive about 28 percent of their average preretirement income in Social Security retirement benefits, while a low-wage earner can expect benefits that replace about 78 percent of their average prior earnings (Herd, 2009c). Although Social Security primarily covers retired workers and their families, the program also provides benefits for survivors and disabled workers. In 2014, 59 million people received Social Security benefits. Of these beneficiaries, 71 percent were retired workers or their spouses and children, 10 percent were the survivors of deceased workers, and 19 percent were disabled workers and their families (CBO, 2014).[1]

Eligibility for Social Security retirement benefits requires a minimum of 40 quarters of contributions, the equivalent of 10 years of Social Security-covered employment. The retirement benefit for workers is then calculated based on lifetime earnings, using the highest 35 years of earnings. As explained above, the progressive benefit formula provides low-wage earners with a higher replacement percentage when compared with high-wage earners. SS benefits account for about 38 percent of income from all sources for all elderly American people (SSA, 2014b). Retired worker benefits may be claimed as early as age 62, but the benefit is permanently reduced to account for the presumed longer receipt of benefits. The retirement age for full benefits ranges from 65 to 67, depending on year of birth (current full retirement age is 66). If an individual waits to claim benefits beyond the full retirement age, monthly benefits increase until age 70 to account for the presumed shorter overall receipt of benefits (Munnell, 2013). The spouse of an eligible retired worker may receive 50 percent of that worker's benefit amount as a dependent, if the dependent amount is higher than the retirement benefit to which they would be entitled based on their own work record. Although spousal dependent benefits can go to husbands or wives, women are overwhelmingly represented among the dependent beneficiary population. Surviving spouses can claim monthly benefits equaling 100 percent of the deceased worker's retirement benefits. Because of their lower lifetime earnings, discussed in greater detail below, two-thirds of older American women currently receive dependent or widow benefits rather than worker benefits in their own right (Harrington Meyer, Wolf, & Himes, 2005).

Brief History of Social Security

The Social Security Act of 1935, Title II, was designed to provide economic security for the nation's workers and prevent extreme poverty in old age through Social Security retirement benefits. At the outset, payroll taxes to finance Social Security were set at 2 percent of wages up to $3,000 in covered employment (1% paid by the worker, 1% paid by the employer). Initially, only about half of all American jobs were covered by Social Security with program assumptions reflecting the expectation that the typical Social Security worker was a white, married, breadwinning man (Mink, 1995; Ginn, Street & Arber, 2001). Occupations excluded from Social Security coverage were those disproportionately held by women and minority workers, with little to no Social Security coverage in the early years for workers employed in teaching, nursing, social work, domestic, and agricultural labor (Quadagno, 1994; DeWitt, 2010). Although the language of Social Security law and regulation was both gender- and race-neutral from the outset, the structure of the Social Security program replicated many of the inequalities of American society and has yielded gendered and raced outcomes from its inception. Program features that disproportionately affect people who vary by gender, marital status, and race/ethnicity have contemporary implications, which are discussed in more detail below.

The Social Security program has a complex history of reform. Even before the program was in full operation, the Social Security Amendments of 1939 expanded coverage to include the dependents and survivors of retired workers, and to establish a minimum benefit. Over the next several decades, legislative changes to the program generally focused on expansion. Over time, covered employment was more broadly defined until coverage became nearly universal. Today 97 percent of older people receive Social Security benefits. Among other major reforms, in 1956 the Disability Insurance (DI) component was added to the Social Security program and in 1972, Congress added an automatic cost-of-living adjustment. Policy makers recognized that, without such an adjustment, inflation eroded the value of the benefit and contributed to higher rates of poverty over time, given that elderly retirees were living longer but losing financial ground when prices rose. Not only were covered employment expanded and benefits inflation-proofed, the payroll tax rate has also increased over the years. From the initial 2 percent, periodic increases in the payroll taxes have led to the current rate of 12.4 percent. The taxable income cap has also increased gradually, from the initial $3,000 to $118,500 in 2015.

Starting in the late 1970s, legislative action on Social Security has taken a different direction. Rather than expanding, legislative efforts have focused primarily on solving persistent funding problems, by increasing revenue (payroll tax rates), and placing limits on future benefit growth. For example, the Social Security Amendments of 1983 gradually raised the full retirement age for future beneficiaries, from the traditional full retirement age of 65 to age 66 for full benefits for individuals born between 1946 and 1955, rising to 67 for individuals born in 1960. The frequency of policy changes demonstrate that the only absolute certainties about Social Security, aside from the millions of bank deposits beneficiaries receive every month, is that the program will continue to evolve in the face of evolving social, demographic, and economic circumstances.

Social Security Financials

Social Security (SS) is the U.S. government's single largest program, accounting for nearly a quarter of all federal spending in fiscal year (FY) 2014. There are currently 59 million people receiving SS, and the program cost $840 billion in FY 2014. Old-age and survivors insurance (OASI) accounted for 83 percent of payments, with the other 17 percent going to DI. For years, payroll taxes exceeded the benefits being paid out, with the surplus invested in Treasury Bonds in the so-called Social Security Trust Fund. Beginning in 2010 current year outlays (payments of benefits and administrative costs) exceeded tax input. Under current law the program is projected to continue to take in less revenue in payroll taxes than it pays out in benefits into the foreseeable future, with the gap growing from 9 percent in 2013 to over 30 percent by the late 2020s (CBO, 2014). Past surpluses were invested in special trust funds created for OASI and DI. Under current law the DI trust fund is estimated to be exhausted in FY 2017 and the OASI fund in FY 2032, as shown in Figure 4.1. If the funds are treated as one, the combined trust fund will be exhausted around 2030 (CBO, 2014). Of course, because payroll taxes would still be collected from workers, there would be current revenue to provide a large fraction of benefits to beneficiaries. However, under most scenarios, at some future date a combination of payroll tax increases, covered earnings income ceilings rises, and benefit decreases—likely through raising the retirement age, or tweaking benefit calculation formulas—will doubtless maintain the integrity of the evolving Social Security program.

In 2004, Social Security benefits cost the federal treasury $492 billion; a decade later annual spending on the program totaled $840 billion (CBO, 2014). The ballooning cost of SS is due to a confluence of factors: an increase in the ratio of retired to working persons, as the baby boomers age, increases in life expectancy, and fertility declines (Palmer, 2006). By 2033, individuals 65 and older will grow from the 46.6 million elderly Americans today to more than 77 million (SSA, 2014b). Currently there are 2.8 workers paying payroll taxes per SS beneficiary, but by 2033 this

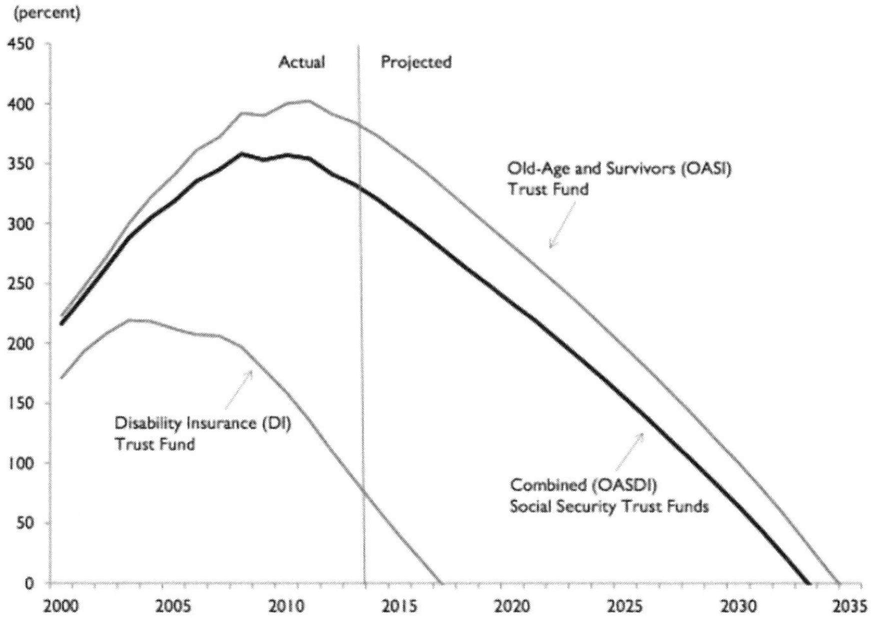

Figure 4.1 Social Security Trust Fund ratios. (Social Security Trustees, 2014 Annual Report of the Board of Trustees of the Federal Old-Age and Survivors Insurance and Disability Insurance Trust Funds, July 28, 2014, Table IV.B3, at http://www.ssa.gov/oact/tr/2014/lr4b3.html)

will decrease to 2.1 workers per beneficiary (SSA, 2014b). One way that legislators have been addressing rising costs is gradually increasing the maximum taxable income that payroll tax is collected on. In 2005, the maximum taxable earnings for SS were $90,000; 10 years later, payroll tax is collected on a maximum of $118,500 (OASDI and SSI Program Rates & Limits, 2005 & 2015). A much discussed option among policy makers to maintain the solvency of the Social Security program is to raise the age for eligibility for full retirement benefits (similar to changes in the 1983 Amendments) to 69 or 70, with the effect of cutting benefits to future Social Security beneficiaries who must wait longer for full benefits. While raising the retirement age across the board on its face seems like an equitable and seemingly inevitable way to share the increased costs of Social Security, many women, minority, and low-paid workers would be disproportionately disadvantaged by such a change. Remaining employed until age 70 is a very different experience, both in terms of capacity to work and sufficiency of income for retirement, for a minimum-wage retail worker who is on his feet all day, a nursing home aide providing personal care to a frail resident, a construction worker in a physically demanding job, or a college professor working in her office.

Race, Class, Gender, and Social Security

While Social Security has reduced income inequality in old age and provided insurance against extreme poverty, it has not done this evenly across all groups. As noted earlier, the aggregate poverty rate for those over 65 is 10 percent, the lowest of any age group in the United States. However, looking at subgroups within the population paints a very different picture. Pockets of elder poverty and near-poverty persist. Older blacks, Hispanics, and unmarried people all entered the twenty-first century with poverty rates over 20 percent (Harrington Meyer, Wolf & Himes, 2005). Some, but not all, women are disadvantaged by the structure of the Social Security Program (Street & Wilmoth, 2001; Harrington Meyer & Herd, 2007; Carr, 2010). For example, one recent study documented the poverty rate for older single black women at around 40 percent, while the poverty rate for married white women the same age was less than 2 percent (Herd, 2009a,b,c). Social Security alone fails to provide a robust safety net for certain groups for several reasons. Often the reason for that failure is because the structure of the program is insufficient to compensate for disadvantages that often occur at the intersection of gender and race (Calasanti & Slevin, 2001) or the vagaries of lifetime low-waged or contingent employment (Ginn, Street & Arber, 2001).

Two key challenges that especially affect the value of women's Social Security benefits are linking noncontributory benefits to marriage and basing benefits on the average earnings over a very long work history. Because SS benefits are based on a long work history (35 years), time out of paid work or many years in low-wage jobs have permanently negative effects on the value of eventual benefits. While the Social Security benefit formula adjusts for this to some extent by providing a great rate of return to low-income earners, the adjustment does not completely remedy the impact of a lifetime of low wages or gaps in paid work. At some point in their life courses many women take time away from paid work or cut their hours to provide care for young children or aging parents, since the normative expectation—and the empirical reality—is that unpaid care and domestic work is mainly women's work (Sayer, 2005). Even when employed consistently, women face a gender wage gap that leaves them with median wages that are considerably less than their male counterparts. Estimates of the gender wage gap range from around 76 cents on the dollar to about 85 cents on the dollar, depending on source (Pew Research Center, 2013). The gender pay gap is long-standing and, despite shrinking somewhat in recent years, it has been stubbornly persistent. Part of the reason women may be paid less than men is because they must work in lower-paid jobs to have sufficient flexibility, through part-time employment or shift work, to meet caregiving responsibilities. Part of the reason may be gender discrimination in the workplace. When women juggle paid and unpaid work, they may not be able to work the longer hours that men can tolerate to earn a raise, or overtime pay, or a promotion (Macpherson & Hirsch, 1995; O'Neill & O'Neill, 2005). The gender wage gap parallels a SS benefit gap, where older women receive about 76 cents on the dollar when compared to similar retired men (Herd, 2009a). While Social Security is redistributive, in reality the program pays very little in retirement benefits to older women who have worked long term in low-paid work and significantly more in spousal dependent benefits to wealthy married women who have worked only sporadically (Harrington Meyer & Herd, 2007). Poverty in early and midlife negatively affects savings, pension eligibility, and also SS benefits. The impact can be seen clearly for single mothers, who are 55 percent more likely to be poor in old age than married mothers (Herd, 2009a). This is a growing problem because the number of households headed by single mothers is increasing, from 10 percent in 1970 to 25 percent by 2005 (Herd, 2009a). In 2013, 40.6 percent of all births were to unmarried women (CDC, 2015). While not all of these women will remain single parents, a sizeable proportion is likely to. When such women reach retirement age, will there be adequate income support for them from Social Security, or will a benefit structure designed in the 1930s condemn them to the struggles of extreme poverty?

As mentioned earlier, Social Security is structured around a male breadwinner model, where a spouse can receive 50 percent of a retired worker's benefit and a surviving spouse receives 100 percent of the deceased worker's benefit. The 1939 Amendments extended coverage in these ways because most married white women were not employed at the time—they took care of the family and household. There was mounting concern that married men's modest SS benefits alone would not be sufficient to support a two-person household in retirement and that many widows, not eligible for benefits, would face extreme poverty.

While a breadwinner system made sense for many women and men in the 1930s, eight decades have dramatically changed patterns of women's workforce participation and changing patterns of family formation. This leaves a system whose eligibility and benefit criteria almost always lag behind social change, with Social Security structured to inadequately protect some of the most vulnerable older people in the United States. Because of the effects of broader social trends, SS is a contributor to racial, gender, and class inequality in old age (Harrington Meyer, Wolf, & Himes, 2005;

Herd, 2005). For many women, marital status matters more than work history in terms of the size of benefit received, with two-thirds of older women receiving spouse or widow SS benefits. Men can also qualify for spousal benefits, but have generally contributed more than they would receive as dependents or widowers because of higher lifetime wages and/or a longer work history, on average, than women. In 2000, 97 percent of recipients of spousal benefits were women (Harrington Meyer, Wolf, & Himes, 2005).[2]

Changing traditional marriage patterns have potentially troubling implications for the economic security of many older women in the future, especially if SS continues the breadwinner system of determining benefits. The current system best supports either women with long, uninterrupted work histories or those who marry, stay married, and never work; few women fit either of these models neatly (Herd, 2005). To receive spousal benefits a person must be currently married or have had a marriage that lasted 10 or more years (Harrington Meyer, Wolf, & Himes, 2005). As marriage rates decline and many marriages are shorter, the group eligible for traditional spousal benefits is shrinking. Despite the obvious disadvantage of women's lower Social Security incomes, it is nonetheless true that Social Security is incredibly important for older women's financial security (Street & Wilmoth, 2001), as it represents more than 80 percent of all retirement income received by over half of elderly American women, and becomes even more important as women age, representing 100 percent of income for a third of women aged 75+ (Fischer & Hayes, 2013).

Different cultural groups in the United States have different experiences associated with family formation and marital status that are eventually expressed in Social Security benefits. While marriage rates in the United States are declining across the board, they are declining dramatically for blacks and those with low educational attainment (Herd, 2009a). In 1970, the percentage of black women 65 and older who were married relative to white women the same age was 87 percent; by 2000 this comparative rate had fallen to 58 percent (Harrington Meyer & Herd, 2007). Only a third (33%) of older black women are married, compared to 57 percent of white women, 52 percent of Asian women, and 48 percent of Hispanic women (Harrington Meyer & Herd, 2007). The marriage rate for younger blacks has continued to decline. In 2010, a quarter of black men and women 35 and older had never married (U.S. Census Bureau, 2012). Marriage rates have also been declining for those with less education. In 2012, 73 percent of those aged 35–39 without a bachelor's degree had never been married, compared to 92 percent of the same group in 1950 (Fry, 2014). Racial minorities and those with less education often have lower lifetime earnings; they are also more likely to be single and unable to benefit from the economies of scale realized in a shared household. Low-wage earners who are also single are constrained in their ability to save for old age. Continuing to tie Social Security income to marriage for future retirees, when the most vulnerable workers are also the least likely to be married, makes little sense if Social Security retirement benefits are to fulfill the original goal of alleviating elder poverty for all Americans.

SS income is critically important for racial minorities because they are less likely to have private pensions and retirement savings than their white counterparts (NASI, 2015). Among those 65 and older, SS was the only source of income for 36 percent of blacks and Hispanics, compared to 19 percent of whites (NASI, 2015). Even though the benefit formula for Social Security is progressive, racial minorities still receive a lower dollar amount due to lower lifetime earnings. Institutional racism is an endemic reality of the American sociopolitical landscape and clearly suppresses income across the life course for blacks and Hispanics. Some of the other factors that reduce lifetime earnings for minorities include higher rates of disability and chronic health conditions, particularly for African Americans, lower levels of education, and high incarceration rates, all of which can lead to intermittent unemployment and low wages (Martin & Murphy, 2014). In 2009, the average annual SS benefit for blacks 65 and older was $10,430, compared with an average benefit of $11,910 for all retirement-age beneficiaries (Martin & Murphy, 2014), more than 10 percent lower monthly Social Security retirement benefits for blacks compared to other beneficiaries. Black SS beneficiaries 62 and older are more than twice as likely to have incomes below the poverty line than all other SS recipients the same age—17.9 percent compared to 8.3 percent in 2009 (Martin & Murphy, 2014). Although SS reduces income inequality in old age to a certain extent, it also reproduces life-course experiences of racial inequality and fails to correct the effects of a lifetime of discrimination, poorer health, higher rates of disability, employment gaps, and lower wages.

When compared with other developed countries, older women in the United States are often more likely to be poor because of the way public and private pensions were designed (Ginn, Street, & Arber, 2001; Herd, 2009c). Elsewhere, adequate retirement income that is less tightly linked to lifetime earnings and marital status, delivered through public pensions, is essential for reducing inequality in old age. Because women have lower attachment to paid labor over the life course, older women fare better in countries where public pensions make up a larger percentage of retirement income, as long the public pension provides adequate benefits. In the United States public pension income is tied to lifetime earnings, although benefit formulas are redistributive, and makes up a smaller share of retirement income than in other developed countries (Herd, 2009c). In Germany and Sweden, more than 70 percent of elderly income comes from public pensions, while only about 50 percent of retirement income in the United States is publicly funded (Herd, 2009c). In Europe, poverty is often defined as less than 40 percent of the median disposable income; by this measure 30 percent of older women in the United States are poor, indicating a failure of our public pension system (SS and SSI) (Herd, 2009c). Social Security makes up two-thirds of the average woman's retirement income in the United States, and is the only source of income for one in five older women (Herd, 2005). Herd (2009a, p. 127) also notes that "the US remains the only industrialized country with non-earnings-related benefits structured primarily around marital status."

Social Security reform is difficult to accomplish, because there are many stakeholders and beneficiaries, as well as a complex and slow-moving political process (Hudson, 2014). Herd (2005) notes that SS reform has the potential to reshape social relations in the United States more than any other policy, because it accounts for almost a quarter of federal spending, compared to about 1 percent spent on traditional welfare (TANF). As SS funding shortfalls become a more immediate challenge, it may even open up an opportunity to debate other creative, progressive, and meaningful policy changes to the program. Three types of reforms aimed at progressive improvements to Social Security are often proposed, based on policies in other developed countries: care credits to offset the costs of raising children, reforms that reduce the impact of divorce, and a universal minimum benefit (Herd, 2005). Projections of how each reform would impact race, class, and gender inequality indicate that a universal minimum benefit would do the most to reduce inequalities across multiple dimensions (Herd, 2005, see also Ginn, Street & Arber, 2001). One example of the way child care credits could improve Social Security records would be through imputing the national median income for a certain number of years for each child, and using the "child-adjusted" record of contributions rather than those years reflecting no or limited earning, to calculate lifetime average income. There are different ways to recognize unpaid care work, but projections indicate that care credit policy changes would make meaningful strides in increasing Social Security benefits to low-asset households and working women, while reducing racial and gender inequality (Herd, 2005). Policies that account for marital dissolution, however, still benefit those at the top of the asset distribution, while doing little for those near poverty or never married. Another possible reform looks at how the tax code, instead of SS payments, could be used to get closer to a minimum benefit. In the United States, the Earned Income Tax Credit (EITC) has been very successful for working-age Americans, providing a refundable tax credit to the working poor. Nearly all of those eligible for the EITC receive it, compared to the 50–60 percent uptake among those eligible for SSI. One proposed reform is to do something similar for the elderly, using the tax code to give a refundable credit to the poorest older individuals (Herd, 2009a). Canada has a program, the Guaranteed Income Supplement (GIS) that works this way and has been successful in reducing poverty among older Canadians (Street & Connidis, 2001; Herd, 2009a).

Supplemental Security Income

The SSI program is a means-tested, federal income assistance program for the poorest elderly, blind, and disabled people in the United States. Social Security Disability Insurance (SSDI) is the largest disability program in the United States, but SSI does not have work history requirements, allowing it to fill in gaps in SS and SSDI (Furtado & Theodoropoulos, 2013). In July 2014, the SSI program distributed $4.7 billion in monthly benefits to 8.4 million recipients. As Figure 4.2 shows, less than 10 percent of SSI recipients qualify on the basis of being poor and elderly, with over 90 percent of recipients qualifying based on disability. However, for elderly beneficiaries receiving SSI benefits, they represent an economic lifeline. The SSI program was not an original part of Social Security; rather, the needs-based safety net program for the poor was created in 1972 under Title XVI of the Social Security Act, with the first benefits paid out in 1974. Prior to the implementation of SSI, the Social Security Act of 1935 had established federal-state needs-based programs of Old Age Assistance and Aid to the Blind, and later in 1950 added Aid to the Permanently and Totally Disabled. Under those programs, states received federal matching dollars

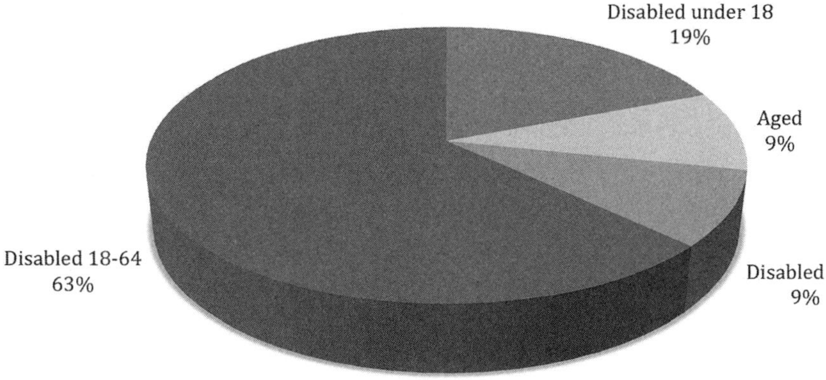

Figure 4.2 Federal SSI payments, 2013, $53.4 billion. (SSA, 2014a, Annual Report of the Supplemental Security Income Program)

to provide cash assistance to eligible needy individuals at a level deemed "practicable." This federal/state policy responsibility resulted in an elaborate patchwork of requirements, provisions, and funding levels that varied substantially across the states. Unlike the retired worker, dependent, and survivor benefits under Social Security, which ensured uniform benefits across the United States, the federal-state partnership guaranteed wildly different experiences among recipients, depending upon the state in which they resided. The 1972 SSI program was established with the goal of providing assurance that the elderly, blind, and disabled across the country would not struggle to subsist on incomes below the poverty line.

SSI is built on the Social Security model (and is administered through the SSA) of federally established and funded monthly income support, although it differs from traditional Social Security benefits in several important respects. First, Social Security is a social insurance entitlement program, whereas receiving SSI benefits is contingent on establishing the need for benefits through extreme poverty (lack of both income and assets) or permanent incapacity to be employed. Second, SSI is funded through general taxation, while SS is funded through a special payroll tax earmarked for the purpose of providing SS benefits. Finally, unlike the uniform national experience of Social Security benefits, individual states have the option of supplementing the base federal SSI payment. In 2015, SSI provided $733 of Federal monthly income to eligible individuals living in their own households with no other countable income; for a couple with two eligible members the benefit was $1,100 per month. Taking into account adjustments that reduce the benefit, the actual average monthly income in 2014 was $535. Since 1975, SSI benefits have increased with the same cost-of-living adjustment applied to Social Security (SSA, 2014a; CWM, 2014).

The SSI program is complex, with layers of requirements determining eligibility and actual benefit levels. Individuals are not eligible for SSI benefits if their countable resources exceed $2,000, or $3,000 for a couple. But what are countable resources? Broadly, anything that can be converted to cash to support oneself, such as bank accounts, stocks, or bonds, is considered a countable resource. Only a few assets are not counted in the means test, including life insurance, burial plots, cars valued at less than $4,500, and the value of an owner-occupied home (McGarry & Schoeni, 2015). Congress has repeatedly amended the law to add new resource exclusions, adding to the complexity. When determining an individual's monthly benefit, all potential sources of income, including occasional cash gifts and living arrangements are also considered and may result in a reduced monthly payment. Income includes cash income, such as wages, Social Security benefits, and unemployment compensation, but also in-kind income, which includes things like food or shelter. Cash and in-kind income are both deducted from the Federal benefit rate. If living arrangements change, the monthly SSI benefit also changes. The complexity of the system adds to administrative costs, creates confusion for recipients, and makes the program difficult to explain to potential beneficiaries (Herd, 2009c).

In essence, SSI was intended to establish the minimum benefit discussed earlier, the lowest monthly income regarded as socially tolerable for elderly people living in the United States. The poorest older Americans should expect to receive additional income from SSI to keep them from living in extreme poverty. The program, however, has failed to establish this minimum benefit because somewhere from 40 percent to 50 percent of individuals eligible for SSI do not apply (Herd, 2009c; McGarry & Schoeni, 2015). Such low levels of participation have persisted throughout the history of the SSI program. Some eligible individuals do not apply simply because they are unaware that they might be eligible for SSI benefits. Others do not apply because they feel stigmatized and ashamed by the humiliating means test, or because they cannot manage the cumbersome eligibility paperwork. McGarry and Schoeni (2015) also found that elderly people who are eligible are less likely to enroll if they have higher-income children or receive transfers from a child. Being married and having higher levels of education also make an eligible individual less likely to enroll, indicating that stigma may play at least as important a role as confusion about whether a person might be eligible for the complex program (McGarry & Schoeni, 2015). When compared with similar programs in other developed countries, the U.S. SSI program offers the lowest minimum benefit, set at around 25 percent of median household income. The United States is also one of the only places that uses an asset test in addition to income guidelines to determine eligibility for a minimum benefit (Herd, 2009c).

SSI does fill in some of the gaps in SS coverage for vulnerable elders, particularly for minority individuals, although coverage is still inadequate. Some of the patterns discussed above, such as lower marriage rates and higher incidence of disability among African Americans, can be seen in SSI uptake. Almost a quarter (22.7%) of working-age SSI recipients are black, reflecting high disability rates, and half of black SSI recipients (50.4%) never married, compared to about a third of all SSI recipients who never married (Martin & Murphy, 2014). At first look, these numbers indicate that SSI is doing what it should to address some of the effects of lifelong disadvantage for minority elders by addressing inadequate coverage and benefits in traditional SS. The benefits actually paid to black beneficiaries, however, show troubling inadequacy. For older SSI recipients (62 and over), average annual SSI payments received by all beneficiaries were about 18 percent higher than those received by blacks (Martin & Murphy, 2014). SSI benefits at the mean and median were about $1,000 less for black recipients than for all recipients ($6,007 vs. $7,097 and $5,300 vs. $6,300, respectively). Black retirement-age SSI recipients were also much more likely to live in poverty than the older SSI population in general, with 43.3 percent of blacks in poverty compared to 32.1 percent overall (Martin & Murphy, 2014). Since SSI is based on need and a federal benefit rate (FBR), not prior work history, consistently lower payments to racial minorities are difficult to explain.

SS and SSI provide inadequate income to alleviate poverty for some of the most vulnerable older people in American society, including many black and Hispanic elders, individuals with low educational attainment, and single mothers. Despite shortcomings, the recent recession, however, shows how critical these income provision programs are. By collectivizing risk and spanning generations, public pensions avoid market volatility and risk that individuals have a difficult time managing (Ginn, Street & Arber, 2001). Herd (2009b) discusses several recent trends that jeopardize income security for older Americans. There has been a trend over the last three decades of shifting risk to the individual, with fewer defined benefit pensions available in any employment sector and a focus on personal savings and matching contributions to retirement accounts. Currently 51 percent of workers have no private pension coverage and 34 percent of workers have no savings for retirement (SSA, 2014b). In the recent recession many middle-class retirees or near-retirees saw huge reductions in their individual retirement accounts; many people in all classes were pushed into foreclosure, losing the most important retirement asset: a home. Housing assets reduce risk in old age, by offsetting the costs associated with the death of a spouse, long-term care, or other medical expenses. This asset, however, is not evenly accessible. Just before the recession, in 2007, nearly 75 percent of whites owned their own home, compared with less than 47 percent of blacks and Hispanics; in addition, the homes owned by blacks and Hispanics have lower average values (Herd, 2009b). Homeowners 65 and older are three times more likely to hold a subprime mortgage than homeowners 35 and younger, placing them at greater risk of foreclosure. Lower-income households and racial minorities are also more likely to hold subprime mortgages (Herd, 2009b). The trend toward individual savings and risk is difficult to manage with limited resources and has the greatest negative effect on blacks, Hispanics, those with limited education, and women. Another trend has been increasing labor-force participation after 65. In previous recessions older workers left paid work in favor of full retirement, opening up jobs for younger workers. However, because retirement risk is so individualized now, this is not an option for many older workers, and the recession has motivated many to continue in employment rather than retire (Herd, 2009b). Through all of the turmoil created by the 2008–2009 recession, Social Security has proven the most stable and secure source of income for older people, demonstrating the importance of collectivizing risk.

Medicare

Medicare is a federal health insurance program for individuals aged 65 and older and younger people with disabilities. Medicare was established in 1965 during the Johnson presidency's Great Society initiatives, designed to provide affordable, quality health insurance for older people where the private insurance market had failed to do so. With the Social Security Amendments of 1972 the program was expanded to cover some younger people with disabilities who become eligible if they receive SSDI benefits for two years, and those with end-stage renal disease. Prior to the passage of Medicare in 1965, only half of people 65 and older had health insurance. Older people who were insured were paying about three times what younger people paid for their health care for insurance premiums and out-of-pocket expenses, despite having only half the income, on average, of working-aged adults (Zainulbhai & Goldberg, 2014). Since 1965, the Medicare program has been instrumental in establishing health security, and by extension greater income stability, for millions of older Americans. In 2013, Medicare covered 43.5 million people 65 and older and 8.8 million individuals under 65 with disabilities; about 20 percent of enrollees are dually eligible for needs-tested Medicaid (Zainulbhai & Goldberg, 2014).

Almost all Americans 65 and older are eligible for Medicare, based on their, or their spouse's, work history. Working at least 40 quarters, or 10 years, in Medicare-covered employment leads to automatic entitlement at 65. Younger disabled individuals who receive SS benefits qualify for Medicare after a 24-month waiting period. Medicare also covers most people who need a kidney transplant or dialysis, regardless of age. The program has four distinct parts: Part A, which provides hospital insurance (HI), Part B, which is Supplementary Medical Insurance (SMI), Part C, also known as Medicare Advantage (MA), and Part D, the prescription drug benefit (see Table 4.1). The program is administered by the Centers for Medicare and Medicaid Services (CMS). In 2014, Medicare cost about $518 billion, which represents 14 percent of the federal budget (CWM, 2014). Medicare Part A covers hospital stays, posthospital care in a skilled nursing facility, limited home health care, and hospice. The patient is responsible for a deductible ($1,216 in 2014) for each hospital admission benefit period. The benefit period begins with hospital admission and ends when the patient has not been in the hospital or a skilled nursing facility for 60 days; patients needing care beyond the 60-day period pay additional daily coinsurance. Medicare Part B is optional, but enrollment is high; in 2014, about 49 million older and disabled people were enrolled in SMI. Enrollees pay a monthly premium on a sliding scale, where premiums are higher for those with higher incomes. SMI covers doctors' visits, laboratory services, durable medical equipment, hospital outpatient care, and other medical services (CWM, 2014). Medicare Advantage (Part C) was introduced in 1985 and allows beneficiaries to obtain a private health plan that agrees to provide all services covered by Medicare Part A and B (with the exception of hospice) for a capitated monthly payment. MA is an attractive alternative to many low-income beneficiaries because it provides care with lower out-of-pocket costs (Newhouse & McGuire, 2014). Medicare Part D was added in 2003 through the Medicare Prescription Drug, Improvement, and Modernization Act and allows beneficiaries to enroll in a private prescription drug plan that is required to meet certain minimum benefit requirements (CWM, 2014). MA beneficiaries may enroll in a plan that covers prescription drugs, rather than maintaining a separate policy. Part D is an important addition to the Medicare program but is structured to have a coverage gap, popularly referred to as the doughnut hole, for some of the neediest beneficiaries (see Figure 4.3). Measures have been taken in the Affordable Care Act (ACA) to phase out this coverage gap by 2020 (Ways and Means Committee Democrats, 2015).

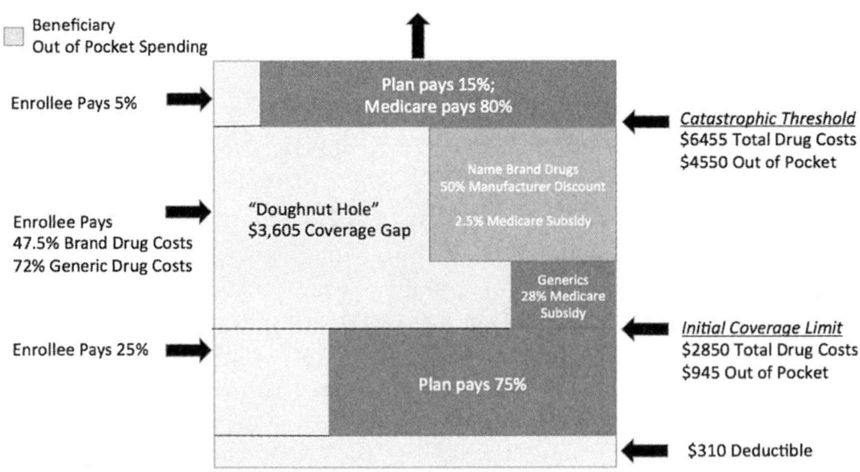

Figure 4.3 2014 Standard Medicare prescription drug benefit. (Congressional Research Service, Medicare Primer [WMC, 2014])

MA has provided an alternative to traditional Medicare (TM, Parts A and B). When the option was added in 1985, only 2 percent of Medicare beneficiaries enrolled; now more than a quarter (28% in 2013) of beneficiaries have chosen MA rather than TM (Newhouse & McGuire, 2014). Many analysts have argued that MA is a policy failure, with problematic selection effects and higher costs than TM, but policy changes in the mid-2000s seem to have resolved some of the key problems (Newhouse & McGuire, 2014). On average MA plans seem to offer higher value than TM at a lower cost, and counties with greater MA penetration also seem to have improved TM performance (Newhouse & McGuire, 2014). MA is preferable for many low-income beneficiaries because it has lower out-of-pocket costs. With average out-of-pocket costs for Medicare beneficiaries around $1,525, MA plans provide an important alternative (Chen et al., 2014). Both TM and MA sometimes overwhelm beneficiaries with choices. When enrolling in TM, a person has to decide if they want to enroll in Part B, if they want to purchase a supplementary plan, and if they want to enroll in Part D, and if so, which prescription drug plan best fits their needs. The choices in MA can be even more overwhelming. As an example, in 2008 in Miami-Dade County, beneficiaries enrolling in MA had to choose from 123 plans; in 2013 if they were in TM, there were 73 supplementary plans offered and 30 Part D plans to choose from (Newhouse & McGuire, 2014).

Medicare faces significant funding challenges as the U.S. population ages. Medicare finances are handled through two trust funds: the Hospital Insurance (HI) Trust Fund, which covers Part A benefits, and the Supplementary Medical Insurance (SMI) Trust Fund, which pays for Part B and Part D benefits (Zainulbhai & Goldberg, 2014). Much like SS, the HI Trust Fund is financed through a payroll tax, set at 2.9 percent in 2015 (OASDI and SSI Program Rates & Limits, 2015). Unlike the ceiling for payroll taxes in Social Security, there is no cap on taxable income for Medicare, and the contributions are split between the employee and employer, 1.45 percent each, with self-employed individuals paying the 2.9 percent. Since 2008 the HI Trust Fund has been running a deficit, and in 2013 expenditures from the HI Trust Fund exceeded revenue by $15 billion (Zainulbhai & Goldberg, 2014). Under current law, the HI Trust Fund will be depleted in 2030, but in the past HI insolvency has been resolved through legislative action. The SMI Trust Fund is always adequately funded because it is financed through general revenue, not payroll tax (Zainulbhai & Goldberg, 2014).

Historically, the perceived high cost of publicly provided Medicare insurance has received a great deal of political attention in the only developed

Table 4.1 Medicare Coverage and Financing

Program Details	Hospital Insurance (HI) Trust Fund (Part A)	Supplementary Medical Insurance (SMI) Trust Fund (Part B and D)
Services Covered	Inpatient hospital stays Skilled nursing facility stays Hospice care Home health visits	Part B: Physician visits, outpatient services, lab test, medical supplies, home health Part D: Prescription drugs
Major Funding Sources	Payroll taxes paid by workers and employers; interest earned on Trust Fund reserves; income taxes on part of Social Security benefits of upper income beneficiaries	Monthly premiums paid by beneficiaries; general revenues composed of federal income taxes; payments from states for premiums
Percentage of Medicare Spending in 2013	46%	Part B: 42% Part D: 12%

Source: Zainulbhai & Goldberg, 2014, National Academy of Social Insurance.

country where most citizens must depend on the private health insurance market for coverage. In general, health-care inflation in the United States has outpaced economic growth for decades. Despite concerns about its cost, Medicare has actually been less expensive and more effective at slowing cost growth than private insurance (Oberlander, 2014). Unsurprisingly, the bulk of Medicare spending is skewed toward a small group of very high-need beneficiaries. In 2009, almost 60 percent of Medicare spending was concentrated on 10 percent of beneficiaries with significant needs (Zainulbhai & Goldberg, 2014). Medicare payments are sensitive to geography, varying dramatically between high- and low-cost areas (Chen et al., 2014). Studies have shown that there is no real improvement in access, mortality, quality, or patient satisfaction in high-cost areas. Surprisingly, however, the Medicare program has been relatively successful at insulating beneficiaries from these spatial cost fluctuations, with no real difference in out-of-pocket expenditures across different geographical areas (Chen et al., 2014).

Medicaid

The Medicaid program provides health coverage to low-income individuals and families. Medicaid covers a variety of people: children and pregnant women in low-income families, low-income individuals, elderly and disabled individuals, and about 1 million American Indians and Alaska natives. The program also funds the vaccines for children program, multiple forms of long-term care, and payments to hospitals that serve a disproportionate share of low-income individuals. In fiscal year 2012, $251 billion was spent on Medicaid. Although Medicaid provides coverage for poor Americans of all ages, the elderly and disabled account for almost two-thirds of payments for benefits (see Figure 4.4). About 32 percent of Medicaid spending was for long-term services and supports, such as nursing home care and in-home care (CBO, 2013).

In 2010, over 9.6 million older or disabled Americans were covered under Medicare and Medicaid (Young et al., 2013). Medicaid fills in gaps in coverage experienced by low-income Medicare recipients, usually referred to as dual-eligibles, in that they are eligible both for Medicare social insurance and needs-based Medicaid support to meet essential health needs. Medicaid pays for a variety of things not covered by Medicare, ranging from help with paying individual Medicare premiums, to covering part or all of the cost of long-term care, to provision of hearing, vision, and dental services (Young et al., 2013). Because Medicaid programs and eligibility criteria vary by state, the percentage of dually eligible Medicaid recipients varies widely across the country, from 9 percent in Utah to 26 percent in Maine. Spending on dual eligible beneficiaries also

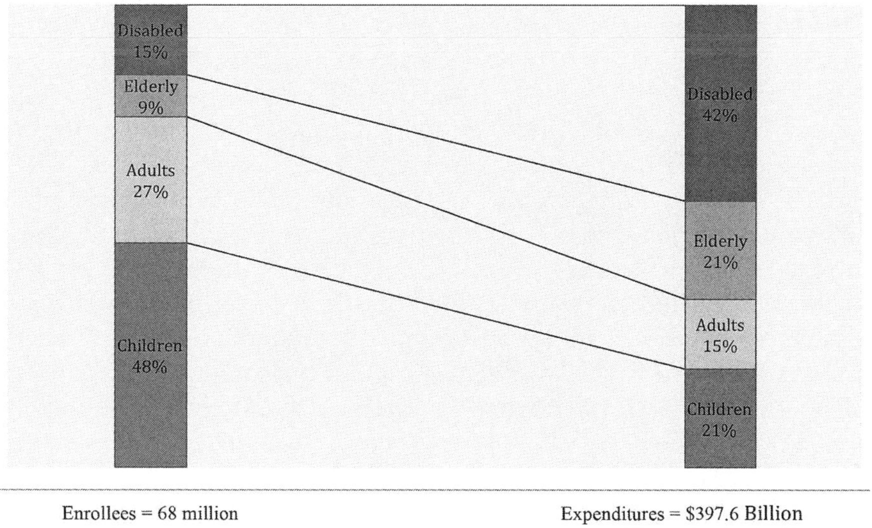

Figure 4.4 Medicaid enrollees and expenditures, FY 2011. (The Henry J. Kaiser Family Foundation, Medicaid Moving Forward, 2015, http://kff.org/health-reform/issue-brief/medicaid-moving-forward/)

varies dramatically, from just 20 percent of Medicaid spending in Arizona to a high of 55 percent of all Medicaid spending in North Dakota (Young et al., 2013). Because Medicare and private insurance provide minimal coverage for long-term care, about two-thirds of the Medicaid spending for dual eligible beneficiaries is for long-term care services (Young et al., 2013). Similar to other health insurance coverage, a small group of high-need dually eligible patients account for a large share of Medicaid spending, particularly when they need long-term services and supports.

The structure of Medicaid eligibility and payment contribute to outcomes that disadvantage some elderly Americans and benefit others. Medicaid reimbursements are lower than private pay for nursing home care in many cases, which can lead to discriminatory admissions processes (Harrington Meyer, 2001). Nursing homes rely on a certain percentage of private payers to maintain cash flow and may be reluctant to admit too many patients who are already Medicaid eligible. Older black and Hispanic individuals are 50 percent more likely to rely on Medicaid at the time of admission to nursing homes than whites, and older single people are about 30 percent more likely than married people to rely on Medicaid at the time of admission (Harrington Meyer, 2001). The bigger the gap between Medicaid payments and private payments in a particular state, the more difficulty those on Medicaid may have quickly getting into a facility.

Marital status is also a structural component of the Medicaid program. Historically, when one spouse became so ill or frail that nursing home admission was unavoidable, the couple would have to spend down virtually all their assets into poverty, so that the spouse who needed long-term care could qualify for Medicaid. This process of getting rid of almost everything the couple owned would leave the community-dwelling spouse in poverty, with no assets to fall back on (Harrington Meyer & Roseamelia, 2007). The 1988 Medicare Catastrophic Coverage Act provided some protection for couples with one spouse entering a nursing home. The community-dwelling spouse's income is no longer included in determining the nursing home resident's eligibility for Medicaid, and if their income is below a federal maintenance allowance (roughly $1,500 / month) then income can be transferred back from the institutionalized spouse's income (Harrington Meyer & Roseamelia, 2007). The community-dwelling spouse is also permitted to retain half of the couple's assets, up to roughly $90,000, a policy change that improves circumstances surrounding Medicaid eligibility for the community-dwelling spouse in long-married couples. However, as discussed above, divorces are more common now than in the past and of particular concern are marriage rates that are declining sharply among specific, already-disadvantaged groups. This is important for Medicaid eligibility because couples who cohabit rather than marry cannot access any of the protections with respect to spending down to eligibility for long-term care, meaning that the community-dwelling spouse may lose access to the couple's home and assets (Harrington Meyer & Roseamelia, 2007).

Discussion: Future Challenges

The long-term financial prospects for Social Security, Medicare, and Medicaid are worrisome for many. The rising costs associated with Social Security and the major health-care programs come from three main sources: an aging population, with proportionately fewer working-age Americans to provide tax revenues for the programs; rising health-care costs per beneficiary; and ACA expansion of federal subsidies for insurance purchased on the exchange and also through Medicaid expansion (CBO, 2014). Historically, cash-flow surpluses in Medicare and SS were invested in special treasury bonds, creating reserves to cover anticipated tax shortfalls in the future. The problem is that these bonds are liabilities of the general fund; over time selling bonds to the Social Security trust fund has created a smaller de facto deficit than would have otherwise been the case, but when redeemed (which started in 2010) they will constrain the ability of the general fund to cover other things (Palmer, 2006). While funding Social Security through baby boomer retirement is problematic and expenditures already make up a quarter of the federal budget, the cost projections for the health-care programs dwarf any challenges presented by SS. Even assuming slowed health-care cost inflation, Medicare spending is expected to double as a percentage of GDP over just two decades (Palmer, 2006). The cost per enrollee in the health-care programs has grown much more quickly than GDP, an average annual rate near 3 percent in excess of the per capita GDP (Palmer, 2006). Palmer (2006) argues that we cannot grow our way out of these funding challenges, as the long-rung growth rate of GDP per worker has averaged around 1.6 percent annually for the past 50 years and there is no reason to expect a huge increase from that. Under current law, the three entitlement programs are projected to equal the entire federal budget (around 18% of GDP) by 2078 (Palmer, 2006).

Separate from these macroeconomic challenges to the solvency of the old-age welfare state are problems associated with predictable vulnerabilities in old age that so far appear to be intractable. Particularly in terms of having an adequate income to fully participate in their social worlds with dignity, for some subgroups of elderly people—disproportionately single elders, race/ethnic minorities, widowed/single women, and the oldest-old—Social Security and SSI are often not up to the task of compensating adequately in old age for lifetimes of disadvantage. Perhaps it is too much to expect any social policy to do that. However, policy makers who will debate and enact changes to the old-age welfare state will serve older Americans well if they take into account ways to provide adequate income and robust access to health care that ameliorates some of life's disadvantages at the same time as they work to ensure the affordability and integrity of these essential public programs. Medicare and Medicaid may become less worrisome budget line items if the promise of universal access to health care under ACA brings health costs under control. The ACA provisions are so recent, however, it is impossible to understand what the contours of Medicare and Medicaid are likely to be in a few years and whether ACA will fulfill its promise of covering more Americans and slowing medical inflation. In terms of income, one certainty is that the institution of retirement—the social expectation that most people will be able to retire one day—depends on Americans having dependable sources income in old age. That underscores the importance of thoughtful Social Security and SSI reform, not just for the most vulnerable older Americans, but for average workers and their families, too.

Notes

1. This chapter focuses mainly on programs specifically designed for older Americans. However, there are many nonelderly Social Security beneficiaries. For example, disabled individuals may be entitled to monthly benefits. To qualify for Social Security disability benefits a worker must have accumulated at least six quarters of Social Security-covered employment. Disability, for the purposes of collecting Social Security, includes medically determined physical or mental impairment that is likely to cause death or last longer than 12 months, which prevents an individual from engaging in any substantial work available in the national economy. It is estimated that more than 1 in 4 of today's 20-year-olds is expected to become disabled before reaching the retirement age of 67 (SSA, 2014b).

2. A recent SS innovation means that more men may qualify for spousal benefits in the future. The June 2015 *Obergefell v. Hodges* Supreme Court decision to recognize same-sex marriage for Social Security benefits, followed by the August 2015 Justice Department decision to incorporate same-sex unions within the SS and SSI system, will offer important new protections to spouses (whether men or women) in those newly recognized unions (SSA 2016).

References

Calasanti T., & Slevin K.F. (2001). *Gender, social inequalities, and aging*. Walnut Creek, CA: Alta Mira Press.

Carr, D. (2010). Golden years? Poverty among older Americans. *Contexts*, 9, 62–63.

Centers for Disease Control and Prevention (CDC). (2015). Births: Final Data for 2013. *National Vital Statistics Reports,* 64(1). Retrieved from http://www.cdc.gov/nchs/data/nvsr/nvsr64/nvsr64_01.pdf

Chen, L.M., Norton, E.C., Langa, K.M., Le, S., & Epstein, A.M. (2014). Geographic variation in out-of-pocket expenditures of elderly Medicare beneficiaries. *Journal of the American Geriatrics Society,* 62(6), 1097–1104.

Committee on Ways and Means U.S. House of Representatives (CWM). (2014). *Green book: Background material and data on the programs within the jurisdiction of the Committee on Ways and Means.* Retrieved from http://greenbook.waysandmeans.house.gov/2014-green-book

Congressional Budget Office (CBO). (2013). *An overview of the Medicaid program.* Retrieved from http://www.cbo.gov/publication/44588

Congressional Budget Office (CBO). (2014). *CBO's 2014 long-term projections for social security: Additional information.* Retrieved from www.cbo.gov/publication/49795

DeWitt, L. (2010). The decision to exclude agricultural and domestic workers from the 1935 Social Security Act. *Social Security Bulletin (2010),* 70(4), 49–68. Retrieved from http://www.ssa.gov/policy/docs/ssb/v70n4/v70n4p49.html

Fischer, J., & Hayes, J. (2013). The importance of social security in the incomes of older Americans: Differences by gender, age, race/ethnicity, and marital status. Institute for Women's Research Briefing Paper IWPR # D503. Retrieved from http://www.iwpr.org/publications/pubs/the-importance-of-social-security-in-the-incomes-of-older-americans-differences-by-gender-age-race-ethnicity-and-marital-status

Fry, R. (2014). New census data show more Americans are tying the knot, but mostly it's the college educated. Pew Research Center.

Furtado, D., & Theodoropoulos, N. (2013). SSI for disabled immigrants: Why do ethnic networks matter? *American Economic Review: Papers & Proceedings 2013,* 103(3), 462–466.

Ginn, J., Street, D., & Arber, S. (Eds.). (2001). *Women, work, and pensions: International issues and prospects.* Buckingham: Open University Press.

Harrington Meyer, M. (2001). Medicaid reimbursement rates and access to nursing homes: Implications for gender, race, and marital status. *Research on Aging,* 23(5), 532–551.

Harrington Meyer, M., & Herd, P. (2007). *Market friendly or family friendly? The state and gender inequality in old age.* New York: Russell Sage Foundation.

Harrington Meyer, M., & Roseamelia, C. (2007). Emerging issues for older couples: Protecting income and assets, right to intimacy, and end-of-life decisions. *Generations,* 31(3), 66–71.

Harrington Meyer, M., Wolf, D.A., & Himes, C.L. (2005). Linking benefits to marital status: Race and social security in the US. *Feminist Economics,* 11(2), 145–162.

Herd, P. (2005). Reforming a breadwinner welfare state: Gender, race, class and social security reform. *Social Forces,* 83(4), 1365–1393.

Herd, P. (2009a). The problem of poverty among older people in America: Options for reform. *Benefits,* 17(2), 125–135.

Herd, P. (2009b). The two-legged stool: The reconfiguration of risk in retirement income security. *Generations,* 33(3), 12–18.

Herd, P. (2009c). Women, public pensions, and poverty: What can the United States learn from other countries? *Journal of Women, Politics & Policy*, 30(2–3), 301–334.

Hudson, R. B. (2014). The future of old age politics and policy. In R. B. Hudson (Ed.), *The New Politics of Old Age Policy* (3rd ed.). Baltimore, MD: Johns Hopkins University Press.

Macpherson, D., & Hirsch, B. (1995). Wages and gender composition: Why do women's jobs pay less? *Journal of Labour Economics*, 13(3): 426–471.

Martin, P. P., & Murphy, J. L. (2014). African Americans: Description of social security and supplemental security income participation and benefit levels using the American Community Survey. U.S. Social Security Administration Office of Retirement and Disability Policy, Research and Statistics, Note No. 2014–01.

McGarry, K., & Schoeni, R. F. (2015). Understanding participation in SSI. University of Michigan Retirement Research Center (MRRC) Working Paper, WP 2015–319.

Mink, G. (1995). *The wages of motherhood: Inequality in the welfare state, 1917–1942*. Ithaca, NY: Cornell University Press.

Munnell, A. H. (2013). Social security's *real* retirement age is 70. Issue Brief 13–15, Center for Retirement Research at Boston College.

Myles, J. (1989). *Old age in the welfare state: The political economy of public pensions*. Lawrence: University Press of Kansas.

National Academy of Social Insurance (NASI). (2015). *Social security and people of color*. Retrieved from https://www.nasi.org/learn/socialsecurity/people-of-color

Newhouse, J. P., & McGuire, T. G. (2014). How successful is Medicare advantage? *The Milbank Quarterly*, 92(2), 351–394.

OASDI and SSI Program Rates and Limits. (2015). Social security administration. Retrieved from http://www.ssa.gov/policy/docs/quickfacts/prog_highlights/index.html

OASDI and SSI Program Rates and Limits. (2005). Social security administration. Retrieved from http://www.ssa.gov/policy/docs/quickfacts/prog_highlights/RatesLimits2005.html

Oberlander, J. (2014). The long struggle for universal health care. In Thomas R. Oliver (Ed.), *Guide to U.S. health and health care policy* (pp. 23–36). New York: Sage/CQ Press.

O'Neill, J. E., & O'Neill, D. M. (2005). What do wage differentials tell us about labor market discrimination? Working Paper 11240, National Bureau of Economic Research, March 2005.

Palmer, J. L. (2006). Entitlement programs for the aged: The long-term fiscal context. *Research on Aging*, 28(3), 289–302.

Pew Research Center (2013). *On pay gap, millennial women near parity—For now*. Retrieved from http://www.pewsocialtrends.org/2013/12/11/on-pay-gap-millennial-women-near-parity-for-now/

Quadagno, J. (1994). *The color of welfare: How racism undermined the war on poverty*. New York: Oxford University Press.

Sayer, L. (2005). Gender, time and inequality: Trends in women's and men's paid work, unpaid work and free time. *Social Forces*, 84, 285–304.

Social Security Administration (SSA). (2014a). *Annual report of the Supplemental Security Income Program.*

Social Security Administration (SSA). (2014b). *Social Security Administration fact sheet.*

Social Security Administration (SSA). (2016). *GN 00210.100—Same-Sex Marriages and Non-marital Legal Relationships—Benefits for Aged Spouses* https://secure.ssa.gov/poms.nsf/lnx/0200210100

Street, D., & Connidis, I. (2001). Creeping selectivity in Canadian women's pensions. In J. Ginn, D. Street, & S. Arber (Eds.), *Women, work and pensions: International issues and prospects* (pp. 158–178). Buckingham: Open University Press.

Street, D., & Wilmoth, J. (2001). Social insecurity: Women and pensions in the US. In J. Ginn, D. Street, & S. Arber (Eds.), *Women, work and pensions: International issues and prospects* (pp. 120–141). Buckingham: Open University Press.

U.S. Census Bureau. (2012). *Historical marriage trends from 1890–2010: A focus on race differences.* Retrieved from http://www.census.gov/library/working-papers/2012/demo/SEHSD-WP2012–12.html

Ways and Means Committee Democrats. (2015). *Medicare.* Retrieved from http://democrats.waysandmeans.house.gov/issue/medicare

Young, K., Garfield, R., Musumeci, M., Clemans-Cope, L., & Lawton, E. (2013). *Medicaid's role for dual eligible beneficiaries. The Kaiser Commission on Medicaid and the uninsured.* Retrieved from http://kff.org/medicaid/issue-brief/medicaids-role-for-dual-eligible-beneficiaries/

Zainulbhai, S., & Goldberg, L. (2014). Medicare finances: Findings of the 2014 trustees report. *National Academy of Social Insurance, Health Policy Brief, No. 11.*

CHAPTER FIVE

Gender, Race, and Ethnicity and the Life Course

Jan E. Mutchler and Ceara R. Somerville

Few characteristics have more significance in shaping the life course than gender, race, and ethnicity—social categories penetrating virtually every aspect of social life (Mayer, 2009). From birth, throughout childhood and young adulthood and on into middle age, gender, race, and ethnicity shape the key elements of well-being. The significance of these social categories stems in part from inequities within the social structure, including racism and sexism, which shape opportunities. As well, these social categories flag differences in values, norms, and orientations that impact outcomes and experiences throughout the life course. When they are devalued by society, behaviors associated with cultural or normative orientations can become a basis not only for *difference* but also for *inequality*, such as the example of low public value assigned to caretaking for children and frail older adults.

The goal of this chapter is to explain how gender, race, and ethnicity shape well-being outcomes in later life, guided by the life-course framework. The key insight of this framework is that behaviors, identities, and inequalities associated with social groupings have implications not only for outcomes at a given point in time, but potentially for a lifetime. The life-course approach describes the temporal processes by which early experiences shape late-life outcomes—for example, how opportunities to obtain high-quality health care in childhood and young adulthood shape longevity and late-life wellness. An additional insight of this framework is that individuals make decisions within the context of primary groups, and that late-life outcomes are shaped by these so-called linked lives—for example, a couple's division of labor regarding paid work and childcare can yield gender differences in late-life income security. While recognizing the importance of human agency—the capacity of each individual to form judgments and act according to his or her own sensibilities—the life-course approach recognizes that choices are constrained not only by social structure in general, but also by the gendered and racialized society within which we live. In our discussion, we also reference theoretical arguments about inequality, especially the cumulative inequality perspective, which has gained traction in recent years. We review literature on selected quality of life issues, including income security, health and health care, and family caregiving and long-term care, as a means of illustrating relevant conceptual themes. Finally, we consider challenges and opportunities for responding to and remediating late-life disparities. We begin our explorations by laying out the demographic context structuring these issues.

The Demographic Context

The gender, race, and ethnic composition of any population are shaped by the confluence of fertility, mortality, and migration. These processes determine both the *number* of people within a population and the demographic *composition* of a population, including the gender, race, and ethnic characteristics of the population at a given time. In the United States, gender composition is shaped primarily by the balance of births and deaths. Currently, the U.S. sex ratio at birth—the ratio of the number of boys to the number of girls born in a given time period—is 1.047, similar to the sex ratio in 1950, which was 1.054, when today's 65-year-olds were born (Martin et al., 2010; Matthews & Hamilton, 2005). Building on these uneven beginnings, gender composition of a cohort is reshaped extensively by mortality. Throughout the life course, males have a higher risk of dying than do females, and as a result, females live longer than men on average; females born in 2013 are expected to live 81 years, on average, compared to 76 years for males (Kochanek et al., 2014). Primarily as a result of these processes, and only minimally shaped by immigration (Fry, 2006), the older population is heavily female. Indeed, the U.S. population includes just 81 men for every 100 women aged 70–79, and only 62 men for each 100 women aged 80–89 (see Figure 5.1).

Race and ethnic composition are also shaped by demographic forces. The terms *race* and *ethnicity* are often used interchangeably, but are thought to describe different attributes. Race typically denotes a status or identity associated with physiological features, especially skin color, while ethnicity reflects an individual's "heritage, nationality group, lineage, or country of birth" (Humes, Jones, & Ramirez, 2011). Racial and ethnic diversity in

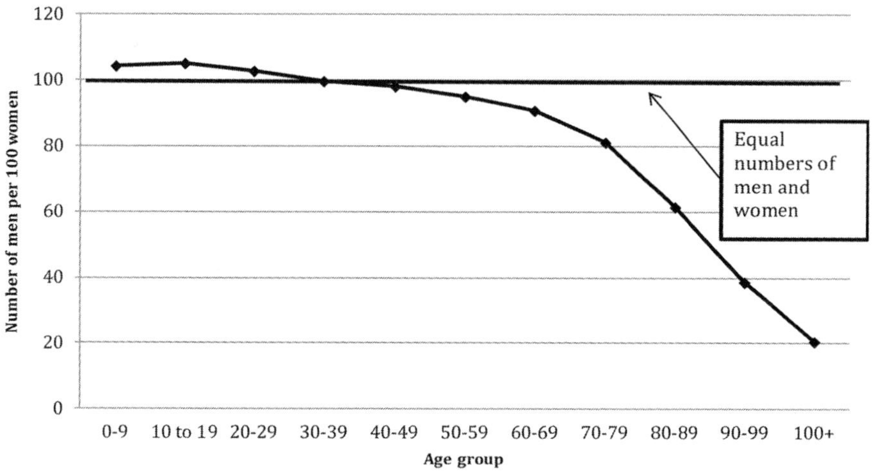

Figure 5.1 Sex ratio by age group, United States, 2010. (U.S. Census Bureau, FactFinder, Census 2010 table QT-P1: [http://factfinder.census.gov/faces/nav/jsf/pages/index.xhtml])

the United States have been fueled in part by fertility differences, as birth rates for Hispanic and African American women are higher than for non-Hispanic white and Asian women. For African Americans, this potential for growth is partially offset by a higher risk of dying throughout the life course (Arias, 2014). Yet, other ethnic groups—including Hispanics and many Asian national origin groups—have expectations of life that are *longer* than that experienced by non-Hispanic whites (Kaiser Family Foundation, 2015; Pollard & Scommegna, 2013).

International migration patterns have an especially significant impact on the diversity of the U.S. population; currently, two-thirds of recent immigrants to the United States are from Asia or Latin America (U.S. Department of Homeland Security, 2013). In recent years, the share of legal immigrants who are aged 50 or older has risen and is now approaching 20 percent; many of these late-life entrants are admitted to the United States as relatives, especially parents, of current U.S. residents or citizens. Because immigration policy provisions give preference to family members of U.S. residents, and allow immediate family members of U.S. citizens, including parents, to be admitted without numerical caps, a gradual increase in the age structure of recent immigrants is expected (Carr & Tienda, 2013).

Together, these demographic influences are reshaping the composition of the U.S. population, decade by decade and cohort by cohort. Looking ahead, what can we expect in terms of racial and ethnic diversity within the older population? Figure 5.2 illustrates the expected transformation.

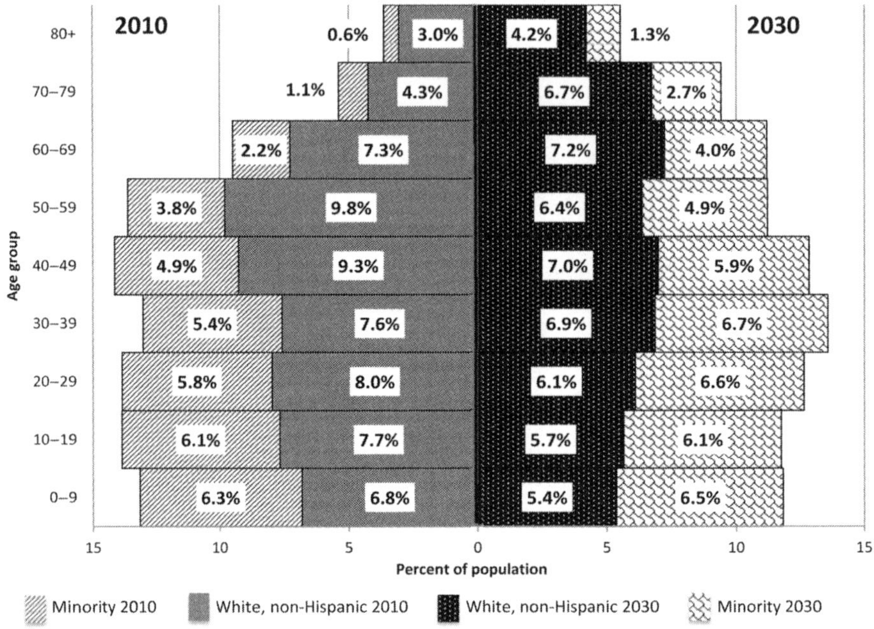

Figure 5.2 Age and ethnicity, United States, 2010 (actual) and 2030 (projected) (2010 data from U.S. Census Bureau, FactFinder, Census 2010 table P12I: [http://factfinder.census.gov/faces/nav/jsf/pages/index.xhtml]. 2030 projections from U.S. Census Bureau http://www.census.gov/population/projections/data/national/2014/downloadablefiles.html)

On the left-hand side of the population pyramid, the age structure based on data from Census 2010 is shown, with each age cohort split into components based on race and ethnicity. For example, 13 percent of the U.S. population in 2010 was under the age of 10, and nearly half of this age group—6 percent of the total population—was either Hispanic, nonwhite, or both. Older cohorts in 2010 include progressively smaller shares who are ethnic minorities and in the 80+ population, a large majority is non-Hispanic white. The right-hand side of the pyramid shows projections for the United States in 2030 and suggests a considerable increase in the share of the U.S. population that is nonwhite or Hispanic. All age groups under the age of 30 are expected to be majority-minority by 2030, and the proportion that is non-Hispanic white will decline relative to the 2010 distribution for all but the oldest age groups. This trend is expected to continue, and in the coming decades even larger shares of the older population will be composed of ethnic minorities. The aging of younger, more diverse cohorts who already live in the United States will drive this process; as well, a continued influx of late-life immigrants will contribute to this trend.

Although the demographic forces depicted here are likely to continue for the foreseeable future, the social and political *significance* of this growing diversity depends on the continuing importance of race and ethnicity as factors that shape well-being in later life. Features of the social and economic climate, as well as evolving public policies, may modify the significance of diversity and group membership. Currently, inequalities in education, income, wealth, and access to high-quality jobs with benefits (such as pension coverage) shape lifelong patterns of resource accumulation. As a result, African Americans and Hispanics enter late adulthood with substantially fewer financial resources than do their white non-Hispanic peers. Although reduced racial and ethnic inequalities in childhood and early adulthood have the potential to bridge late-life differences in well-being, among today's older and middle-aged adults, race, and ethnic inequalities persist at a high level.

The Life Course and Late-Life Outcomes: Disparities in Later Life by Gender, Race, and Ethnicity

The scientific literature documents sharp contrasts in the aggregate characteristics of older men and women, as well as contrasts by race and ethnicity. The life-course processes leading to these disparities have been extensively explored; yet debate continues regarding the social, economic, or policy modifications that would be most successful in reducing disparities in later life. Processes relating to identity, culture, and discrimination each shape how and why gender, race, and ethnicity matter in distinctive and sometimes competing ways. For example, gender identity may shape health behaviors (Calasanti, 2010), which, in turn, has consequences for successful management of chronic disease. Cultural factors play a role as well. Examples include health behaviors and beliefs, norms regarding intergenerational support and caretaking, and English language proficiency—all of which shape trajectories into later life, as well as experiences as an older adult. Dynamics of sexism and racism may limit lifelong opportunities for education and subsequent career advancement, resulting in lower economic security in later life among women and some ethnic minorities. Bias and discrimination against individuals based on their membership in given gender, race, or ethnic groups can also limit access to high-quality health care, increasing the risk of accumulating chronic conditions and causing people to enter late-life sicker and more disabled than their more privileged peers.

The life-course perspective offers a well-developed foundation for understanding the ways in which gender, race, and ethnicity shape the dynamics of the aging process. By providing rich conceptualization of the twists and turns of an individual's life, the life-course approach draws our attention to transitions and trajectories relating to roles and statuses (Hagestad, 1990; Settersten, 2006), which are subject to factors relating to gender, race, and ethnicity. While incorporating the importance of *human agency*—free will and the unique choices made by each individual—the life-course perspective emphasizes that broad social forces, including those linked to gender and race, influence those choices. In addition, gender or ethnic groups may be impacted by the *interconnected lives* of family members and significant others in distinctive ways. Features of the broader social structure relating to educational and work organizations, labor markets, and public policies lend significance to the *timing* at which transitions occur, the *sequence* of transitions relative to one another, and the *duration* of time spent in given statuses (Elder, 1985).

The life-course approach yields insight regarding group-based differentiation in experiences (Settersten, 2006). An expanded theoretical understanding of how inequality throughout the life course impacts late-life disparities requires attention not only to features of the life course at the microlevel—such as individual decision making—but also to social structural processes shaping inequality throughout one's lifetime. Life experiences are shaped by membership in gender, race, or ethnic groups and are carried into later life, where they influence strengths and vulnerabilities with respect to resources, health, and social support (O'Rand, 2006). For example, barriers to obtaining schooling or training associated with group membership contribute to disparities in lifelong accumulation of occupational and economic benefits; these disparities, in turn, have implications for later-life resources in the form of wealth accumulation, pension eligibility and values, Social Security credits, and health outcomes (see Walsemann, Geronimus, & Gee, 2008).

Cumulative advantage/disadvantage (CAD) theory is a useful and well-known approach to explaining how early advantage or disadvantage contributes to trajectories of accumulation (Dannefer, 2003). In recent years, insights from CAD theory have been refined and reformulated into cumulative inequality (CI) theory by Ferraro and colleagues (Ferraro & Shippee, 2009; Ferraro, Shippee, & Schafer, 2009). Blending insights from the life-course approach and cumulative advantage/disadvantage theory, the CI theory offers a nuanced understanding of how social structural inequalities intersect with life changes and trajectories, noting that "age is an index of life changes and the accumulation of inequality" (Ferraro & Shippee, 2009:2).

Although not framed exclusively in terms of gender, race, and ethnicity, several elements of CI theory are especially informative to understanding disparities relating to these attributes. As one example, Ferraro and Shippee (2009) note that both *risks* and available *resources* are socially structured, allowing for the accumulation of both advantage and disadvantage. Group differences in exposure to risk (hazards to health or finances, for example) and in access to resources are important, but they do not entirely determine trajectories. Individual choices matter too—even when those choices are also structured to an extent by group membership, through norms and socializing influences. As another example, Ferraro and Shippee draw attention to the important role of *perception* of life trajectories, noting that "people view and evaluate their trajectories in comparison to significant others and reference groups" (2009:4). As individuals navigate their own life-course trajectories, progress and success are measured relative to the experience of others. Yet to the extent that reference groups are structured by gender, race, and ethnicity, as well as by age group, those perceptions may be shaped by perceived inequalities as well as reinforced by lived experience. For example, England (2010) argues that women may track their own "success" in reference to that of their mothers, or older women with similar educational accomplishments, rather than to men with similar characteristics.

In the remainder of this section, we will discuss, in more depth, these issues with respect to three topics of key importance to late-life disparities in well-being: economic security, health and health-care access, and caregiving and long-term care. Space limitations prevent extensive review of these topics; as a result, we focus our discussion on key conceptual issues and provide only illustrative citations. We describe selected disparities by gender and across racial and ethnic groups, focusing on key characteristics relating to well-being (see Table 5.1). We acknowledge a high degree of differentiation within the specified groups profiled here; for example, substantial differences in characteristics and resources are evident across national origin groups within the Asian (e.g., Vietnamese vs. Japanese), Hispanic (e.g., Mexican vs. Cuban), and black (e.g., U.S. black vs. Caribbean black) populations. Moreover, we focus our attention on the largest groups; data for Native Americans, seniors reporting multiple races, and other relatively small categories are not presented.

Economic security and the life course. Economic security is achieved when the financial resources to support an acceptable quality of life are stably in place. Among older adults, economic security depends in large part on access to pension income, including both public and private pensions, and on personal savings, financial investments, and other forms of wealth, such as real estate, which either generate income or could serve as a source of funds, if liquidated. Economic security is further promoted when capacity to work at least part time is maintained. Statistics on the amounts and sources of income among older adults highlight that all else equal, having more *sources* of income is associated with having higher *amounts* of income, and consequently greater economic security. Older adults living exclusively on a Social Security pension typically have substantially less income than older adults who also have a private pension, income from savings or investments, and wage or salary income. Recent data suggest that among

Table 5.1 Selected Characteristics of U.S. Older Adults Aged 65+, by Gender, Race, and Ethnicity (2013–2014)

	Non-Hispanic				Gender	
	White	Black	Asian	Hispanic	Men	Women
Socioeconomic resources						
College graduate (%)	26.4	14.8	34.1	9.9	30.2	19.8
Household income[a] (median)	$46,700	$35,700	$67,000	$38,700	$51,400	$40,900
Poor (%)	7.4	18.3	13.3	19.8	7.4	11.3
Homeowner[b] (%)	77.7	56.5	44.9	48.7	77.2	68.3
With pension income[c] (%)	33.1	28.1	17.2	15.7	39.2	23.7
Health and health-care access						
Health status[c]:						
– Excellent/ very good (%)	38.1	25.2	27.6	25.0	36.6	34.5
– Good (%)	34.7	36.1	38.8	34.0	34.7	35.3
– Fair/poor (%)	27.1	38.6	33.6	41.1	28.7	30.1
With a disability (%)	35.3	41.2	32.0	40.3	35.5	36.7
Insurance coverage[c]:						
– No insurance	1.0	2.4	5.1	5.2	1.9	1.5
– Public only	36.1	55.3	52.6	63.6	38.3	42.5
– Private (with or without public)	62.9	42.3	42.3	31.2	59.8	56.0
Limited English proficiency (%)	2.2	2.9	58.2	55.0	8.0	8.9
Linguistically isolated (%)	1.3	1.2	29.4	27.6	4.3	4.5
Living arrangements and long-term care						
Living in an institution (%) (age 75+)	5.4	7.2	2.8	3.4	3.5	6.4

	Non-Hispanic				Gender	
	White	Black	Asian	Hispanic	Men	Women
Living in an intergenerational household (%)	17.4	36.1	49.2	46.4	19.7	24.8
Living alone (%)	28.2	32.2	13.4	19.0	18.5	34.1

Note: Except for % in an institution, all figures exclude group quarters population and are based on adults aged 65 and older.

[a]Household income is based on all households including residents aged 65 and older. The older adult may or may not be the householder.

[b]Homeowners include both householders and their spouses living in an owned home.

[c]The source for these data is the 2014 Current Population Survey microdata, retrieved from the IPUMS website.

Sources: Calculated by authors from data retrieved from the Integrated Public Use Microdata Series (IPUMS; Ruggles et al., 2010). Except as noted, original data source is the 2013 American Community Survey.

older adults with an income of $63,648 or higher in 2012—representing the highest income quintile—half of all income was from earnings (Social Security Administration, 2014). Financial resources in later life, including both income and wealth, are a function of lifelong opportunities and choices relating to both paid and unpaid work, to human capital investments, and to intergenerational transfers of wealth. Because gender, race, and ethnicity are associated with these key dimensions, differences in economic security in later life are substantial.

Decades of research on gender inequality at work and at home documents the ways in which disparate gender roles, socializing influences, and bias combine to yield differences between men and women in access to financial resources and benefits. Most girls growing up in the United States during the 1950s—including today's 65-year-olds—were socialized to expect that they would prioritize family roles over work roles. Indeed, today's older women are less likely than their male counterparts to have completed college (see Table 5.1). Moreover, they are more likely to have experienced interrupted careers as a result of caring for children and other family members (Calasanti, 2010). Perhaps in part due to dominant gender roles at the time, but also as a result of gender discrimination and the devaluation of "women's work" (England, 2010), the jobs most of today's older women held when they did work had lower pay than those held by men and were less likely to provide benefits in the form of pension coverage (Calasanti, 2010). The tension between paid and unpaid work continues into later life, with older women being more likely than men to reduce work hours in order to care for a disabled or frail loved one (Pleau, 2010), or to care for a grandchild (Harrington Meyer, 2014).

For many women entering late life, these experiences and trajectories have resulted in low economic security. As shown in Table 5.1, older women are considerably more likely to be poor than are older men and less likely to have a pension or to own a home. They are more likely than men to rely largely or exclusively on Social Security as a source of retirement income (Social Security Administration, 2014), making them especially reliant on a single source of income and vulnerable to threats to the Social Security system (Harrington Meyer & Herd, 2007).

Socioeconomic disparities across race and ethnic groups are also substantial. Completing a college degree typically occurs in young adulthood, but the implications of completion and the associated accumulation of economic resources are considerable over a lifetime. Table 5.1 shows that one-third of Asian and one-quarter of non-Hispanic white older adults are college graduates, but only 15 percent of black and 10 percent of Hispanic older adults have completed college. Corresponding disparities in income, poverty, and financial assets are also evident; older blacks and Hispanics live in households with less income and a higher risk of poverty. Older non-Hispanic whites are far more likely than the other ethnic groups to own a home and to have income from a pension. Indeed, African American, Asian, and Hispanic seniors are less likely than their white counterparts to receive Social Security, asset, or pension incomes (Social Security Administration, 2014). These disparities may be partially a result of the high prevalence of immigrants among older Hispanics and Asians, many of whom worked in lower-paying jobs with fewer benefits. Immigrants arriving in the United States at older ages have especially low incomes, having had few opportunities to build an employment history in the United States that provides access to Social Security or a pension (O'Neil & Tienda, 2015). Discrimination throughout the life course undoubtedly plays a role as well, with ethnic minority group members encountering fewer opportunities to pursue higher education and well-paid employment.

Much has changed in recent decades, and some disparities in economic security may be narrowing. Young women now enter adulthood with different expectations and experiences than what was common among their mothers and grandmothers. For example, women are currently more likely than men to enroll in college (Lopez & Gonzalez-Barrera, 2014). Delays in marriage and childbearing, increases in the share of women who remain childless, and increasing involvement of men in household and childrearing activities suggest that men's and women's life-course trajectories may be converging, at least to some extent (Treas & Marcum, 2011). It is likely that current cohorts of young women will convert these new experiences into stronger economic security in later life, with diminishing gaps between older men and women. Yet there is reason to be cautious in these expectations. Continued wage gaps between working men and women will result in late-life disparities in income indexed to lifetime earnings, including Social Security pension benefits, private pension income, and other forms of wealth (Harrington Meyer & Herd, 2007). Moreover, gender asymmetry at home and work continues (England, 2010). For example, Cha (2010) reports that in dual-earner households, a wife has an increased likelihood of quitting work when her husband works long hours, especially when the couple has children. In contrast, husbands do not respond in a similar way when their wives work long hours. In these and numerous other ways, the lives of men and women remain in partially separate spheres, with powerful implications for late-life disparities in income security.

Disparities in economic security by race and ethnicity may also be narrowing. While acknowledging far lower levels of net worth among older African Americans than whites, a report on well-being among older Americans identifies a narrowing of this gap in recent decades (Federal Interagency Forum on Aging-Related Statistics, 2012). And disparities in high school graduation rates and college attendance are narrowing as well, despite persistent gaps in educational attainment (Fry & Taylor, 2013; Kena et al., 2015). More equitable access to education and jobs would be expected to result in greater parity in late-life resource profiles in coming decades. Yet immigration trends that shape the number and characteristics of new arrivals, along with policies that determine immigrants' access to opportunities and supports that shape economic security, will contribute to disparities moving forward.

Health status and access to medical services. Life-course influences on later-life health are well established in the literature (Pearlin et al., 2005); these findings are largely consistent with the cumulative inequality framework offered by Ferraro and Shippee (2009). A growing literature documents the many ways in which opportunities, risks, and exposures stemming from childhood shape health trajectories, ultimately leading to lower survivorship and poorer health outcomes in later life among some individuals and groups. Gender, race, and ethnic inequality, as well as social and cultural factors that shape health-related experiences in childhood and beyond, have long-lasting impacts on health. Poor late-life health outcomes result from a matrix of exposures throughout the life course, including participating in unhealthy behaviors, being exposed to unhealthy environments, and experiencing poor access to appropriate medical services. Indeed, gender, race, and ethnic differences in health profiles and survivorship are stubborn reminders of the complex inequalities that continue to permeate American society.

Health disparities. Although women live longer than men on average, health disparities by gender are evident in women's having more chronic illnesses and higher levels of disability (Crimmins, 2004). Health disparities are substantial across race and ethnic groups as well. Members of some groups, most notably African Americans and Native Americans, are less likely to survive to old age and more likely than whites and Asian Americans to be disabled as they enter later life (e.g., Goins et al., 2007; Hayward & Heron, 1999). Fewer blacks, Asians, and Hispanics report their health status as "excellent" or "very good," compared to whites (see Table 5.1). Rates of *frailty*—a cluster of symptoms and deficits occurring especially in later life, and predictive of mortality—are higher among women than men and are substantially higher among African Americans than among whites (Hirsch et al., 2006; Xue, 2011).

A considerable amount of research suggests that populations with lower socioeconomic status—including African Americans and some other ethnic groups—have poorer health and higher death rates; indeed, Link and Phelan (1995) refer to socioeconomic status as a fundamental cause of disease. Yet, the scientific literature highlights the complex matrix of factors shaping health-related outcomes. For example, despite having lower income and education levels, and contrary to the expectation that low-income populations are at higher risk of mortality, U.S. Hispanics have a life expectancy that is *higher* than their non-Hispanic white peers—an observation referred to as the "Hispanic paradox" (Lariscy, Hummer, & Hayward, 2015). Explanations abound as to the source of this anomaly, but a firm conclusion is elusive. Some researchers speculate that health behaviors such as quality of diet and smoking behavior may play a role. Currently, the most likely explanation relates to migration selectivity, as Hispanic immigrants to the United States may be selected for good health, which could in turn confer a measure of advantage for later-life health and survivorship. Moreover, some speculate that Hispanic immigrants may return to their country of origin when their health declines—the so-called salmon bias—thus removing those most at risk of dying from the pool of Hispanics in the United States (Pollard & Scommegna, 2013).

An active area of research in recent years has focused on detecting and measuring *under the skin* mechanisms by which disadvantage leads to health consequences. For example, some evidence suggests that stress associated with low socioeconomic and minority status increases the pace of biological aging such that African Americans and Hispanics take on biological features of later life more rapidly than whites (Diez Roux et al., 2009; Geronimus et al., 2010). As one example of how this might work, we consider high blood pressure, or hypertension—a dangerous condition for older adults as it is a precursor to a number of deadly heart and health conditions. Nearly two-thirds of Americans who are 60 and older have hypertension (Nwankwo et al., 2013), but prevalence of hypertension is not equally distributed by race. Age-adjusted prevalence rates of hypertension are substantially higher among non-Hispanic blacks than among others. Factors that contribute to high blood pressure include socioeconomic status, health and lifestyle behaviors, environmental factors, and stress; higher levels of exposure to these risks would be expected to produce higher rates of hypertension. But even when controlling for such risk factors, blacks still have a significantly higher prevalence of hypertension compared to their white counterparts (Quinones, Liang, & Ye, 2012). The persistence of higher blood pressure among black Americans is thought to be a result of long-term inequality that has manifested itself biologically (Rooks & Thorpe, 2014)—an example of *under the skin* mechanisms by which social exposures have physiological consequences. Enduring a life course conditioned by chronic and eventful stressors linked to racial disadvantage takes a toll on the physiological response to stress, so by middle- and late-age stages of life, the body functions at a lower capacity than it might have otherwise.

Another active area of research links early-life events—even conditions occurring in childhood and adolescence—to late-life health consequences. Literature exploring this linkage considers both *under the skin* processes and the accumulation of disadvantageous social and economic circumstances into later life (Kuh & Ben-Shlomo, 2004). Evidence has been offered suggesting that childhood disadvantage is associated with higher risk of late-life disability (Montez & Hayward, 2014), greater risk of functional limitations and serious health conditions such as cancer, diabetes, heart disease, hypertension, stroke (Brown, O'Rand, & Adkins, 2012), and poorer physical performance (Haas, Krueger, & Rohlfsen, 2012). Gruenewald et al. (2012) report substantial effects of childhood socioeconomic situation on later-life allostatic load—a concept capturing the wear and tear on the body associated with the experience of and response to stress. How these early-life conditions lead to late-life health outcomes is not fully understood. However, it is clear that populations at higher risk of experiencing poverty, low educational attainment, and other childhood disadvantages disproportionately experience negative health outcomes in older adulthood as a result.

Access to appropriate medical services. Gender, race, and ethnicity shape access to health care in later life and throughout the life course. In part, this relates to the affordability of medical care. Many women are poorly equipped to seek adequate health care in later life, as a result of poor economic security levels and greater reliance on public forms of health insurance, including Medicare and Medicaid (see Table 5.1). Socioeconomic barriers to obtaining needed care disproportionately impact populations that have lower average levels of education and income, including racial and ethnic minorities. Health-care access may be lower among Asians and Hispanics, both of whom are more likely to lack health insurance coverage. Non-Hispanic whites are more likely to have supplemental coverage through private insurance, which adds a layer of protection and access not shared by other ethnic groups.

The Affordable Care Act (ACA) appears to be having a positive impact on medical care coverage rates, especially among low-income and ethnic minorities (Collins, Rasmussen, & Doty, 2014), but many working-age Americans (and some older adults) still are uninsured. Moreover, many seniors lacked health insurance for substantial periods of time during youth and adulthood, resulting in inadequate preventive care and poor management of chronic disease. These health consequences of early-life disparities in health insurance coverage are carried into later life.

The lack of linguistically or culturally appropriate medical services may also contribute to health disparities, especially for ethnic groups with sizable numbers of immigrants. Many older adults, especially Hispanics and Asians, speak a language other than English at home. Many of them speak English poorly or not at all and more than one-quarter live in linguistically isolated households—that is, households in which no adult member speaks English well (see Table 5.1). For these individuals, limited English proficiency (LEP) may serve as a barrier to obtaining medical services. Medical facilities and practitioners have responded by devising ways to access and use medical interpreters in clinical settings (Chen, Youdelman, & Brooks, 2007). Indeed, using professional medical interpreters improves the quality of care for patients with LEP (Ngo-Metzger et al., 2007), but the use of interpreters across medical settings is uneven (Karliner et al., 2011; Schenker et al., 2011). In practice, family members and other acquaintances are often used as interpreters, despite federal rulings that require providers to ensure language access to all patients (Ginde et al., 2010).

Racism and discrimination in health care also negatively shape health outcomes (Williams, 2012). Institutional racism may contribute to poorer health outcomes among racial minorities; for example, evidence suggests that hospitals that disproportionately serve African Americans yield significantly higher rates of mortality following acute myocardial infarction among Medicare patients (Skinner et al., 2005). Empirically, differences in treatment patterns, and in the process of decision making related to treatment, are well documented across ethnic groups (see, e.g., Freedman et al., 2009; Prehn et al., 2002), although the extent to which these differences are related to bias, to cultural (in)competence in the provision of care, or to communication barriers is not fully understood.

Looking ahead: health disparities resolved? A considerable amount of past research indicates that disability levels in later life have declined in recent decades (Crimmins, 2004; Manton, Gu, & Lamb, 2006). These declines have been traced to changes in health-related behaviors and to cohort succession, whereby younger, healthier cohorts are moving into later life and replacing less healthy and less affluent persons from earlier cohorts. With the implementation of the ACA, we might expect that access to health-promoting medical care will be more widely and evenly available across racial, ethnic, and socioeconomic groups. Yet looking ahead, we suspect that some disparities in health outcomes are likely to persist, despite improvements across cohorts as a whole. Many chronic conditions, including hypertension, arthritis, and diabetes, continue to be more prevalent among African Americans on the brink of later life (Mutchler & Burr, 2007). Unhealthy behaviors, including excess alcohol consumption, smoking, and physical inactivity, are unevenly distributed across gender, race, and ethnic groups as well (Adams & Schoenborn, 2006; Hummer & Hayward, 2015). Group differences in health behaviors and resources, including appropriate medical care, are likely to persist to some degree in coming years and disparities in health outcomes are expected to result.

Family caregiving and formal long-term care. Long-term services and supports (LTSS), including both formal and informal long-term care, demand growing attention as the population becomes older. Among those who survive to age 85, it is estimated that half need some form of long-term care (Rogers & Komisar, 2003). The majority of care for older adults is provided on an unpaid basis by family members and friends (Scan Foundation, 2012), many of whom are themselves older. The extent to which care needs are met informally, versus formally in a nursing home or other type of facility, depends partly on an older adult's level of frailty; some care demands are so great that they cannot be effectively managed at home. Yet the availability of potential informal caregivers, and the predisposition of those individuals to engage in care activities, can be a deciding factor in determining the extent to which care will be provided formally or informally.

Features of the life course shape the likelihood of an older adult needing long-term care, as well as the type of care accessed. As described earlier in this chapter, assaults to health and well-being early in the life course accumulate throughout a lifetime, and may result in a high risk of needing long-term care. In comparing group-risk profiles, both those who live the longest on average and those who become frail at the youngest ages, women and African Americans, respectively, will experience the highest risk of needing these supports. Receiving supports informally at home or formally in a facility will be shaped in part by characteristics of one's social network. Recalling the principle of linked lives, care can only be provided informally when one's network includes people who have the capacity to provide care and are willing to do so. Differences by gender, race, and ethnicity in use of formal and informal long-term care result from life-course processes shaping the need for care, as well as the networks available to provide care. As shown in Table 5.1, gender, race, and ethnic groups differ in their relative propensities to live in nursing homes as well as in multigenerational households, which are common platforms for exchange of support, including caregiving. These living arrangement differences may be a result of divergent familistic values regarding coresidence, but also reflect resource differences that make living alone unaffordable for an older adult as well as for others in his or her social network. These differences are significant in shaping the extent to which informal caregivers are relied upon in later life, as well as the degree to which older adults provide care and support to others in their close networks.

Women make up a large majority of both caregivers and care recipients. The most typical informal care provider is either a spouse—most commonly a wife—or an adult child—most commonly a daughter. As well, a large majority of paid care providers—such as homecare workers and CNAs in nursing homes—are female. The most typical care *recipient* is also a woman, both among older adults receiving care at home and those in a long-term care setting. Women are at higher risk than men of frailty, and they are more likely to need support with activities of daily living. As well, because they are more likely to outlive their spouses, women are at increased risk of needing care from another family member or through formal services. Indeed, as shown in Table 5.1, a larger share of women than men live in an intergenerational household or in an institution.

Formal long-term supports and services have long been underutilized by minority families, in part due to strong familial norms associated with caregiving, as well as distrust of large institutions. African Americans tend to focus on the family as a unit rather than the individual, yielding a sense of obligation to care for senior members at home (Bradley et al., 2002). Moreover, some African Americans express mistrust in nursing facility staff (Bradley et al., 2002); when they do choose a nursing facility they prioritize characteristics such as neighborhood location and the race and ethnic background of staff members and other residents (Howard et al., 2002). African Americans who enter a nursing facility may experience a different quality of care compared to non-Hispanic whites, because many live in highly segregated, lower-tier facilities, characterized by a greater number of Medicaid residents, poorer structural characteristics—such as lighting and cleanliness—and a smaller number of nurses and certified nursing assistants compared to the number of residents (Mor et al., 2004). Since the nursing home is a last resort care option for African American elders, many in nursing facilities have much higher needs for help managing activities of daily living, instrumental activities of daily living, diabetes, and stroke, compared to non-Hispanic whites (Borrayo et al., 2002).

Older Hispanics face similar issues in nursing home utilization as those faced by older African Americans in terms of access and quality of care, but may experience additional obstacles to securing informal care due to acculturation of younger generations. Traditionally, caregiving responsibilities have fallen to the young women in a Hispanic family (Herrera et al., 2008). Young Latinas, however, have begun to seek higher levels of education and enter the workforce rather than remain in the household, thus leaving a gap in care for older members of the family who may then be required to seek formal long-term care services.

Although the proportion of older minorities in nursing homes is growing (Feng et al., 2011), white older adults are at higher risk of entering a nursing home, all else equal. Thomeer, Mudrazija, and Angel (2014) report that African Americans and Hispanics experience a risk of entering a nursing home that is lower than what would be expected based on need for support, relative to non-Hispanic whites, which could be evidence of either cultural preference or health-care inequity. Obstacles to obtaining nursing home care may include the availability of geographically proximate facilities, the availability of linguistically concordant services, or other barriers. These authors also find that the availability of future help—family or friends who would be willing to provide support if needed—does not impact the probability of entering a nursing home for whites or blacks, although it does reduce the risk of nursing home admission for Hispanics, once again highlighting the principle of linked lives.

Challenges and Solutions

Gender, race, and ethnicity exert powerful and enduring influences on virtually every element of the life course, resulting in late-life experiences and opportunities that are highly differentiated across these groups. As discussed in this chapter, many factors condition these differences, including cultural beliefs and practices, socialization, and social norms, as well as discriminatory features of organizations and social institutions. Because circumstances of later life result from experiences, investments, and accumulations throughout the life course, it is unlikely that late-life disparities will be remedied by focusing exclusively on late-life interventions.

Disadvantageous experiences in childhood and young adulthood may set young people on course to uncertain futures in midlife and older adulthood. Despite the potential of choice and human agency for redirecting individual pathways, there is little question but that the accumulation of advantages and disadvantages over time result in later-life experiences and profiles that are distinctively shaped by gender, race, and ethnicity.

How might we remedy this unequal progression? Certainly disrupting patterns of childhood inequality would be beneficial. Programs and policies directed toward leveling the playing field in education, healthcare access and quality, and career entry for youth and young adults will impact late-life inequality. Yet policies and interventions directed toward older adults have potential to remediate inequalities as well. Policy modifications could make a difference in reducing gender disparities in old-age economic security. For example, Social Security policy linking benefits strongly to marital history could be modified, reshaping the implications of marriage for income security in later life and taking important steps toward reducing the gender gap in pension benefits (Harrington Meyer & Herd, 2006). Yet initiatives focusing exclusively on older adults will not reshape the likelihood that older women will bring with them into later life substantially fewer financial resources in the form of private pensions, savings, and investment wealth. For those disparities to be minimized, more fundamental changes to the organization of work, availability and affordability of childcare, and societal support for caregiving will be required.

Policy modifications can also impact disparities in health and healthcare access by broadening access to health insurance and promoting more stable access to health care. The ACA appears to be making progress in securing improved health trajectories for low-income people (Collins et al., 2014), a disproportionate share of whom are ethnic and racial minorities. With time, this improved access should translate to better health, avoidance of disease, and improved management of chronic conditions—all of which should result in reduced disparities in later-life health profiles. Yet additional broad-based policies will be needed. Strategies for increasing the number of medical clinicians who speak a second language in addition to English may reduce current barriers to obtaining high-quality medical care among patients with limited English proficiency, including many elders. Targeting health promotion messages more effectively to racial and ethnic minorities is an important means of remedying gaps in healthy behaviors that account for some health disparities in later life. To the extent that low socioeconomic status is indeed a fundamental cause of poor health (Link & Phelan, 1995), breaking the association between ethnic status and low-SES is a challenging and necessary step.

Securing access to appropriate LTSS will become increasingly important as the older population becomes larger, older, and more diverse. In past decades, formal services (e.g., nursing homes) were primarily used by white elders, with African American, Hispanic, and other ethnic minority older adults relying largely on informal care from family members or close others. In recent years, this has been shifting, in part, through new policies relating to financing long-term care. Feng et al. (2011) suggest that recent efforts to rebalance LTSS (institutional vs. home and community-based services) have not closed the majority/minority gap in nursing home use, but instead have shifted it such that institutions have seen an increase in Medicaid expenditures and reimbursements far greater than has occurred for home-based care (Woodcock et al., 2011). This shift has made institutional care more accessible to lower-income seniors. At the same time, other more costly LTSS options have developed, such as continuing-care retirement communities, assisted living options, and additional home-based care options. White seniors are far more likely to be able to afford these services compared to nonwhites. So as minority seniors are moving into nursing homes, white seniors are staying at home or moving to other LTSS options. Indeed, as shown in Table 5.1 and reported elsewhere (Feng et al., 2011), African Americans are now more represented in nursing homes, a departure from patterns observed in the recent past.

Most elders and their families would prefer informal and community-based options for LTSS over institutional settings. Moreover, noninstitutional supports save payers—including families, insurers, as well as the Medicaid system and taxpayers—billions of dollars annually (Feinberg et al., 2011). Yet these cost savings are secured at the expense of millions of informal, unpaid, family caregivers who quit their jobs, reduce their hours, and in turn, jeopardize their own economic security in order to provide support for loved ones, challenging their ability to prepare for their own old age. Women and members of some ethnic groups are far more likely to participate in unpaid caregiving, incurring the long-term financial implications of those experiences. Strategies and policies are sorely needed to help caregivers reconcile the competing demands of caregiving and paid work, potentially reducing the financial costs of caring (Lee et al., 2014).

A majority of the older population will continue to be female for the foreseeable future. Moreover, demographic trends ensure that the older population will become increasingly diverse in terms of race and ethnic composition. Through cohort succession, we can be sure that the *significance* of being male or female, white or nonwhite, a member of one ethnic minority group or another will be different for older adults in the future than they are today. These differences are ensured in large part because each cohort entering later life has encountered a unique set of experiences that are relevant to late-life outcomes. Reducing gender-, race-, and ethnic-based risks for poor outcomes in later life requires attention to the ways in which membership in these social groupings shapes life trajectories from the moment of birth, as well as the ways in which social institutions and policies value some pathways over others. Recalibrating old-age policy in anticipation of these new, more diverse cohorts is needed.

References

Adams, P., & Shoenborn, C. (2006). *Health behaviors of adults: United States, 2002–04. Vital Health Statistics, 10* (230). Hyattsville, MD: National Center for Health Statistics.

Arias, E. (2014). *United States life tables, 2009. National vital statistics reports, 62* (7). Hyattsville, MD: National Center for Health Statistics.

Borrayo, E., Salmon, J., Polivka, L., & Dunlop, B. (2002). Utilization across the continuum of long-term care services. *The Gerontologist, 42*, 603–612.

Bradley, E., McGraw, S., Curry, L., Buckser, A., King, K., Kasl, S., & Andersen, R. (2002). Expanding the Andersen model: The role of psychosocial factors in long-term care use. *Health Services Research, 37*, 1221–1242.

Brown, T., O'Rand, A., & Adkins, D. (2012). Race–ethnicity and health trajectories: Tests of three hypotheses across multiple groups and health outcomes. *Journal of Health and Social Behavior, 53*, 359–377.

Calasanti, T. (2010). Gender relations and applied research on aging. *The Gerontologist, 50*, 720–734.

Carr, S., & Tienda, M. (2013). Family sponsorship and late-age immigration in aging America: Revised and expanded estimates of chained migration. *Population Research and Policy Review, 32*, 825–849.

Cha, Y. (2010). Reinforcing separate spheres: The effect of spousal overwork on men's and women's employment in dual-earner households. *American Sociological Review, 75*, 303–329.

Chen, A., Youdelman, M., & Brooks, J. (2007). The legal framework for language access in healthcare settings: Title VI and beyond. *Journal of General Internal Medicine, 22* (Suppl. 2), 362–367.

Collins, S., Rasmussen, P., & Doty, M. (2014). Gaining ground: Americans' health insurance coverage and access to care after the Affordable Care Act's first open enrollment period. *The Commonwealth Fund*. Retrieved from http://www.commonwealthfund.org/~/media/files/publications/issue-brief/2014/jul/1760_collins_gaining_ground_tracking_survey.pdf

Crimmins, E. (2004). Trends in the health of the elderly. *Annual Review of Public Health, 25*, 79–98.

Dannefer, D. (2003). Cumulative advantage/disadvantage and the life course: Cross-fertilizing age and social science theory. *Journal of Gerontology: Social Sciences, 58*, S327–S338.

Diez Roux, A., Ranjit, N., Jenny, N., Shea, S., Cushman, M., Fitzpatrick, A., & Seeman, T. (2009). Race/ethnicity and telomere length in the multi-ethnic study of atherosclerosis. *Aging Cell, 8*, 251–257.

Elder, G., Jr. (1985). Perspectives on the life course. In G. Elder (Ed.), *Life course dynamics: Trajectories and transitions, 1968–1980* (pp. 23–49). Ithaca, NY: Cornell University Press.

England, P. (2010). The gender revolution: Uneven and stalled. *Gender & Society, 24*, 149–166.

Federal Interagency Forum on Aging-Related Statistics. (2012). *Older Americans 2012: Key indicators of well-being.* Washington, DC: U.S. Government Printing Office. Retrieved from http://www.agingstats.gov/agingstatsdotnet/Main_Site/Data/2012_Documents/docs/EntireChartbook.pdf

Feinberg, L., Reinhard, S., Houser, A., & Choula, R. (2011). *Valuing the invaluable: 2011 update. The growing contributions and costs of family caregiving.* AARP Public Policy Institute. Retrieved from http://assets.aarp.org/rgcenter/ppi/ltc/i51-caregiving.pdf

Feng, Z., Fennell, M., Tyler, D., Clark, M., & Mor, V. (2011). Growth of racial and ethnic minorities in US nursing homes driven by demographics and possible disparities in options. *Health Affairs, 30*, 1358–1365.

Ferraro, K., & Shippee, T. (2009). Aging and cumulative inequality: How does inequality get under the skin? *The Gerontologist, 49*, 333–343.

Ferraro, K., Shippee, T., & Schafer, M. (2009). Cumulative inequality theory for research on aging and the life course. In V. Bengtson, D. Gans, N. Putney, & M. Silverstein (Eds.), *Handbook of theories of aging* (pp. 413–434). New York: Springer.

Freedman, R., He, Y., Winer, E., & Keating, N. (2009). Trends in racial and age disparities in definitive local therapy of early-stage breast cancer. *Journal of Clinical Oncology, 27*, 713–719.

Fry, R. (2006). *Gender and migration.* Washington, DC: Pew Hispanic Center.

Fry, R., & Taylor, P. (2013). *Hispanic high school graduates pass Whites in rate of college enrollment.* Washington, DC: Pew Research Hispanic Center. Retrieved from http://www.pewhispanic.org/files/2013/05/PHC_college_enrollment_2013-05.pdf

Geronimus, A., Hicken, M., Pearson, J., Seashols, S., Brown, K., & Cruz, T. (2010). Do US Black women experience stress-related accelerated biological aging? A novel theory and first population-based test of Black–White differences in telomere length. *Human Nature: An Interdisciplinary Biosocial Perspective, 21*, 19–38.

Ginde, A., Sullivan, A., Corel, B., Caceres, J., & Camargo, C. Jr. (2010). Reevaluation of the effect of mandatory interpreter legislation on use of professional interpreters for ED patients with language barriers. *Patient Education Counseling, 81*, 204–206.

Goins, R., Moss, M., Buchwald, D., & Guralnik, J. (2007). Disability among older American Indians and Alaska Natives: An analysis of the 2000 Census Public Use Microdata Sample. *The Gerontologist, 47*, 690–696.

Gruenewald, T., Karlamangla, A., Hu, P., Stein-Merkin, S., Crandall, C., Koretz, B., & Seeman, T. (2012). History of socioeconomic disadvantage and allostatic load in later life. *Social Science and Medicine, 74*, 75–83.

Haas, S., Krueger, P., & Rohlfsen, L. (2012). Race/ethnic and nativity disparities in later life physical performance: The role of health and socioeconomic status over the life course. *The Journals of Gerontology, Series B: Psychological Sciences and Social Sciences, 67*, 238–248.

Hagestad, G. (1990). Social perspectives on the life course. In R. Binstock, & L. George (Eds.), *Handbook of aging and the social sciences* (3rd ed., pp. 151–168). San Diego, CA: Academic Press.

Harrington Meyer, M. (2014). *Grandmothers at work: Juggling families and jobs*. New York: New York University Press.

Harrington Meyer, M., & Herd, P. (2007). *Market friendly or family friendly? The state and gender inequality in old age*. New York: Russell Sage Foundation.

Hayward, M., & Heron, M. (1999). Racial inequality in active life among adult Americans. *Demography, 36*, 77–91.

Herrera, A., Lee, J., Palos, G., & Torres-Vigil, I. (2008). Cultural influences in the patterns of long-term care use among Mexican American family caregivers. *Journal of Applied Gerontology, 27*, 141–165.

Hirsch, C., Anderson, M., Newman, A., Kop, W., Jackson, S., Gottdiener, J., . . . Cardiovascular Health Study Research Group. (2006). The association of race with frailty: The cardiovascular health study. *Annals of Epidemiology, 16*, 545–553.

Howard, D., Sloane, P., Zimmerman, S., Eckert, K., Walsh, J., Burle, V., . . . Koch, G. (2002). Distribution of African Americans in residential care/assisted living and nursing homes: More evidence of racial disparity? *American Journal of Public Health, 92*, 1272–1277.

Humes, K. R., Jones, N. A., & Ramirez, R. R. (2011). Overview of race and Hispanic origin: 2011. *2011 census briefs, C2010BR-02*. Available online at: http://www.census.gov/prod/cen2010/briefs/c2010br-02.pdf

Hummer, R. A., & Hayward, M. D. (2015). Hispanic older adult health and longevity in the United States: Current patterns and concerns for the future. *Daedalus, 144*(2), 20–30.

Kaiser Family Foundation. (2015). *Life expectancy at birth by race/ethnicity*. Retrieved from http://kff.org/other/state-indicator/life-expectancy-by-re/#notes

Karliner, L., Hwang, E., Nickleach, D., & Kaplan, C. (2011). Language barriers and patient-centered breast cancer care. *Patient Education Counseling, 84*, 223–228.

Kena, G., Musu-Gillette, L., Robinson, J., Wang, X., Rathbun, A., Zhang, J., Wilkinson-Flicker, S., Barmer, A., & Dunlop Velez, E. (2015). *The condition of education 2015 (NCES 2015–144)*. Washington, DC: U.S. Department of Education, National Center for Education Statistics. Retrieved from http://nces.ed.gov/pubsearch

Kochanek, K., Murphy, S., Xu, J., & Arias, E. (2014). *Mortality in the United States, 2013. NCHS Data Brief (No. 178)*. Hyattsville, MD: National Center for Health Statistics.

Kuh, D., & Ben-Shlomo, Y. (2004). *A life course approach to chronic diseases epidemiology*. New York: Oxford University Press.

Lariscy, J., Hummer, R., & Hayward, M. (2015). Hispanic older adult mortality in the United States: New estimates and an assessment of factors shaping the Hispanic paradox. *Demography, 52*, 1–14.

Lee, Y., Tang, F., Kim, K., & Albert, S. (2014). The vicious cycle of parental caregiving and financial well-being: A longitudinal study of women. *The Journals of Gerontology, Series B: Psychological Sciences and Social Sciences*. Advance online publication. doi:10.1093/geronb/gbu001

Link, B., & Phelan, J. (1995). Social conditions as fundamental causes of disease. *Journal of Health and Social Behavior, 35* (Extra Issue), 80–94.

Lopez, M., & Gonzalez-Barrera, A. (2014). Women's college enrollment gains leave men behind. *Pew research center fact tank*. Retrieved from http://www.pewresearch.org/fact-tank/2014/03/06/womens-college-enrollment-gains-leave-men-behind/

Manton, K., Gu, X., & Lamb, V. (2006). Change in chronic disability from 1982 to 2004/2005 as measured by long-term changes in function and health in the U.S. elderly population. *Proceedings of the National Academy of Sciences of the United States of America, 103*, 18374–18379.

Martin, J., Hamilton, B., Sutton, P., Ventura, S., Mathews, T., Kirmeyer, S., & Osterman, J. (2010). *Births: Final data for 2007. National Vital Statistics Reports, 58* (24). Hyattsville, MD: National Center for Health Statistics.

Matthews, T., & Hamilton, B. (2005). *Trend analysis of the sex ratio at birth in the United States. National Vital Statistics Reports, 53* (20). Hyattsville, MD: National Center for Health Statistics.

Mayer, K. (2009). New directions in life course research. *Annual Review of Sociology, 35*, 413–433.

Montez, J., & Hayward, M. (2014). Cumulative childhood adversity, education, and active life expectancy among U.S. adults. *Demography, 51*, 413–435.

Mor, V., Zinn, J., Angelelli, J., Teno, J., & Miller, S. (2004). Driven to tiers: Socioeconomic and racial disparities in the quality of nursing home care. *The Milbank Quarterly, 82*, 227–256.

Mutchler, J., & Burr, J. (2007). Varieties of wellbeing: Race, class, gender, and age. In B. Hudson (Ed.), *Boomer bust? Economic and political dynamics of the graying society* (pp. 23–46). New York: Praeger.

Ngo-Metzger, Q., Sorkin, D., Phillips, R., Greenfield, S., Massagli, M., Clarridge, B., & Kaplan, S. (2007). Providing high-quality care for limited English proficient patients: The importance of language concordance and interpreter use. *Journal of General Internal Medicine, 22*(Suppl. 2), 324–330.

Nwankwo, T., Yoon, S., Burt, V., & Gu, Q. (2013). Hypertension among adults in the United States: National health and nutrition examination survey, 2011–2012. *NCHS Data Brief* (133). Hyattsville, MD: National Center for Health Statistics.

O'Neil, K., & Tienda, M. (2015). Age at immigration and the incomes of older immigrants, 1994–2010. *Journals of Gerontology, Series B: Psychological Sciences and Social Sciences, 70*, 291–302.

O'Rand, A. (2006). Stratification and the life course: Life course capital, life course risks, and social inequality. In R. Binstock & L. George (Eds.), *Handbook of aging and the social sciences* (pp. 145–162). San Diego, CA: Elsevier.

Pearlin, L., Schieman, S., Fazio, E., & Meersman, S. (2005). Stress, health, and the life course: Some conceptual perspectives. *Journal of Health and Social Behavior, 46*, 205–219.

Pleau, R. (2010). Gender differences in postretirement employment. *Research on Aging, 32*, 267–303.

Pollard, K., & Scommegna, P. (2013). The health and life expectancy of older blacks and Hispanics in the United States. *Today's Research on Aging* (Issue 28, June). Retrieved from http://www.prb.org/pdf13/TodaysResearchAging28.pdf

Prehn, A., Topol, B., Stewart, S., Glaser, S., O'Connor, L., & West, D. (2002). Differences in treatment patterns for localized breast carcinoma among Asian/Pacific Islander women. *Cancer, 95*, 2268–2275.

Quinones, A., Liang, J., & Ye, W. (2012). Racial and ethnic differences in hypertension risk: New diagnoses after age 50. *Ethnicity and Disease, 22*, 175–180.

Rogers, S., & Komisar, H. (2003). Who needs long-term care? *Long-term care financing project fact sheet*. Retrieved from http://hpi.georgetown.edu/ltc/papers.html#Briefs

Rooks, R., & Thorpe, R. (2014) Understanding age at onset and self-care management to explain racial and ethnic cardiovascular disease disparities in middle- and older-age adults. In K. Whitfield & T. Baker (Eds.), *Handbook of minority aging* (pp. 471–486). New York: Springer.

Ruggles, S., Sobek, M., Alexander, M., Fitch, C., Goeken, R., Hall, P., . . . Ronnander, C. (2010). *Integrated public use microdata series: [Machine-readable database]*. Minneapolis: Minnesota Population Center [producer and distributor].

Scan Foundation. (2012). Who provides long-term care in the U.S.? (Updated). *Fact sheet* (October). Retrieved from http://www.thescanfoundation.org/sites/thescanfoundation.org/files/us_who_provides_ltc_us_oct_2012_fs.pdf

Schenker, Y., Perez-Stable, E., Nickleach, D., & Karliner, L. (2011). Patterns of interpreter use for hospitalized patients with limited English proficiency. *Journal of General Internal Medicine, 26*, 712–717.

Settersten, R., Jr. (2006). Aging and the life course. In R. Binstock & L. George (Eds.), *Handbook of aging and the social sciences* (6th ed., pp. 3–19). New York: Academic Press.

Skinner, J., Chandra, A., Staiger, D., Lee, J., & McClellan, J. (2005). Mortality after acute myocardial infarction in hospitals that disproportionately treat black patients. *Circulation, 112*, 2634–2641.

Social Security Administration. (2014). *Income of the aged chartbook, 2012*. Washington, DC: Social Security Administration. Retrieved from http://www.ssa.gov/policy/docs/chartbooks/income_aged/2012/

Thomeer, M., Mudrazija, S., & Angel, J. (2014). How do race and Hispanic ethnicity affect nursing home admission? Evidence from the Health and Retirement Study. *Journals of Gerontology, Series B: Psychological Sciences and Social Sciences*. Advance online publication. doi:10.1093/geronb/gbu114

Treas, J., & Marcum, C. (2011). Diversity and family relations in an aging society. In R. Settersten & J. Angel (Eds.), *Handbook of sociology of aging* (pp. 131–141). New York: Springer.

U.S. Department of Homeland Security. (2013). *Yearbook of immigration statistics: 2012*. Washington, DC: U.S. Department of Homeland Security. Retrieved from http://www.dhs.gov/immigration-statistics

Walsemann, K., Geronimus, A., & Gee, G. (2008). Accumulating disadvantage over the life course: Evidence from a longitudinal study investigating the relationship between educational advantage in youth and health in middle age. *Research on Aging, 30*, 169–199.

Williams, D. (2012). Miles to go before we sleep: Racial inequities in health. *Journal of Health and Social Behavior, 53*, 279–295.

Woodcock, C., Stockwell, I., Tripp, A., & Milligan, C. (2011). *Rebalancing long-term services and supports: Progress to date and a research agenda for the future*. Baltimore, MD: The Hilltop Institute, UMBC. Retrieved from http://www.hilltopinstitute.org/publications/RebalancingLTSS-ProgressToDateAndResearchAgendaForFuture-June2011.pdf

Xue, Q. (2011). The frailty syndrome: Definition and natural history. *Clinical Geriatric Medicine, 27*, 1–15.

CHAPTER SIX

Poverty, Income, and Wealth across the Life Course

Andrea E. Willson and Nicole Etherington

The economic status of the older population in the United States has improved over recent decades; however, levels of economic inequality remain highest in later life (Crystal & Shea, 1990; O'Rand & Henretta, 1999; Reno & Veghte, 2011). Some groups, including women and racial-ethnic minorities, are much more likely to experience poverty (Bastos et al., 2009; Hogan & Perrucci, 2007). Economic well-being, measured by income, wealth, and experiences of poverty over the life course, is shaped by complex and diverse life events as well as interactions with social institutions. Therefore, inequality in economic status among older Americans is the result of long-term processes that unfold over the life course that have both systematic and random aspects (Crystal & Shea, 2002). When faced with the task of explaining heterogeneity among older persons, gerontologists came to recognize the value in studying unequal access to resources that resulted in inequalities that persisted and accumulated over time (O'Rand, 1996). Social relations that produce inequality are reinforced by institutions and social policy and change with age, leading to varying levels of economic inequality over the life course (e.g., McDonough & Berglund, 2003). At the aggregate level, inequality within a population can be viewed as the end product of an accumulative process of exposure to risks and opportunities that unfold across the life course.

In this chapter, we focus on the connection of later-life economic outcomes to earlier stages in the life course. We first review key elements of the life-course perspective (Elder & Johnson, 2003), which has proven useful for understanding economic outcomes and the inequality that is evident in the aging process. Next, we discuss poverty, income, and wealth dynamics across the life course in the United States and how inequality in each is shaped by age, gender, and race-ethnicity. Economic outcomes influence many aspects of well-being over one's life course, but in the last decade, perhaps none has received as much attention from the social sciences as health. We, therefore, briefly introduce research on the relationship between socioeconomic status and health across the life course. We conclude with a discussion of the changing dynamics of poverty, income, wealth, and inequality in later life and challenges to its study. Our intent is not to provide an exhaustive review of the literature on the poverty status, income, and wealth of older Americans, but instead to provide a framework for understanding economic outcomes over the life course and to highlight examples that demonstrate the potential of life-course approaches to the study of inequality in later life.

The Life-Course Perspective, Economic Outcomes, and Inequality in Later Life

The life-course perspective provides an analytical framework for studies of the processes that shape inequality in economic outcomes in old age, as well as the effects of pathways of economic advantage and disadvantage on a variety of other outcomes, such as health. The life-course perspective generally refers to "the age-graded sequence of roles, opportunities, constraints, and events that shape biography from birth to death" (Shanahan & Macmillan, 2008:40). Foremost, the life-course perspective is grounded in the recognition that individual lives are embedded in both historical and biographical context. There are five key principles of the life course that are useful for our understanding of economic outcomes and inequality in later life (Elder & Johnson, 2003).

First, the life-course perspective offers a longitudinal view of economic security, not only based on income or wealth at a particular life stage, such as old age, but rather as a process that begins in childhood through to old age. Human development and aging are lifelong processes; thus, no single stage of an individual's life can be understood without its antecedents and consequences (Dannefer et al., 2005). The magnitude of intracohort economic inequality by statuses such as gender and race-ethnicity varies over the life course, and studies in the social sciences have focused on the individual and social patterning of trajectories of income and wealth over time (e.g., Crystal & Shea, 1990; Pampel, 1994; Willson, 2003) as well as movement in and out of poverty over the life course (see Western et al., 2012 for a review).

Second, to understand economic outcomes, individual agency within the constraints of structure/history must be considered, as pathways of economic hardship or advantage are not fixed. While considerable research demonstrates the impact of structural variables on economic outcomes, there still exists the possibility of individual resilience or agency in changing life-course trajectories. At the individual level, agency can be understood as willful action or choices undertaken on the actor's own behalf to shape his or her life trajectory, in response to macro-, meso-, or micro-level constraints (Hitlin & Elder, 2007). The interaction between the state, the market, and the family as systems of resource distribution determine opportunities and constraints across the individual life course and create social inequality between groups and individuals (O'Rand, 1996).

Turning points may also change pathways and may occur as the result of individual action (Sampson & Laub, 1996). Life events, such as divorce or widowhood, or changing economic environments, such as the Great Recession, may moderate life-course pathways of advantage, while positive events such as mentoring in adolescence may offer compensatory resources for disadvantaged youth (Erickson, McDonald, & Elder, 2009).

Third, the idea that human lives are linked to others recognizes the importance of taking into consideration the interdependence of lives and the intergenerational context of life-course processes (Elder & Johnson, 2003). These tenets are rooted in the classical social stratification literature, for which a central problematic is the intergenerational transmission of social inequality. Research in sociology on the transmission of inequality across generations has historically focused on class mobility, often by examining educational attainment and occupational location (for a review see Erikson & Goldthorpe, 2002). Most sociological studies have focused on the linkages between childhood socioeconomic status and educational attainment (e.g., Duncan et al., 1998; Wagmiller et al., 2006).

Fourth, the life course is embedded in historical time and place, which shapes unique experiences for each cohort. The experience and effects of historical events differ across birth cohorts based on the distinct point in the life course at which they occur. For example, as a result of the Great Recession and plummeting home values, the wealth of younger households was hit harder than that of older households because their homes constituted a larger share of their wealth portfolio (Wolff, 2014). On the other hand, many older workers were forced to delay retirement due to enormous losses to retirement plans that were market-based (McFall, 2011). Thus, the effects of the Great Recession varied by birth cohort.

Fifth, the timing of particular transitions in the life course affects both their meaning and their consequences. For example, early educational achievements allow for higher occupational status at entry into the labor force, the subsequent compounding effects of wages and asset accumulation, and other resources such as occupational benefits and social capital (Elman & O'Rand, 2004). Elder's (1987) study on the impact of war mobilization on the lives of men which revealed that men recruited in World War II at later ages were more negatively affected than younger men, as their lives were more likely to be disrupted in terms of both family and career. And findings that adolescent childbirth increases a mother's risk of dropping out of school and working in low-paying jobs with less job security, which has long-term implications for income security, also highlight the importance of timing (Teti & Lamb, 1989).

Overall, these principles call attention to the flexible and continuous nature of human lives and serve as a guide to life-course research. Accordingly, life-course research on stratification and inequality strives to take into account time, context, and process (Shuey & Willson, 2014). Cumulative advantage/disadvantage theory (CAD) is a key framework that emerged from the life-course perspective and is used to inform studies that examine social mobility at the individual level and changing dynamics of inequality as cohorts age (Dannefer, 2003; O'Rand, 1996). The CAD framework, rooted in the theoretical literature on stratification and status attainment, suggests an intraindividual accumulative process through which initial relative advantage associated with structural location and resources generates further gains across the life course. This, in turn, results in systematic divergence in life-course outcomes across individuals or groups over time and increases interindividual inequality, particularly within cohorts. Time is the complex organizing principal of CAD, as it emphasizes the process of change over the life course, both in terms of human development and in levels of resources, such as income, and the cumulative consequences of the timing of life transitions (O'Rand, 2002).

Various forms of life-course capital, or resources that can be used to "meet human needs and wants" (O'Rand, 2006:146), interact over the life course to shape divergent pathways of poverty, income, and wealth. Life-course capital can take various forms and includes one's accumulating stock of human capital, or skills and productive knowledge; social capital, which includes direct and indirect social ties; psychophysical capital, one's health and well-being; and personal capital, including efficacy and confidence (O'Rand, 2001:200). Further, the accumulation and depletion of life-course capital occurs at variable rates across social groups based on statuses such as social class and race-ethnicity with early and high attainments in education and the labor market supporting the accumulation of life-course capital and the compounding of economic advantage with age (O'Rand, 1996).

Life-course risks are associated with the unequal exposure to adverse conditions or structural opportunities (DiPrete, 2002; O'Rand, 2006). Emanating from structural sources, these risks shape exposure to opportunities and risks that begin in childhood and accumulate across the life course. Among them, the first of life-course risks experienced stems from an individual's social origins (Currie, 2011). Early-life advantage provides opportunities to obtain access to additional resources as well as to avoid many sources of adversity, while disadvantage increases exposure to risk (O'Rand, 2006). Early dis/advantage does not, however, predetermine one's life experiences as trajectories can change or reverse course. Educational attainment can mediate the impact of childhood disadvantage (Hayward & Gorman, 2004), and psychosocial resources can enhance one's ability to cope with adversity (Ferraro & Shippee, 2009). Conversely, although advantage may send an individual on an upward trajectory of increased advantage, transitions related to family structure and employment, such as divorce or job loss, increase the risk of downward mobility and poverty (Western et al., 2012). Moreover, turning points resulting from human agency, random structural opportunities, or some other cause can trigger a reverse in the direction of a trajectory (Sampson & Laub, 1996).

Economic well-being and mobility is determined by the interrelation of various dynamic forms of life-course capital and life-course risks which are shaped by opportunity structures that are stratified by race and gender (DiPrete, 2002; Vandecasteele, 2011; Western et al., 2012). Life events and transitions across the life course can have different implications for later-life outcomes depending on dimensions of social location, including social class, race/ethnicity, and gender, and these dimensions intersect to shape economic vulnerability over the life course (Vartanian & McNamara, 2002). Negative life-course risks, such as job loss, have differential effects on subgroups of the population, and vulnerable and disadvantaged populations endure the highest relative costs of these events (e.g., Vandecasteele, 2011). The lifelong poverty, income, and wealth disadvantage experienced by women and racial-ethnic minorities in the United States reflect processes of CAD and result in women and racial minorities facing increasing disadvantage with age (Angel, Prickett, & Angel, 2014).

Life-Course Influences on Gender and Racial-Ethnic Disparities in Income, Poverty, and Wealth in Later Life

Poverty, income, and wealth are highly stratified by gender and race-ethnicity. Discrimination in employment as well as in housing and mortgage markets, coupled with the fact that racial-ethnic minorities are less likely than whites to obtain inheritances (Shapiro, 2004), results in racial-ethnic inequality in income and wealth accumulation and composition (Campbell & Kaufman, 2006). Figure 6.1 displays U.S. poverty rates in 2013 by selected characteristics, and Figure 6.2 graphs median household income in 2013 for various groups. The percentage of African Americans living in poverty was more than twice that of whites in 2013 (27% vs. 10%) (DeNavas-Walt & Proctor, 2014). In 2013, the median income for white households was $58,270 compared to $34,598 for black households (DeNavas-Walt & Proctor, 2014). The racial wealth gap is especially pronounced and wealth disparities are larger than income inequalities (Campbell & Kaufman, 2006). The average wealth of white families was over $500,000 higher than that of African American and Hispanic families in 2013 (Bricker et al., 2014), and racial-ethnic inequality in wealth has widened in the years following the Great Recession (Wolff, 2014). The

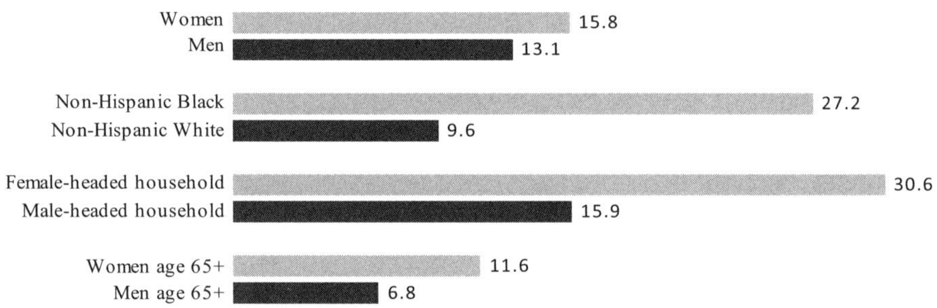

Figure 6.1 Poverty rates by selected characteristics, United States, 2013. (U.S. Census Bureau, Current Population Survey, 2014 Annual Social and Economic Supplement)

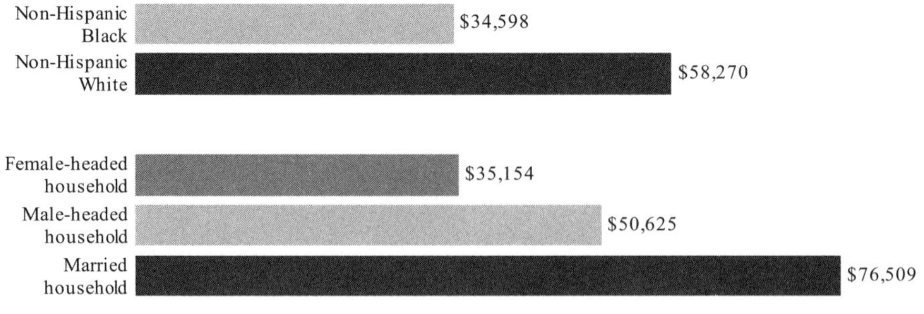

Figure 6.2 Real median household income by selected characteristics, United States, 2013. (U.S. Census Bureau, Current Population Survey, 2014 Annual Social and Economic Supplement)

race gap in wealth remains after taking into account various demographic and socioeconomic factors (Shapiro, 2004).

Because racial-ethnic minorities have lower average incomes they must therefore allocate a greater proportion of their income to essential items, such as housing and food, leaving less to invest in savings and other portfolios (Oliver & Shapiro, 1997). Hispanics and blacks are less likely to own stocks or bonds or to have any cash savings (Kochhar, 2004). Moreover, although home equity comprises a major part of net worth, less than half of Hispanics and blacks own their own homes compared to 74 percent of whites (Kochhar, 2004). The average home equity value for whites is double that of blacks, as blacks are more likely to reside in poorer neighborhoods, to experience devaluation of home values, and to face limited access to mortgage loans, resulting in asset inequality between middle-class blacks and whites (Shapiro, 2004). Not surprisingly, blacks experience less wealth growth than whites, and the racial wealth gap increases dramatically with age (Gittleman & Wolff, 2004).

Gender differences in poverty, income, and wealth are pronounced as well. As shown in Figure 6.1, although the poverty rate for women and men is similar (approximately 16% vs. 13%), the rate for female-headed family households is almost twice that of male-headed households with no wife present: 31 percent compared to 16 percent (DeNavas-Walt & Proctor, 2014). In 2013, the median household income for female-headed family households was $35,154, compared to $50,625 for male-headed households with no wife present, and $76,509 for married couples (Figure 6.2; DeNavas-Walt & Proctor, 2014).

Evidence suggests that gender disparities in income contribute to the gender gap in wealth; however, wealth is typically measured as a household rather than an individual characteristic, and analyses of gender differences in wealth are relatively rare (Deere & Doss, 2006). As a household measure, the effect of gender on wealth accumulation must be examined in combination with marital status and parenthood status (Yamokoski & Keister, 2006). Among young baby boomers, single females and single males are almost equally disadvantaged compared to married couples (Yamokoski & Keister, 2006). Single mothers and fathers also are economically disadvantaged compared to their married counterparts and to adults without children, but unmarried women with children experience the most severe disadvantage in household wealth accumulation (Yamokoski & Keister, 2006).

The one form of wealth data collected at the individual level is pension information, and from that we know women are less likely than men to have a pension plan or retirement savings account, and have lower levels of pension wealth when they do have pension plans (O'Rand & Shuey,

2007). A lack of wealth accumulation contributes to the high rate of poverty experienced by women in later life, and gender disparities in poverty rates are particularly evident among those individuals 65 years of age and older. Approximately 12 percent of women 65 and older live in poverty compared to 7 percent of men (DeNavas-Walt & Proctor, 2014). Older minority women, in particular, face serious economic insecurity given the lack of substantial wealth accumulation by minority couples despite great improvement to the overall economic situation of older Americans in recent decades (Angel, Jiménez, & Angel, 2007; Brown, 2012). As a result, poverty rates among older African American and Hispanic women are more than double the rate for white women (Lee, 2009).

In sum, gender, racial-ethnic, and class relations result in interlocking inequalities in economic resources over the life course (Reskin, 2012; Ruel & Hauser, 2013). We next discuss the importance of employment and marital history in shaping access to life-course capital and exposure to risks that are uniquely impacted by the intersection of gender and race-ethnicity.

Gender, Race-Ethnicity, and Employment History

Poverty, income, and wealth levels in old age are largely determined by employment histories. Significant differences exist in employment rates and returns between women and men as well as among women and men of various race-ethnicities. The ratio of women's to men's earnings varies by race and ethnicity (Bureau of Labor Statistics, 2015a). For example, in 2014 women's median weekly earnings were 81 percent as much as white men's and compared to 90 percent as much as black men's. Black women's earnings are about 82 percent that of white women, while median earnings of Hispanics who worked full time are the lowest (Bureau of Labor Statistics, 2015b). Women earn less than men even after controlling for education, work experience, employment status, and marital status, providing evidence of gender discrimination in compensation (Hogan & Perrucci, 2007).

In addition to the wage gap, employment rates and exposure to nonstandard and precarious employment is also gendered and racialized. Blacks are twice as likely as whites to be unemployed (Bureau of Labor Statistics, 2015a), and African American and Hispanic women are less likely to be employed than white women (Lee, 2009). Research highlights the greater precariousness of nonstandard employment arrangements, which are often defined in juxtaposition to the standard employment relations typical of the postwar period involving full-time work with a single employer that provided statutory benefits and job security (Kalleberg, 2000). In contrast, nonstandard arrangements that have grown over time are associated with greater job insecurity, reduced access to training, lower and less stable wages, and the absence of pensions and other forms of compensation (Kalleberg, 2000, 2009; Vosko, 2006). The stratification of precarious work mirrors other patterns of labor-market inequality, with women and racial-ethnic minority workers dominating temporary and part-time jobs and disproportionately affected by the risks of nonstandard employment, such as low wages (Prokos, Padavic, & Schmidt, 2009; Fuller & Vosko, 2008; Vosko, 2006).

Women's lives are inextricably linked to the lives of others, the effects of which manifest predominantly in employment trajectories. Due to their role as primary caregivers, women are more likely to experience discontinuity in employment over the life course (Moen, Robison, & Fields, 1994). Women are more likely than men to work part time and to work in jobs that do not include fringe benefits such as employer pensions and health insurance, and even women with access to pension plans receive significantly lower benefits (O'Rand & Shuey, 2007). Later in the life course, elder care affects women's labor-force attachment and wages as well. The negative effects of caregiving on employment are especially pronounced for married women with low levels of education (Wakabayashi & Donato, 2006). Women in midlife are more likely than noncaregivers to reduce hours of employment or leave the labor force once they start caregiving for an ill or disabled family member (Pavalko & Artis, 1997). Therefore, annual earnings are substantially reduced when women begin caregiving, and it is difficult for women to recover employment losses once caregiving is terminated (Wakabayashi & Donato, 2006).

This disadvantage in employment is in turn associated with further economic insecurity over time, as labor-market participation shapes access to pensions, Social Security, and other related benefits. Consequently, women do not accumulate as much wealth as men over the life course and do not obtain the same economic benefits from the Social Security system (Ruel & Hauser, 2013). The Social Security system is particularly important for economic security in later life. It is a contribution-based, nearly universal social insurance program, funded through a flat tax on workers' earnings that is matched by employers (Social Security Administration, 2010). It is especially important for women and racial-ethnic minorities, who rely on Social Security for 60 percent and 90 percent or more of their income, respectively (Social Security Administration, 2010). Most strikingly, one in five older women depends on Social Security for 100 percent of their income (Social Security Administration, 2010). However, black and Hispanic women less often qualify for Social Security because they have not made the requisite 10 years of contributions (U.S. General Accounting Office, 1997), and if they do receive Social Security they often receive only the minimum payment (Social Security Administration, 2010). As a result of these compounding disadvantages, older black women, in particular, face poverty and economic insecurity over the life course (Brown & Warner, 2008).

Gender, Race-Ethnicity, and Marital History

Although unmarried women are more likely than married women to live in poverty across all racial-ethnic groups, there are important racial-ethnic differences within each marital status (Lee, 2009). For example, a larger percentage of married African American and Hispanic women are poor compared to married white women. The decline in household income and assets following marital disruption is far greater for black and Hispanic widowed women than for whites (Angel, Jiménez, & Angel, 2007). Marriage rates are lower among Hispanics and blacks compared to whites, and rates of marital dissolution are higher (Angel, Jiménez, & Angel, 2007). African American women therefore spend more of their lives single than white women and are less likely to live with a partner in old age (Harrington Meyer, Wolf, & Himes, 2005). Disadvantages in Social Security benefits occur as a result, given the requirement of at least a 10-year marriage for spousal benefits eligibility. This also contributes to racial disparities in wealth given much higher per capita levels of wealth among married couples. Further, unmarried older black women are more likely to take in younger family members who are also experiencing financial difficulties, resulting in a high risk of poverty when living in an extended household (Lee & Shaw, 2008).

Widowhood is the most common marital transition faced by older women. For many widows, retirement security is dependent upon their husband's employment history and asset accumulation (Angel, Prickett, & Angel, 2014). Currently, the majority of older women receive Social Security spouse or widow benefits, which equals 50 percent of their spouse's benefit, or 100 percent of their husband's benefit if widowed, rather than benefits based on their own work histories (Harrington Meyer, Wolf, & Himes, 2005). Therefore, racial-ethnic disparities in women's spouse and widow benefits are reflective of racial-ethnic differences in men's wages. High unemployment among black men means marriage offers less financial security for married black women than white women (Willson, 2003). African American and Hispanic women are more likely to rely on Social Security income after retirement, and lower earnings among them as well as their husbands result in much less sufficient levels of benefits and a greater risk of poverty (Lee, 2009).

The Importance of Poverty, Income, and Wealth for Health over the Life Course

Economic advantage and disadvantage influence many aspects of well-being over the life course, but perhaps the clearest and most documented relationship is to health. The strong and enduring influence of economic status on health has been long established, and recent research demonstrates that economic conditions in childhood have enduring effects throughout the life course (see Pavalko & Caputo, 2013 for a review). Mortality and morbidity rates are inversely related to income, wealth, and poverty across all age groups (see Robert Wood Johnson Foundation, 2011 for a review) and individuals with lower socioeconomic status are more likely to experience chronic disease and functional limitations at younger ages (House, Lantz, & Herd, 2005). Poor adults are almost five times more likely to report fair/poor health as those with family incomes at or above 400 percent of the federal poverty line and three times more likely to experience activity limitations as the result of chronic illness (Robert Wood Johnson Foundation, 2011).

According to Fundamental Cause Theory, high socioeconomic status offers a broad range of flexible resources that can be used to protect against health threats in any given historical period. Thus, the link between socioeconomic status and health has persisted despite changes in causes of mortality and morbidity (Phelan, Link, & Tehranifar, 2010). Research on the social determinants of health from a life-course perspective has emphasized that health inequality in later life is the result of an accumulative process of exposure to risks and opportunities that operate across the individual life course and generates diverging trajectories of health and widening disparities (see Ferraro, 2011; Willson, Shuey, & Elder, 2007 for reviews). A recent focus on the childhood origins of health inequality has revealed the importance of when and how this accumulative process begins and emphasizes the effects of the timing, duration, and transitions in economic hardship in childhood on health in adulthood (Shuey & Willson, 2014). This growing literature demonstrates the importance of focusing on long-term processes to inform our understanding of the mechanisms through which stratification affects individual well-being over the life course.

Changes in Life-Course Poverty, Income and Wealth, and Challenges to Research

The dynamics of poverty, income, and wealth over the life course, and subsequent inequality in these outcomes, evolve over time with changes in demographic, social, and political trends. In the United States, poverty in old age declined dramatically in the 1960s and 1970s as more older

Americans had worked long enough to qualify for Social Security benefits, Supplemental Security Income for the elderly was implemented, and the level of benefits was increased (Burkhauser, Holden, & Feaster, 1988). However, as discussed earlier, these gains were not experienced universally, as many older people, particularly unmarried women, African Americans, and Latinos, remain more likely to be in poverty or near-poverty, and income inequality is at its highest among older Americans.

Economic inequality is complex but systematic due to the interaction of individual biography with social institutions (Crystal & Shea, 2002). Today, several trends—in demography, family structure, and women's employment—coincide to influence the late-life economic well-being of future generations in ways that are not yet completely clear. Because these trends have been discussed in depth elsewhere (e.g., Martin, 2011), rather than provide a thorough review, we focus on their implications for poverty, income, and wealth in later life. In addition, we highlight the importance of the role of the welfare state and the current trend toward the devolution of risk for economic well-being in later life. We conclude this section with a discussion of several challenges to research on poverty, income, and wealth from a life-course perspective.

Demographic Trends

For some time now, social gerontologists and social scientists from almost every discipline have investigated the implications of population aging. Population aging, defined as the growth in the proportion of the population over age 65 (see Martin, 2011 for a review) is occurring worldwide, in both more- and less-developed countries (United Nations: Department of Social and Economic Affairs, 2013). The United States, and many rich countries, experienced high fertility rates following World War II, and subsequent birth cohorts were significantly smaller. Because many social programs, including Social Security, depend on current workers to fund the retirement income of retirees through tax contributions, an imbalance in the ratio of the number of people aged 65 and older to those of traditional working age, referred to as the old-age dependency ratio, provides insight into the implications of population aging. This ratio has changed over time from 15 in 1955, to 22 in 2010 and is projected to rise to 35 in 2030 (Vincent & Velkoff, 2010). Although dependency ratios provide only a rough indicator of the extent to which one group in a population is dependent on another, trends in the old-age dependency ratio may be useful in understanding the implications of population aging on the viability of Social Security.

Compared to other OECD countries that face greater population aging and more urgent and severe challenges to maintaining the solvency of public pension systems, the United States is expected to be only moderately affected (Reno & Veghte, 2011). Population aging and debates over the future of Social Security are relevant to the economic security of older Americans because Social Security benefits are critical for keeping many retirees above the poverty line. Social Security comprises a substantial portion of household income for most households, including middle- and upper-middle income households; however, it represents a much larger proportion of the retirement income of disadvantaged groups. Because a larger proportion of women and racial-ethnic minorities retire due to poor health or as the result of a period of unemployment before they are eligible for full benefits, increases to the age of eligibility and concurrent increases in the penalty for taking early benefits function to increase disadvantage for these already vulnerable groups (Harrington Meyer & Parker, 2011). In sum, disadvantaged elders are most likely to be negatively impacted by any reduction in Social Security benefits that occurs in response to population aging.

Trends in Family Structure and Women's Employment

Although some social and demographic changes in the United States in recent decades have led to a narrowing of gender inequality in wages and labor-force participation, other trends may lead to greater financial vulnerability for women in later life. Since the 1970s, the proportion of women, particularly young mothers, in the labor force has increased and occupational segregation based on gender has decreased (Dunn & Skaggs, 2006). Average and median female earnings have increased at the same time that male wages have fallen or stagnated resulting in the narrowing of the gender wage gap (Wolff et al., 2012). Greater labor-force attachment also has increased women's participation in occupational pensions and eligibility for Social Security benefits (O'Rand & Shuey, 2007). Nonetheless, women continue to earn less than men, are more likely to work part time, and experience considerable time out of the labor force due to unpaid caregiving responsibilities, which will contribute to economic vulnerability in old age.

Additionally, younger Americans are experiencing more complex family arrangements and marital histories than previous generations (Manning & Brown, 2011). There are higher levels of divorce and remarriage (Kennedy & Ruggles, 2014), which tend to negatively affect the accumulation of assets (O'Rand & Shuey, 2007). Increases in nonmarital childbearing have been dramatic; for example, among women under 40, the share of births to unmarried mothers—single or cohabiting—doubled between 1980 and 2013 (Manning, Brown, & Stykes, 2015). As single parenting is linked to poverty, and particularly so for black and Hispanic mothers, these women are at a high risk of poverty or near-poverty in old age (Harrington Meyer & Parker, 2011).

Two other nontraditional trends in living arrangements have emerged in recent decades: cohabitation and the rise of same-sex families. Because access to a partner's Social Security benefits and other entitlements in old age are linked to marital status, these trends have implications for the economic well-being experienced in old age by growing numbers of Americans. First, rates of cohabitation have increased dramatically in the United States, with the percentage of women who have ever cohabited doubling to almost two-thirds over the 25-year period ending in 2013 (Manning & Stykes, 2015). Currently, over one-fourth of all unions among young to middle-aged women are cohabiting unions (Manning & Stykes, 2015). Cohabitation is common across all demographic subgroups; however, important gaps in economic well-being exist among cohabiters based on educational attainment. While among the college-educated the median-adjusted household income of cohabiters is slightly higher than that of married couples, it is lower among adults without college degrees. College-educated cohabiters are much less likely to live with children in the household than their counterparts without college degrees, and both partners are more likely to be employed (Fry & Cohn, 2011).

Second, historically, same-sex couples have been economically vulnerable in old age due to the lack of legal rights afforded by marriage, as marriage determines access to a partner's pension and Social Security benefits, as well as tax rates on inheritance and the ability to remain in one's home following a partner's move to a nursing home or death (Manning & Brown, 2011). As same-sex couples gain legal recognition in the United States, the security of these families has improved; however, rights remain state specific, and benefits at the federal level, such as Social Security, are not yet universally available. As of this writing, 37 states allow same-sex marriage, with judicial rulings pending in others and the U.S. Supreme Court poised to decide whether or not nationwide marriage equality will become law.

In sum, changes in family structure and in women's labor-force participation potentially have both potentially positive and negative implications for the future financial security of disadvantaged groups. Women have made gains in the labor force that could lead to greater income and wealth in later life; however, earnings inequality and continued employment disruptions make the magnitude of these gains unclear. Because current policies regarding income in later life assume a stable history of marriage over the life course, recent cohorts' shift away from marriage to more diverse family forms could lead to greater insecurity in old age for women and racial-ethnic minorities. However, one historically disadvantaged family form, same-sex families, continues to achieve greater recognition under the law, which, in turn, could lead to greater economic security for these families in old age.

The Role of the Welfare State and the Devolution of Risk

As these examples demonstrate, welfare states help mitigate unexpected and unavoidable risks, such as sickness, unemployment, and old age through risk-sharing and risk-spreading mechanisms, such as Social Security (O'Rand, 2011). Welfare state benefits reduce uncertainty and buffer the influence of the market, and most individuals and families make their long-term plans for old age within the context of the welfare state entitlements in place during their working years (Weymann, 2009). Welfare states also function as "mechanisms of social stratification" as, depending on the structure of entitlements, social programs can reduce market-driven inequality over the life course. Welfare state entitlements also mean inclusion for some individuals and groups and exclusion for others, as eligibility for benefits such as pensions are tied to earnings, work history, and marital status (O'Connor, Orloff, & Shaver, 1999; Weymann, 2009).

While the first part of the twentieth century witnessed an expansion of welfare state programs, a trend toward retrenchment of welfare state entitlements has emerged in recent decades. At the same time, private employer pensions are increasingly shifting to individualized, market-based plans that place more responsibility for managing risk on workers and their families, and some families have greater resources to absorb these risks than others (O'Rand, 2011; Quesnel-Vallée, Willson, & Reiter-Campeau, 2015). In sum, although Social Security and occupational pensions have reduced poverty among the older population, the current trend toward the "devolution of risk" from states to individuals will potentially result in greater inequality (O'Rand, 2011).

These rapidly changing social and demographic trends require us to monitor the implications of macrolevel change on the individual life course and the influence of social policy and the welfare state on patterns of economic inequality by gender, race-ethnicity and family structure. In the following section, we highlight methodological challenges to research on poverty, income, and wealth over the life course.

Challenges to Research in on Poverty, Income, and Wealth over the Life Course

At least three challenges are faced by researchers studying poverty, income, and wealth from a life-course perspective: measurement of key concepts, data and modeling requirements, and theoretical and methodological incorporation of both the individual and institutions into research. First, determining the most appropriate measure has been the subject of much debate (for a review, see Haveman, 2009). The official U.S. poverty measure has stood nearly unchanged since 1964, and despite efforts almost since its inception, there has been no commonly accepted improved approach to measuring poverty. Income only provides a partial picture of the relative well-being of one demographic group compared to another (Wolff et al., 2012) and, ideally, measures of poverty would move beyond the concept of income poverty to include other measures of material hardship and of deprivation, such as social exclusion (Haveman, 2009). However, this is both conceptually and methodologically challenging, as ideally, detailed survey data including a wide range of living conditions over a long period of time would be required (Haveman, 2009). In addition, variations in measurement across countries make comparative research difficult. Beyond these basic problems with measuring poverty, official poverty rates, and much academic research, measure poverty rates at a single point in time, which does not distinguish temporary from persistent poverty (Western et al., 2012). Most poverty at the household level is temporary, lasting for two years or less, so that point-in-time measures capture only a small fraction of people who experience poverty at some time in their lives (Western et al., 2012). The long-term effects of these varying experiences remain largely unknown.

Problems with the measurement of other key concepts, such as income, wealth, and retirement are almost equally vexing. Income is notoriously difficult to measure in surveys, as respondents may be reluctant to reveal their income, and it is difficult to remember income from many different sources accurately (Smith, 2002). As a result, income is often not reported at all and survey data is plagued with high levels of missing income data, making it unreliable. Estimates of levels of household wealth vary depending on how comprehensive the measure of wealth is—the inclusion of housing wealth, a variety of financial assets, business equity, wealth that generates annuity income are all wealth components that influence estimates of the extent of wealth and therefore inequality (Smith, 2002).

Finally, women's historically sporadic work patterns challenge the utility of conventional measures of retirement. Traditional stratification research has assumed a male-model of work and family based on white, middle-class men's experiences consisting of a stable work history, with a clear beginning and end, followed by retirement income (Calasanti, 1996). Research demonstrates that these assumptions do not hold for a substantial minority and fail to adequately capture the experience of many older people (Hardy, 2011). Conceptualizing and measuring retirement is becoming even more difficult as employment patterns become increasingly complex and variable and the transition to retirement becomes more blurred. Today, definitions of retirement are moving beyond categories of employment status to emphasize patterns of changing sources of income over the life course, health transitions, and employment histories that are experienced jointly (Hardy, 2011).

As our concepts become more comprehensive and complex, so do our data requirements and statistical models. For example, CAD postulates that the duration, timing, and sequencing of children's exposure to economic hardship during childhood are important for developmental processes and outcomes such as socioeconomic attainment in young adulthood and midlife (Wagmiller et al., 2006). In most analyses, however, changes in individual circumstances, such as whether childhood conditions are improving or deteriorating, or issues of timing—whether disadvantage occurs early or later in childhood—are not captured. A primary difficulty for life-course researchers lies in the lack of adequate data sources that allow such observations, and the challenges associated with developing models that measure more than average effects and normative patterns (Shuey & Willson, 2014). Life-course researchers continue to employ creative data and analysis techniques to address these challenges.

Finally, the life-course perspective emphasizes the interaction of micro-, meso- and macrolevels of society, and this is particularly difficult for research to incorporate (Mayer, 2009). One example is the challenge of incorporating macrolevel processes into models of individual behavior and outcomes (Mayer & Schoepflin, 1989). With its stronger "state tradition" (Leisering, 2003), Europe has been at the center of life-course investigations of the impact of governmental policies on the life course of individuals (e.g., Allmendinger & Hinz, 2003) while the North American approach has tended to focus on the individual life course. As possibilities improve for linking longitudinal microdata with policy data and cross-country comparable data, opportunities for analyses of the role of social policies in shaping work and family experiences and relationships between life-course experiences and socioeconomic outcomes continue to emerge (Corna, 2013).

Conclusion

Existing disparities in economic outcomes based on relations of gender and race-ethnicity culminate in a greater risk of disadvantage for racial-ethnic minority women across the life course and in later life. Examining poverty, income, and wealth from a life-course perspective allows us to better understand the variability in individual outcomes by recognizing that later life is shaped by cumulative experiences, such as labor-force participation and marital history that produce distinctive life patterns. Assumptions regarding gender roles and family structure reflected in institutions and policies contribute to the structuring of inequality in old age and are often not reflective of the realities of older Americans (Apfel, 2011). As a result of processes of social change, new social risks have emerged. The transition from an industrial to postindustrial mode of production has led to new labor-market uncertainties and higher unemployment; family instability has grown, and the aging of the population places increasing pressure on families and states. Coupled with these processes is a trend toward the devolution of risk, placing greater responsibility on workers and their families to absorb life-course risks associated with income security (O'Rand, 2011). Life-course research focusing on the influence of social institutions and policies on life-course outcomes provides a framework for understanding the dynamic interplay of social policy and cumulative advantage/disadvantage over the life course, in contrast to the view of social exclusion and poverty as a deviation from the normal life course (Dewilde, 2009). As new opportunities arise from long-term studies of individuals and families as they age, as well as advances in the availability of statistical tools to analyze complex data, social scientists continue to further our understanding of unanswered questions regarding the stability of socioeconomic conditions and dynamics of life trajectories, and long-term effects of childhood conditions on middle and later adulthood.

References

Allmendinger, J., & Hinz, T. (2003). Occupational careers under different welfare regimes. In W.R. Heinz, A. Weymann, & J. Huinink (Eds.), *The Life Course Reader: Individuals and Societies Across Time* (pp. 234–251). New York: Campus Verlag.

Angel, J.L., Prickett, K.C., & Angel, R.J. (2014). Retirement security for Black, non-Hispanic White, and Mexican-origin women: The changing roles of marriage and work. *Journal of Women, Politics & Policy*, *35*(3), 222–241.

Apfel, K. (2011). Policy foreword. In R.A. Settersten & J.L. Angel (Eds.), *Handbook of Sociology of Aging* (pp. ix–xii). New York: Springer.

Bastos, A., Casaca, S.F., Nunes, F., & Pereirinha, J. (2009). Women and poverty: A gender-sensitive approach. *Journal of Socio-Economics*, *38*, 764–778.

Bricker, J., Dettling, L.J., Henriques, A., Hsu, J.W., Moore, K.B., Sabelhaus, J., & Windle, R.A. (2014). *Changes in US family finances from 2010 to 2013: Evidence from the Survey of Consumer Finances. Federal Reserve Bulletin* (Vol. 100). Washington, DC. Retrieved from http://www.federalreserve.gov/pubs/bulletin/2012/PDF/scf12.pdf

Brown, Tyson H. (2012). The intersection and accumulation of racial and gender inequality: Black women's wealth trajectories. *The Review of Black Political Economy*, *39*, 239–258.

Brown, T.H., & Warner, D.F. (2008). Divergent pathways? Racial/ethnic differences in older women's labor force withdrawal. *The Journals of Gerontology, Series B: Psychological Sciences and Social Sciences*, *63*(3), S122–S134.

Bureau of Labor Statistics. (2015a). Table A-2. *Employment status of the civilian population by race, sex, and age*. Retrieved March 1, 2015, from http://www.bls.gov/news.release/empsit.t02.htm

Bureau of Labor Statistics. (2015b). *Usual weekly earnings of wage and salary workers: Fourth Quarter 2014*. Washington, DC.

Burkhauser, R.V., Holden, K.C., & Feaster, D. (1988). Incidence, timing, and events associated with poverty: A dynamic view of poverty in retirement. *Journal of Gerontology*, *43*(2), S46–S52.

Calasanti, T. (1996). Incorporating diversity: Meaning, levels of research, and implications for theory. *The Gerontologist*, *36*(2), 147–156.

Campbell, L.A., & Kaufman, R.L. (2006). Racial differences in household wealth: Beyond Black and White. *Research in Social Stratification and Mobility*, *24*(2), 131–152.

Corna, L.M. (2013). A life course perspective on socioeconomic inequalities in health: A critical review of conceptual frameworks. *Advances in Life Course Research*, *18*(2), 150–159.

Crystal, S., & Shea, D.G. (1990). Cumulative advantage, cumulative disadvantage, and inequality among elderly people. *The Gerontologist*, *30*(4), 437–443.

Crystal, S., & Shea, D.G. (2002). Introduction: Cumulative advantage, public policy, and inequality in later life. In S. Crystal, D. Shea, & K.W. Schaie (Eds.), *Annual Review of Gerontology and Geriatrics: Focus on Economic Outcomes in Later Life* (22nd ed., pp. 1–13). New York: Springer Publishing Company.

Currie, J. (2011). Inequalities at birth: Some causes and consequences. *Ungleichheiten Bei Der Geburt: Einige Ursachen Und Folgen*, *12*, 42–65.

Dannefer, D. (2003). Cumulative advantage/disadvantage and the life course: Cross-fertilizing age and social science theory. *Journal of Gerontology*, *58B*(6), S327–337.

Dannefer, D., Uhlenberg, P., Foner, A., & Abeles, R.P. (2005). On the shoulders of a giant: The legacy of Matilda White Riley for gerontology. *The Journals of Gerontology, Series B: Psychological Sciences and Social Sciences*, *60*(6), S296–S304.

Deere, C.D., & Doss, C.R. (2006). The gender asset gap: What do we know and why does it matter? *Feminist Economics*, *12*(1–2), 1–50. doi:10.1080/13545700500508056.

DeNavas-Walt, C., & Proctor, B.D. (2014). *Income and poverty in the United States: 2013 Current Population Reports* (No. P60–249). Washington, DC.

Dewilde, C. (2009). A life course perspective on social inclusion and poverty. In W.R. Heinz, J. Huinink, & A. Weymann (Eds.), *The Life Course Reader: Individuals and Societies Across Time* (pp. 252–269). Frankfurt: Campus Reader.

DiPrete, T.A. (2002). Life course risks, mobility regimes, and mobility consequences: A comparison of Sweden, Germany, and the United States. *American Journal of Sociology*, *108*, 267–309.

Duncan, G.J., Yeung, W.J., Brooks-Gunn, J., & Smith, J.R. (1998). How much does childhood poverty affect the life chances of children? *American Sociological Review*, *63*(3), 406–423.

Dunn, D., & Skaggs, S. (2006). Gender and paid work in industrial nations. In J. Saltzman Chafetz (Ed.), *Handbook of the Sociology of Gender* (pp. 321–342). New York: Springer.

Elder, G.H., Jr. (1987). War mobilization and the life course: A cohort of World War II veterans. *Sociological Forum*, 2(3): 449–472.

Elder, G.H., Jr., & Johnson, M.K. (2003). The life course and aging: Challenges, lessons, and new directions. In R. A. Settersten (Ed.), *Invitation to Life Course: Toward New Understandings of Later Life* (pp. 1–52). Amityville, NY: Baywood.

Elman, C., & O'Rand, A.M. (2004). The race is to the swift: Socioeconomic origins, adult education, and wage attainment. *American Journal of Sociology*, *110*(1), 123–160.

Erickson, L.D., McDonald, S., & Elder, G.H. (2009). Informal mentors and education: Complementary or compensatory resources? *Sociology of Education*, *82*, 344–367.

Erikson, R., & Goldthorpe, J.H. (2002). Intergenerational inequality: A sociological perspective. *The Journal of Economic Perspectives*, *16*(3), 31–44.

Ferraro, K. F. (2011). Health and Aging: Early origins, persistent inequalities? In R. A. Settersten and J. Angel (Eds.), *Handbook of Sociology of Aging* (pp. 465-475). New York: Springer.

Ferraro, K.F., & Shippee, T.P. (2009). Aging and cumulative inequality: How does inequality get under the skin? *The Gerontologist*, *49*(3), 333–343.

Fry, R., & Cohn, D. (2011). *Living Together: The Economics of Cohabitation*. Washington, DC. Retrieved from http://www.pewsocialtrends.org/2011/06/27/living-together-the-economics-of-cohabitation/

Fuller, S., & Vosko, L.F. (2008). Temporary employment and social inequality in Canada: Exploring intersections of gender, race, and migration. *Social Indicators Research*, *88*(1), 31–50.

Gittleman, M., & Wolff, E.N. (2004). Racial differences in patterns of wealth accumulation. *Journal of Human Resources*, *39*(1), 193–227.

Hardy, M.A. (2011). Rethinking retirement. In R.A. Settersten & J.L. Angel (Eds.), *Handbook of the Sociology of Aging and the Life Course* (pp. 213–227). New York: Springer Publishing Company.

Harrington Meyer, M., & Parker, W.M. (2011). Gender, aging, and social policy. In R.H. Binstock & L.K. George (Eds.), *Handbook of Aging and the Social Sciences* (7th ed., pp. 323–336). New York: Elsevier.

Harrington Meyer, M., Wolf, D. A, & Himes, C.L. (2005). Linking benefits to marital status: Race and social security in the US. *Feminist Economics*, *11*(2), 145–162.

Haveman, R. (2009). What does it mean to be poor in a rich society? *Focus*, *26*(2), 81–86.

Hayward, M.D., & Gorman, B.K. (2004). The long arm of childhood: The influence of early life social conditions on men's mortality. *Demography*, *41*(1), 87–107.

Hitlin, S., & Elder, G.H., Jr. (2007). Time, self, and the curiously abstract concept of agency. *Sociological Theory*, 25, 170–191.

Hogan, R., & Perrucci, C. C. (2007). Black women: Truly disadvantaged in the transition from employment to retirement income. *Social Science Research, 36*, 1184–1199.

House, J. S., Lantz, P. M., & Herd, P. (2005). Continuity and change in the social stratification of aging and health over the life course: Evidence from a national representative longitudinal study from 1986 to 2001/2002 (Americans' Changing Lives Study). *The Journals of Gerontology, 60B*, 15–25.

Kalleberg, A. L. (2000). Non-standard employment relations: Part-time, temporary, and contract work. *Annual Review of Sociology, 26*, 341–365.

Kalleberg, A. L. (2009). Precarious work, insecure workers: Employment relations in transition. *American Sociological Review, 74*, 1–22.

Kennedy, S., & Ruggles, S. J. (2014). Breaking up is hard to count: The rise of divorce in the United States, 1980–2010. *Demography, 51*(2), 587–598. doi:10.1007/s13524–013–0270–9.

Kochhar, R. (2004). *The wealth of Hispanic households: 1996 to 2002*, (October), 1–44. Retrieved from http://www.sas.upenn.edu/~dludden/HispanicWealth REPORT.pdf

Lee, S. (2009). Racial and ethnic differences in women's retirement security. *Journal of Women, Politics & Policy, 30*, 141–172.

Lee, S., & Shaw, L. (2008). *From Work to Retirement: Tracking Changes in Women's Poverty Status*. Washington, DC.

Leisering, L. (2003). Government and the life course. In M. J. Shanahan & J. Mortimer (Eds.), *Handbook of the Life Course* (pp. 205–228). New York: Springer Publishing Company.

Manning, W. D., & Brown, S. L. (2011). The demography of unions among older Americans 1980-present: A family change approach. In R. A. Settersten & J. L. Angel (Eds.), *Handbook of the Sociology of Aging* (pp. 193–212). New York: Springer.

Manning, W. D., Brown, S. L., & Stykes, B. (2015). *Trends in Births to Single and Cohabiting Mothers, 1980–2013*. Bowling Green, OH: National Center for Marriage and Family Research.

Manning, W. D., & Stykes, B. (2015). *Twenty-Five Years of Change in Cohabitation in the U.S., 1987–2013*. Bowling Green, OH: National Center for Marriage and Family Research.

Martin, L. G. (2011). Demography of aging. In R. H. Binstock & L. K. George (Eds.), *Handbook of Aging and the Social Sciences* (7th ed., pp. 33–46). New York: Elsevier.

Mayer, K. U. (2009). New directions in life course research. *Annual Review of Sociology, 35*, 413–433.

Mayer, K. U., & Schoepflin, U. (1989). The state and the life course. *Annual Review of Sociology, 15*(1), 187–209.

McDonough, P., & Berglund, P. (2003). Histories of poverty and self-rated health trajectories. *Journal of Health and Social Behavior, 44*(2), 198–214.

McFall, B. H. (2011). Crash and wait? The impact of the Great Recession on the retirement plans of older Americans. *American Economic Review, 101*, 40–44.

Moen, P., Robison, J., & Fields, V. (1994). Women's work and caregiving roles: A life course approach. *Journal of Gerontology, 49*(4), S176–S186.

O'Connor, J., Orloff, A., & Shaver, S. (1999). *States, Markets, Families: Gender, Liberalism and Social Policy in Australia, Canada, Great Britain, and the United States*. Cambridge, England: Cambridge University Press.

O'Rand, A. M. (1996). The precious and the precocious: Understanding cumulative disadvantage and cumulative advantage over the life course. *The Gerontologist*, *36*(2), 230–238.

O'Rand, A. M. (2001). Stratification and the life course: The forms of life-course capital and their interrelationships. In R. H. Binstock & L. K. George (Eds.), *Handbook of Aging and the Social Sciences* (5th ed., pp. 197–210). San Diego, CA: Academic Press.

O'Rand, A. M. (2002). Cumulative advantage and gerontological theory. In S. Crystal & D. Shea (Eds.), *Annual Review of Gerontology and Geriatrics* (Vol. 22, pp. 14–30). New York: Springer Publishing Company.

O'Rand, A. M. (2006). Stratification and the life course: Life course capital, life course risks, and social inequality. In R. H. Binstock & L. K. George (Eds.), *Handbook of Aging and the Social Sciences* (6th ed., pp. 145–162). Burlington, MA: Academic Press.

O'Rand, A. M. (2011). The devolution of risk and the changing life course in the United States. *Social Forces*, *90*(1), 1–16.

O'Rand, A. M., & Henretta, J. C. (1999). *Age and Inequality: Diverse Pathways through Later Life*. Boulder, CO: Westview.

O'Rand, A. M., & Shuey, K. M. (2007). Gender and the devolution of pension risks in the US. *Current Sociology*, *55*, 287–304.

Oliver, M. L., & Shapiro, T. M. (1997). *Black Wealth/White Wealth: A New Perspective on Racial Inequality*. New York: Routledge.

Pampel, F. C. (1994). Changes in income inequality during old age. *Research in Social Stratification and Mobility*, *13*, 239–263.

Pavalko, E. K., & Artis, J. E. (1997). Women's caregiving and paid work: Causal relationship in late midlife. *Journal of Gerontology*, *52B*(4), S170–S179.

Pavalko, E. K., & Caputo, J. (2013). Social inequality and health across the life course. *American Behavioral Scientist*, *57*(8), 1040–1056.

Phelan, J. C., Link, B. G., & Tehranifar, P. (2010). Social conditions as fundamental causes of health inequalities: Theory, evidence, and policy implications. *Journal of Health and Social Behavior*, *51 Suppl.*, S28–S40.

Prokos, A. H., Padavic, I., & Schmidt, A. (2009). Nonstandard work arrangements among women and men scientists and engineers. *Sex Roles*, *61*, 653–665.

Quesnel-Vallée, A., Willson, A. E., & Reiter-Campeau, S. (2015). Health inequalities among older adults in developed countries: Reconciling theories and policy approaches. In L. K. George & K. F. Ferraro (Eds.), *Handbook of Aging and the Social Sciences* (8th ed., pp. 483–498). New York: Elsevier.

Reno, V. P., & Veghte, B. (2011). Economic status of the aged in the United States. In R. H. Binstock & L. K. George (Eds.), *Handbook of Aging and the Social Sciences* (7th ed., pp. 175–192). Boston: Elsevier.

Reskin, B. (2012). The race discrimination system. *Annual Review of Sociology*, *38*, 17–35.

Robert Wood Johnson Foundation. (2011). *Income, Wealth, and Health*. San Francisco, CA: Author.

Ruel, E., & Hauser, R. M. (2013). Explaining the gender wealth gap. *Demography*, *50* (December 2012), 1155–1176.

Sampson, R.J., & Laub, J.H. (1996). Socioeconomic achievement in the life course of disadvantaged men: Military service as a turning point, circa 1940–1965. *American Sociological Review*, *61*(3), 347–367.

Shanahan, M.J., & Macmillan, R. (2008). *Biography and the Sociological imagination*. New York: W.W. Norton and Company.

Shapiro, T. M. (2004). *The Hidden Cost of Being African American: How Wealth Perpetuates Inequality*. New York: Oxford University Press.

Shuey, K.M., & Willson, A.E. (2014). Economic hardship in childhood and adult health trajectories : An alternative approach to investigating life-course. *Advances in Life Course Research*, *22*, 49–61.

Smith, J.P. (2002). Measurement of late-life income and wealth. In S. Crystal, D.G. Shea, & K.W. Schaie (Eds.), *Annual Review of Gerontology and Geriatrics: Focus on Economic Outcomes in Later Life* (Vol. 22, pp. 95–115). New York: Springer Publishing Company.

Social Security Administration. (2010). *Annual Statistical Supplement to the Social Social Security Bulletin*. Washington, DC.

Teti, D.M., & Lamb, M.E. (1989). Socioeconomic and marital outcomes of adolescent marriage, adolescent childbirth, and their co-occurrence. *Journal of Marriage and the Family*, *51*(1), 203–212.

U.S. General Accounting Office. (1997). *Social Security Reform: Implications for Women's Retirement Income*. Washington, DC: Author.

United Nations: Department of Social and Economic Affairs. (2013). *World Population Prospects: The 2012 Revision*. Retrieved from http://esa.un.org/unpd/wpp/Excel-Data/population.htm

Vandecasteele, L. (2011). Life course risks or cumulative disadvantage? The structuring effect of social stratification determinants and life course events on poverty transitions in Europe. *European Sociological Review*, *27*(2), 246–263.

Vartanian, T.P., & McNamara, J.M. (2002). Older women in poverty: The impact of midlife factors. *Journal of Marriage and Family*, *64*(2), 532–548.

Vincent, G.K., & Velkoff, V.A. (2010). *The Older Population in the United States: 2010 to 2050*. Washington, DC. Retrieved from https://www.census.gov/prod/2010pubs/p25–1138.pdf

Vosko, L. F. (2006). *Precarious Employment: Understanding Labour Market Insecurity in Canada*. Montreal and Kingston: McGill-Queen's University Press.

Wagmiller, R.L., Lennon, M.C., Kuang, L., Alberti, P.M., & Aber, J.L. (2006). The dynamics of economic disadvantage and children's life chances. *American Sociological Review*, *71*(5), 847–866.

Wakabayashi, C., & Donato, K.M. (2006). Does caregiving increase poverty among women in later life? Evidence from the Health and Retirement Survey. *Journal of Health and Social Behavior*, *47*(3), 258–274.

Western, B., Bloome, D., Sosnaud, B., & Tach, L. (2012). Economic insecurity and social stratification. *Annual Review of Sociology*, *38*, 341–359.

Weymann, A. (2009). The life course, institutions, and life course policy. In W.R. Heinz, J. Huinink, & A. Weymann (Eds.), *The Life Course Reader: Individuals and Societies Across Time* (pp. 139–158). Frankfurt: Campus Reader.

Willson, A. E. (2003). Race and women's income trajectories: Employment, marriage, and income. *Social Problems*, *50*(1), 87–110.

Willson, A. E., Shuey, K. M., & Elder, G. H. (2007). Cumulative advantage processes as mechanisms of inequality in life course health. *American Journal of Sociology*, *112*(6), 1886–1924.

Wolff, E. N. (2014). *Household Wealth Trends in the United States, 1962–2013: What Happened over the Great Recession?* (No. 20733). Cambridge, MA: National Bureau of Economic Research.

Wolff, E. N., Zacharias, A., Masterson, T., & Eren, S. (2012). *A Comparison of Inequality and Living Standards in Canada and the United States using an Expanded Measure of Economic Well-Being* (No. 703). Annandale-on-Hudson, NY: Levy Economics Institute.

Yamokoski, A., & Keister, L. A. (2006). The wealth of single women: Marital status and parenthood in the asset accumulation of young baby boomers in the United States. *Feminist Economics*, *12*(1), 167–194.

CHAPTER SEVEN

Work and Retirement

Jeanette M. Zoeckler and Michael Silverstein

The aging workforce is redefining both work and retirement. Older workers are remaining in the labor force longer, and the process of retirement is becoming messier. This chapter characterizes the demographics of the workforce with an emphasis on variation by age, gender, race, ethnicity, and nativity. We explore key sociological theories that assist in understanding the links between employment, health, and well-being. We then assess the risks and accommodations necessary for older workers. Finally, we analyze the factors that shape retirement decisions and satisfaction.

Demographics of the Aging Workforce

The U.S. labor force has been growing steadily, and much of the increase has been among older workers. Employment patterns vary significantly by age, gender, race, ethnicity, and nativity. Some groups are more likely to work full time while others are more likely to work part time or to be unemployed. Even though wages are rising, persistent patterns in wage inequality remain. These disparities can be partially explained by differential exposure to unstable jobs in the New Economy, which is related to different levels of education and different returns on educational investments.

Labor-Force Participation

The total labor force has grown from approximately 60 million in 1950 to 154 million in 2011 (Hayutin et al., 2013; p. 11). But labor-force participation, defined as the proportion of the population that is either employed or seeking to be employed, has declined for everyone except older workers in recent decades. Figure 7.1 shows labor-force participation by age since 1992. While employment declined slightly between 1992 and 2013 for those aged 25–54, it increased, and is expected to continue increasing, for all workers aged 55 and older (Toossi, 2013). From 2002 to 2014, the steepest increase in labor-force participation occurred for workers aged 65–74, and this rate of increase is expected to be maintained through 2022 (Toossi, 2013). These are unprecedented levels of labor-force participation among middle- and older-aged workers, and they are helping to redefine the golden years.

Among those in the labor force, the amount of hours worked varies dramatically. Roughly 80 percent work full time and 20 percent work part time. Younger workers and older workers are both more likely than middle-aged workers to be employed part time (Toossi, 2015a,b). Moreover, many in the labor force are actually unemployed. Persons are classified as unemployed in the Current Population Survey if they do not have a job, have actively looked for work in the prior four weeks, and are currently available for work. Unemployment rates soared from 4.4 percent in May of 2007 to a high of 10 percent in October 2009 due to the Great Recession. Overall, unemployment remained high for 2010 and 2011 and then began to gradually decrease to 5.5 percent in 2015 (Toossi, 2015a,b).

Teen labor-force participation has been on the decline for many years. Additionally, teens have the highest rates of unemployment, and those rates increased even further during the recessionary period. Workers aged

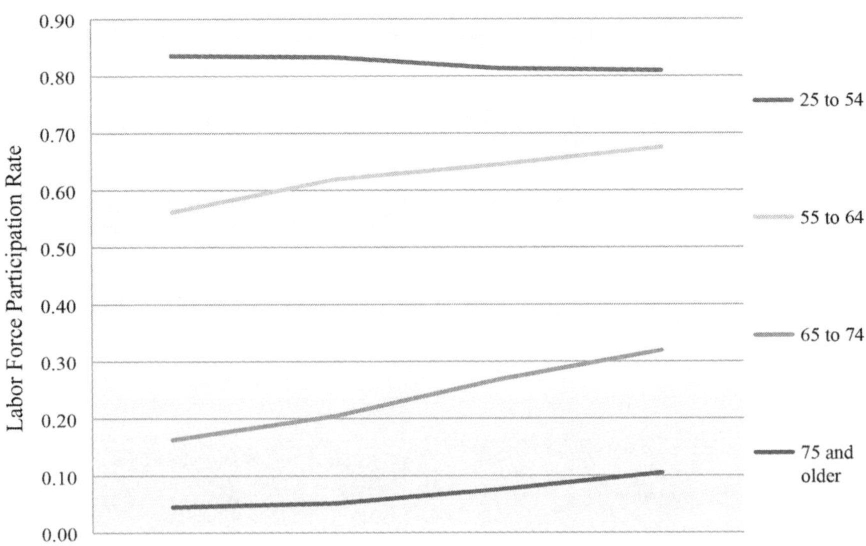

Figure 7.1 Percentage participating in the labor force, by age, 1992–2022. (BLS, 2013)

20–24 experience relatively high unemployment rates, but in the last year, the unemployment rate for this group dropped from 12.7 percent to 10.6 percent. Workers aged 55 and over consistently report lower unemployment rates, between 4.2 and 4.5 percent; however, those statistics are interpreted with caution because older workers tend to retire rather than become unemployed (Toossi, 2015a,b).

Historically, men's labor-force participation rates have been significantly higher than women's but the gap is closing. The most dramatic increase in labor-force participation rate occurred in women aged 55–64, which increased from 47 percent to 55 percent between 1992 and 2002, representing a 9 percentage point increase in just a decade. During that same time frame, men's participation rate rose only from 67 to 71 percent. As Figure 7.2 shows, labor-force participation rates vary by gender and age.

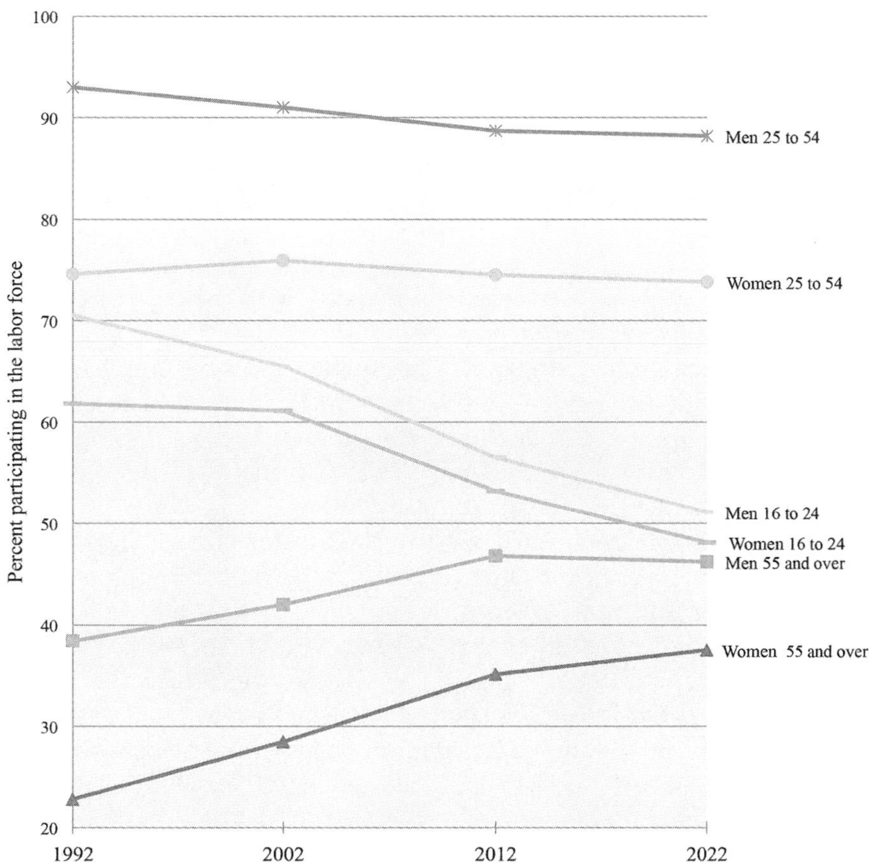

Figure 7.2 Percentage participating in the labor force, by age and gender, 1992–2022. (BLS, 2013)

Young workers, aged 16 to 24, have declining labor-force participation rates. In 2013, these rates declined from 71 percent to 51 percent for men and, less dramatically, from 61 percent to 48 percent for women. The gender gap in participation rates between men and women are the smallest in this group.

The highest labor-force participation rates are for adults aged 25 to 54 and this group has also been experiencing a slow decline since 1992. This decline is expected to continue through 2022 with both men and women declining. Men's participation rate is expected to drop from 93 percent in 1992 to 88 percent in 2022, while women's participation rate is expected to remain fairly stable, from 75 percent in 1992 to 74 percent in 2022 (Toossi, 2013).

Labor-force participation rates for workers aged 55 and older have risen substantially. Men's participation rates rose from 38 percent in 1992 to 47 percent in 2012 and is projected to taper off to a projected 46 percent in 2022. Women's labor-force participation rate for that age group is expected to rise from 23 percent to 38 percent over that same period. Furthermore, the Bureau of Labor Statistics projects that by 2022, fully 36 percent of men and 28 percent of women will be working at ages 65–74 (Toossi, 2013).

Part-time work is defined as usually working less than 35 hours per week by the Bureau of Labor Statistics, and women are more likely to work part time than men. In 2013, 26 percent of all working women worked part time, compared to only 13 percent of men (BLS, 2014a). In May 2015, for example, there were 9 million men 20 years of age and older working part time, compared to 16 million women (Toossi, 2015a,b). Though there are marked gender differences in part-time work rates, there is little gender difference in unemployment rates. Over the last two years, the seasonally adjusted unemployment rate for men averaged 5.4 percent and women 5.2 percent (Toossi, 2015 a,b).

Labor-force rates are similar, and declining, for all race and ethnic groups, but unemployment rates vary starkly by race and ethnicity. For whites aged 16 and over, labor-force participation rates are expected to drop from 67 percent in 1992 to 62 percent in 2022 (Toossi, 2013). During the same period, rates for blacks are expected to fall from 64 percent to 60 percent. Labor-force participation for Asians is projected to decline from 67 percent in 1992 to 63 percent in 2022. Hispanic labor-force participation is expected to decline the least, from 67 percent in 1992 to 66 percent in 2022.

With respect to full- or part-time work, there are only very small differences by race or ethnicity (Shaefer, 2009); however, unemployment rates vary markedly by race and ethnicity. Generally all ethnicities have trended in the same pattern of seasonally adjusted unemployment rates with historic lows prior to the recession and high spiking unemployment in 2010, followed by a slow decline as the economy began to recover. But the rates are dramatically higher for some groups than others. Asians experienced the lowest average unemployment rate from 2005 to 2014 at 5 percent (BLS, Current Population Survey, 2014). During the same period, the average unemployment rate for whites was 6 percent, for Latinos was nearly 9 percent, and for blacks was over 12 percent. Historically black unemployment rates have been consistently double those of whites. Moreover, black workers experienced the most dramatic rise in unemployment during the Great Recession. In March of 2010, blacks experienced a striking 17 percent unemployment rate (Toossi, 2015a,b).

Foreign-born workers comprised nearly 11 percent of the labor force in 1992 and nearly 17 percent in 2014 (BLS, 2014b). Latinos account for 48 percent and Asians account for 24 percent of all foreign-born workers. Recent immigrants are more likely than those who have been here for more years to be working only part time or for only part of the year (Seghal, 1985; Rose & Hartmann, 2008). Also, foreign-born workers are more likely than native-born workers to be employed in service occupations, which tend to have lower pay and offer fewer benefits. In general, the unemployment rate for foreign-born is very similar to native-born people (BLS, 2014b).

Wages

Wages have been rising for men and women of all ages in the United States, but they vary markedly by age, gender, race, ethnicity, and nativity. Generally wages increase across the life course, until age 65 when many reduce hours or change jobs and therefore accrue lower earnings. Until recently, workers, aged 65 and older, have reported lower weekly earnings than other adults. But as Figure 7.3 demonstrates, workers over 65 caught up with 25–54-year-olds in 2014. While this is good news for older workers' incomes, it may result in some pressure from employers for older workers to retire earlier than they may desire. Employers value the experience of older workers but may be reluctant to have such high-paying workers on the payroll for increasing numbers of years.

Though median earnings rose between 2000 and 2014 for men and women alike, Figure 7.3 shows that women's median earnings are well below men's at all ages. In 2014, among workers aged 25–54, men's median weekly earnings are 20 percent higher than women's; among workers aged 55–64, they are 26 percent higher than women's; and among those aged 65 and older, they are 24 percent higher (BLS, 2014a). The

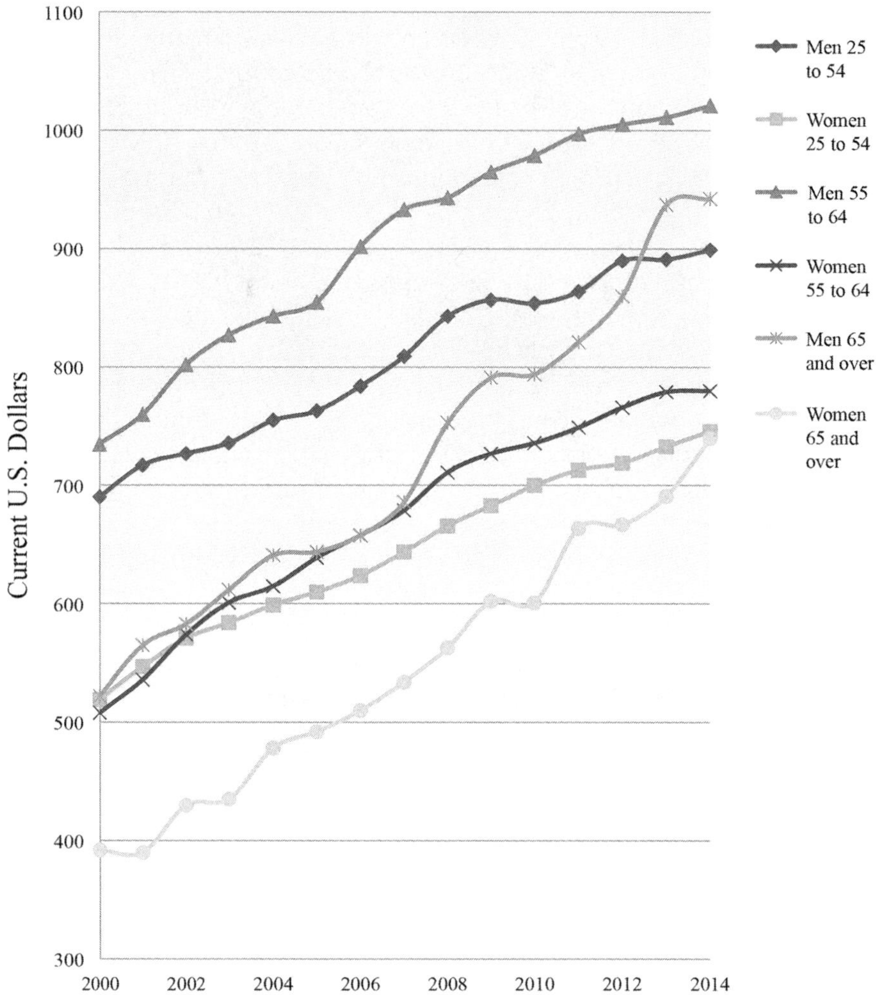

Figure 7.3 Median usual weekly earnings, by age and gender, 2000–2014. (BLS, 2014)

stubborn gender gap in wages leaves women more economically vulnerable than men in old age. The gender gap in wages is linked to gender differences in responsibilities for unpaid care work and housework, gender differences in full- and part-time status, and gender discrimination (Harrington Meyer & Parker, 2012). There is little pay equity in the labor force. Women tend to be segregated into lower-paying jobs, they tend to earn less than men when they work jobs traditionally held by men, and even when women are employed in comparable jobs, they tend to earn significantly less than men (Rose & Hartmann, 2008; Hegewich & Ellis,

2015). Thus at any point in time, women's earnings average just 70 percent of men's, but over the course of the 15 years between ages 25 and 40, Hartmann, Rose, & Lovell (2006) found women's cumulative wages averaged just 38 percent of men's.

Median usual weekly earnings differ significantly by race and ethnicity, with whites of all ages significantly out-earning blacks and Latinos (BLS, 2014c). Figure 7.4 shows that from 2000 to 2014, whites aged 55 and over earned the most, followed by whites aged 25 to 54. Median weekly earnings for whites aged 55 were 22 percent more than for comparable blacks and 32 percent more than for comparable Latinos (BLS, 2014c). Similarly, median weekly earnings for whites aged 25 to 54 were 21 percent more than for comparable blacks and 29 percent more than for comparable

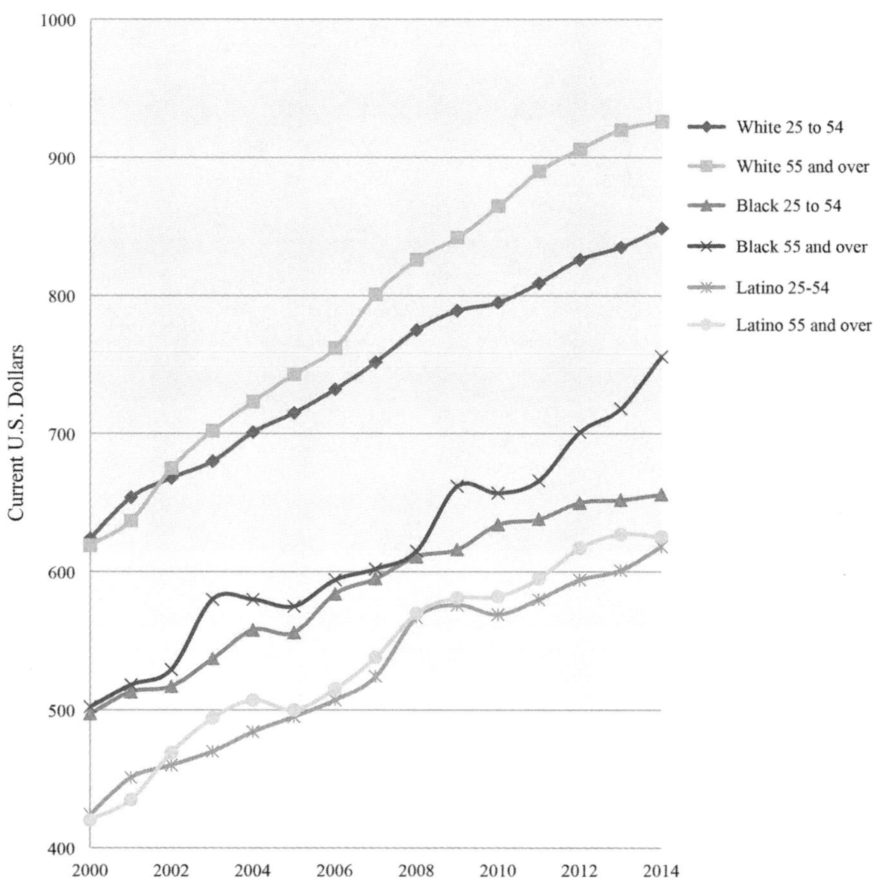

Figure 7.4 Median usual weekly earnings, by age and ethnicity, 2000–2014. (BLS, 2014)

Latinos (BLS, 2014c). Blacks and Latinos both experienced wage stagnation, particularly during the Great Recession, but Latinos consistently experienced the lowest levels of earnings. Moreover, Latinos 55 years of age and older experienced decreasing wages between 2013 and 2014, the only group to experience such losses (BLS, 2014c).

Those emigrating to the United States from other countries generally earn less than native-born members of the workforce. Although the flow of unauthorized immigrants slowed during the economic downturn of 2008, the United States has in excess of 11 million immigrants without official documentation (Passel et al., 2014). In 2014, the median usual weekly earnings of foreign-born were $664, compared with $820 for workers born in the United States (BLS, 2014b).

As would be expected, those with more education earn significantly more than those with less education. Figure 7.5 displays the dramatic impact that education has on earning potential. For example, those with bachelor's degrees earn 2.4 times as much, and those with an advanced degree earn 2.8 times as much, as those with less than a high school diploma (BLS, 2014). Perhaps even more importantly, returns on investments in

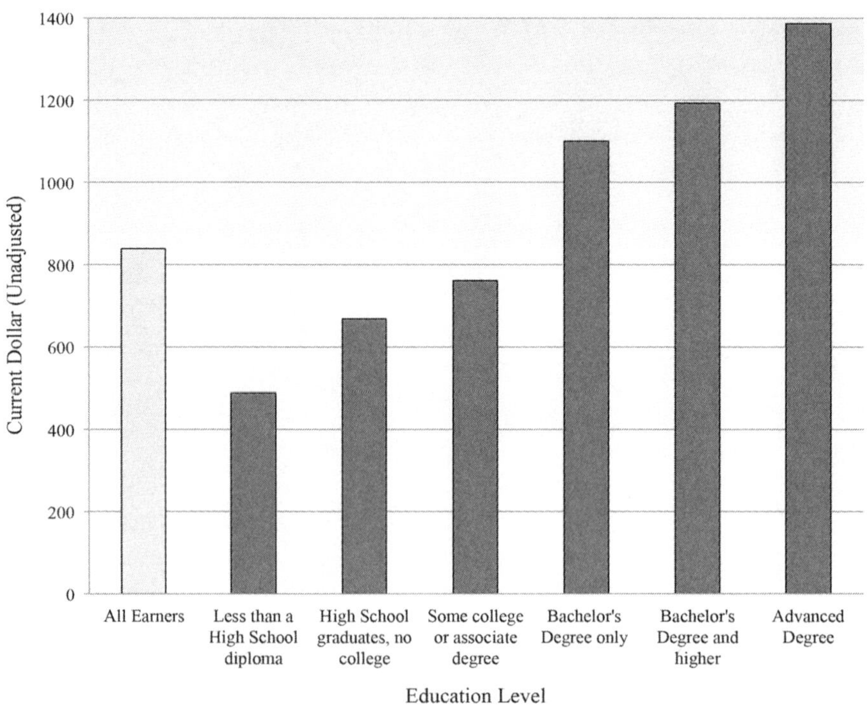

Figure 7.5 Median usual weekly earnings, by education, 2014. (BLS, 2014)

education vary substantially by gender, race and ethnicity, and socioeconomic status. For example, even though women are more likely than men to complete high school, B.A., M.A., and most PhD degrees, they often receive substantially less than equally educated men. Women with less than a high school diploma earn 81 percent, with a BA earn 78 percent, with an MA earn 74 percent, and with a PhD earn 79 percent of what comparably educated men earn (BLS, 2014a).

Not all jobs are good jobs. Some provide high salaries and generous fringe benefits, while others provide neither. The financial crisis of 2008 led to a recession, decreased demands for labor, and a sluggish recovery. It also led to the creation of more bad jobs. Fewer jobs hold the promise of long-term commitment on the part of the employer. Rising numbers of bad jobs with short-term work arrangements in the temporary work industry have generated low pay, low benefit, and low-security jobs (Quinlan, Mayhew, & Bohle, 2001; Kalleberg, 2013). These bad jobs change the landscape for workers of all ages by increasing the supply of low wage and unstable work. Their impact is even greater, however, for older workers because it is within that context that they make decisions about whether to work or retire (Clarke et al., 2007; Cahill, Giandrea, & Quinn, 2012).

Major globalization trends have been impacting U.S. workers through vast economic, technological, legal, and political changes (Sauter et al., 2002; Phillipson, 2004a, 2004b, 2013). These changes not only influence labor-force participation rates (Downs et al., 2006), but they have redefined the types of work available and the way work is organized. Increasingly liberal trade regulations have given rise to more global operations, intensifying competition, and tightening labor markets. For workforce members, declines in manufacturing jobs and changing technologies have led to the development of a menu of lower-paying jobs, mostly in the service sector. Many of these jobs are devoid of meaning or satisfaction while at the same time posing health and safety risks. Amidst rapid deunionization, corporations have become more intent on reengineering their business processes to shed experienced workers in favor of just-in-time hiring, favoring flexibility over retention (Cappelli, 1995). So, both middle-aged and older workers face problems maintaining wages and increasing job insecurity (Cahill et al., 2012). Even through median usual weekly earnings have been slowly increasing, substantial numbers of workers of all ages are not able to garner a living wage (Leigh, 2012). Experts fear that the proliferation of low-wage jobs may become fixed at a level that has not been evident since before the Great Depression. In the New Economy, incomes have been rising and more people are working, but patterns of inequality are striking, and there is little discussion of implementing policies that would protect workers from the rising insecurities of the New Economy.

Theoretical Links between Work, Retirement, Health, and Well-Being

The relationship between work and retirement on health is central to individual, family, and community life. Research on this relationship requires the assistance of many fields and a wide variety of theoretical gazes. Ideally, information should flow freely between the biological sciences such as epidemiology, medicine, environmental science, and the social sciences such as psychology, sociology, and political economy. Taken together, these professional domains clarify the socioeconomic and political pathways between the economy, work organization, work and retirement patterns, and health.

Many researchers have adopted a rosy picture that older workers have better physical health, mental health, and more meaning in their lives by working longer (Butrica, 2011; Freund & Baltes, 1998). These empirical studies demonstrate that older workers experience improved well-being and stave off physical, cognitive, and mental health declines by remaining in the workforce longer (Soumerai & Avorn, 1983; Mein et al., 2003; Andel et al., 2007; Wickrama et al., 1997, 2013). There is evidence that prolonged work life and gradual retirement increase sense of control and increase future happiness (Calvo, Haverstick, & Sass, 2009). For example, Successful Aging theories emphasize how older people might maximize the potential of the golden years (Baltes & Smith, 2003; Robson & Hansson, 2007). Selection, optimization, and compensation theories advance similar arguments (Abraham & Hansson, 1995; Unson & Richardson, 2013). From these perspectives, lengthening labor-force attachment and engagement tends to lengthen healthier and more productive living.

Not all researchers' findings create such optimism about the links between work and old-age health and well-being, particularly in light of the cumulative effects of certain types of work on health over time. Among those raising questions about older workers' occupational health, some have relied upon epidemiological traditions (Kuh et al., 2003). Others have drawn from more sociological traditions (George, 1993; Mirowsky & Ross, 1999; Elder, Johnson, & Crosnoe, 2003; Dannefer, 2003) and from demographical standpoints (McDonough and Berglund, 2003). Longitudinal cohort studies have given rise to important findings elucidating the social determinants of health. Occupational and environmental factors do impact health over time. Much of the research regarding aging and work-related health is focused on injury rates. This data is easy to collect because it is frequently acute trauma and easily recorded and quantified. On average, older workers have lower rates of injury, but they have more severe injuries and lengthier recoveries. Falls at work are more likely to result in fractures or fatality for workers over 65 (Rogers & Wiatrowski, 2005).

The complex nature of establishing work-relatedness causes occupational disease to be underappreciated. Occupational cancers such as mesothelioma can express decades after exposure to the hazardous substance. Job type is the strongest predictor of poor occupational health outcomes in old age, and there are emerging concerns about older workers who increasingly work in service sectors especially because of the financial vulnerability an injury may cause (Zwerling et al., 1996; Kenny et al., 2008; Bohle, Pitts, & Quinlan, 2010). Because work-related illness and injury must be considered in the context of a life history, longitudinal work in these areas is especially important for determining the impact of work on health for the long term.

Life-course researchers have analyzed health inequalities from the perspective that "retirement is a complex process that occurs over individuals' working lives" (Szinovacz, Martin, & Davey, 2014, p. 245). Life-course research emphasizes trajectories and supports the idea that decisions are embedded deeply in contextuality. Life-course researchers think about work and retirement decisions in terms of pivotal junctures. For example, they examine the way unexpected poor health, changing options emanating from the employer, and historical and/or economic events such as the Great Recession influence the retirement experience (Dannefer, 2003; Moen, 1996; Szinovacz et al., 2014). From the life-course approach, "individuals' retirement plans will balance a lifetime of retirement preferences with the mandates of current events both at the individual and societal levels" (Szinovacz et al., 2014, p. 246). Empirical studies on work and health find that wealth accumulation and upward social mobility are inversely related to the incidence of coronary heart disease (Hallqvist et al., 2004; Loucks et al., 2009). Chronic pain, on the other hand, is related to lower socioeconomic status and manual work (Lacey, Belcher, & Croft, 2013). Certainly occupational trajectories have critical life junctures and cumulative effects on health, shaping worker health very differently for older workers from different socioeconomic classes.

Finally, gerontologists examine power relations originating from political and economic frameworks to more fully explain gerontological patterns. While many studies focus intently and almost exclusively on econometric measures, critical theorists examine social location and social stratification to question the status quo. By considering the impacts of global changes on local economies (Calasanti, 2002), work in these areas not only acknowledges the inherent disempowerment found in the heterogeneous workforce, but also acknowledges the interdependence of formal and informal economies, migration patterns, and the impact of profit-seeking policies of private business on local working populations (Estes, 2001; Estes & Phillipson, 2002; Phillipson, 2013). With regard to analyzing the impact of work and retirement on health and well-being, gerontologists identify sources of alienation and changing social structures that foster displacement and marginalization of vulnerable groups. They explore how macrolevel political and economic decisions shape individual-level physical, mental, and social well-being. These theorists generally view redistributive features of economic programs like Social Security as essential policies for offsetting the inequalities generated by the labor market and for supporting an aging population in need of material means to prevent deep poverty and poor health (Quadagno, 2004; Harrington Meyer & Herd, 2007; Harrington Meyer, 2013).

The Occupational Health of Older Workers

Work in middle and old age can be good for health, but that is certainly not always the case. Work has the potential to provide deep engagement, social identity, and basic satisfaction. Generally older Americans are in better health than they have been at any time in history and many are considered healthy enough to work. However, many researchers have questioned just how healthy work is at old ages. How do aging, health, and work intersect (Behncke, 2012; Bohle et al., 2008; Bohle, Pitts, & Quinlan, 2010)? Health inequalities are systematically being created or reinforced because older workers are working more frequently in low-wage work, and education levels limit work opportunities (Baron et al., 2014; Zajacova, Montez, & Herd, 2014). Older workers face a plethora of common worrisome circumstances. High quality of work life is not guaranteed as older workers face changes in technology with accompanying skill set requirements. Often poor attitudes toward older workers and outright discrimination persist in the workplace (Posthuma & Campion, 2009; Roscigno et al., 2007; McMullin & Bereger, 2006). Though older workers tend to work safer, when they are injured, recovery is slower (Wegman, 1999; Wegman & McGee, 2004; Silverstein, 2008). Older workers often manage multiple chronic health concerns such as arthritis or depression while on the job (Lee & Smith, 2009). Low-wage work picked up for extra income in retirement can be demeaning or dangerous. Most occupational health researchers suggest that accommodation is a necessary component of keeping older workers in the labor force. Too often, the workplace creates or sustains health inequalities, and meaningful accommodation of older workers may not be a high priority for employers.

Remaining engaged in the labor force has many important potential benefits. Some remain in lifelong careers, while others change careers entirely. The later practice, known as creating encore careers, is growing increasingly popular as an exit strategy. In any case, working during older ages brings generativity and social ties (MorBarak, 1995; Freedman, 2006). Creating alternative income streams often provides new flexibility in later life (Platman 2004; McNamara et al., 2012, 2013). Work gives identity, and attachment to work is often reassessed in the complex process of retirement (Strangleman, 2012). Satisfaction may come from the realization that the workers' lengthy experience may be valuable to their employer given that it helps the company to retain knowledge that might otherwise be lost (Voelpel & Dous, 2006). Providing assistance in the employer's transition to the next generation is likely beneficial to all involved (Taylor et al., 2010). Finally, adapting to the ever-changing demands of the workplace may create new challenges and new types of activities that are highly valued (Moen, Flood, & Louis, 2011).

Older workers with lower socioeconomic status have greater economic incentives to remain working past traditional retirement age, but they tend to be in worse health and have less healthy work options available to them. Less-advantaged workers tend to have higher rates of chronic conditions including arthritis and heart disease, mobility problems, and mental health problems such as depression (Smith, Bielecky, & Mustard, 2012). Moreover, lower-paying jobs tend to include more physical stress and strain, repetition, supervision, and other characteristics that can take a toll on health (Krause, Scherzer, & Rugulies, 2005). In recent decades, the quality of low-wage work has diminished as union influence waned and the economy reconfigured. This combination set the stage for increased health and safety risks at a time when older people began to work even longer (Mulatu & Schooler, 1999; Mutchler et al., 1999; Quinlan, Mayhew, & Bohle, 2001; Pransky, Benjamin, & Savageau, 2005; Peeters & van Emmerik, 2008). Given their reliance on high turnover to keep wages low, employers of low-wage workers have few incentives to create workplaces that accommodate older workers (Head et al., 2006). Older workers are often viewed as problems to be managed properly (Morrow, 2011; Brooke & Taylor, 2005). Aging workers under chronic financial strain are already at risk for poorer physical and mental health and reliance on low-wage work may exacerbate that tendency.

Older workers with higher socioeconomic status may have less financial incentive to keep working at old ages, but they tend to have better health and healthier options for work. Indeed, occupational health is not experienced equally across socioeconomic groups and those from higher classes have a decided health advantage (Steege et al., 2014; Baron et al., 2014). In 2008, some estimate that 73 percent of those who had retired or were not working for some other reason were actually healthy enough to work (Hayutin et al., 2013). Because a high percentage of workers entering their 60s remain healthy enough to work, even more older men and women may elect to remain employed longer (Hayutin, Beals, & Borges, 2013). Of less concern are those whose life paths have afforded them education and attainment in ways that enhance their approach to health and aging (Ross & Wu, 1996). These are workforce members who have numerous work and retirement options (Cahill, Giandrea, & Quinn, 2006) and may freely elect to make decisions about continuing to work in well-paying jobs with elevated social benefits. The relatively affluent person may see a convergence of good health, pleasing opportunities for generating later stages of life. The three planes of their health, work, and aging are intersecting well for them (Kim & Durden, 2007), whereas those who have accumulated less advantage face fewer options.

Older workers are more vulnerable than younger workers to layoffs and firings during economic downturns and that may adversely affect psychological well-being (Hao, 2008; Dave, Rashad, & Spasojevic, 2008). Older workers were hit hard by the recent recessionary period. Almost 13 million workers were displaced from their jobs between 2009 and 2012. Older workers comprised nearly 20 percent; however, only 15 percent were reemployed (BLS, 2014d). Recurring involuntary job loss is deleterious to mental health, bringing on persistent depression (Gallo et al., 2003, 2006) and/or increasing alcohol consumption (Gallo et al., 2001). Work is thought to be protective against depression (Christ et al., 2007), cognitive declines, memory loss (Wickrama et al., 2013), intellectual functioning (Schooler, Mulau, & Oates, 1999), and cognition. That said, the impact of work depends on primary lifetime occupation (Frisoni et al., 2007; Andel et al., 2007). There is little doubt that working longer in meaningful and rewarding positions, for those who are healthy enough, stimulates social connection, reduces physical decline, and increases mental acuity. Though it is also clear that working for pay is not the only way to generate these gains. It some instances, volunteering or caregiving may be as effective (Moen et al., 2011; Moen, Robinson, & Fields, 1994) and more accommodating.

The benefits to working in old age may be elusive, however, for those who are unable to secure or retain employment. Older workers may be particularly valuable to employers, but their labor-force attachments may be tenuous because employers may be reluctant to train them properly. Recent findings indicate that while older workers are more loyal, conscientious, and possess strong interpersonal skills, these soft skills are not valued as highly as hard skills such as technical knowledge or ability to produce specific deliverables required by the job. Many employers prefer to hire younger workers (Brooke et al., 2013). More comprehensive technological training would enhance the ability of older workers to remain engaged and to reap the associated health rewards. Experts emphasize the need for employers to develop appropriate training models for the intergenerational transfer of technology (Lazazzara, Karpinska, & Henkens, 2013), particularly related to Internet use, product adoption, information environment, and skill acquisition among older workers (Nair, Czaja, & Sharit, 2007; Sharit et al., 2008).

Accommodating Aging Workers

Understanding what it means to accommodate older workers in the workplace is in its infancy even though simple solutions might enhance the work experience. Specific forms of accommodation may include changes to workplace lighting to account for normal changes in vision among older workers; recognizing that older workers may require elder care rather than childcare; or allowing more frequent opportunities to work from a seated rather than standing position (Head et al., 2006; Hill et al., 2008; Lynch, 2012). Occupational health risks faced by older workers are challenging to measure. Aging itself is a highly variable process and reductions in capacities are often compensated for by efficient use of resources and well-established skills. It is not surprising that jobs requiring heavy lifting produce the highest injury rates with increasing age. Falls from the level are more likely in older workers (Kenny et al., 2008; Wegman & McGee, 2004). Common work arrangements such as contingency work or shift work have caused increased risks (Costa & Di Milia, 2008). Certain fields, such as construction, agriculture, and/or truck driving, generate problems for older workers (Choi, 2009; Arcury et al., 2014). Physical and cognitive changes predispose older workers to injury, but poor work organization or working conditions also create preventable exposures. Meeting the physical, mental, and social demands of any given job leads to better health outcomes for older workers.

Although workers of all ages have similar occupational health and safety issues, older workers sustain fewer injuries. However, when they become injured, older workers are more likely to sustain fatal injuries and more severe injuries (Kenny et al., 2008; Algarni et al., 2015). In addition, older workers require longer recovery times and therefore have poorer return-to-work rates than younger workers (Kiss, DeMeester, & Braeckman, 2008). Occupational health issues may be harder to address especially if access to quality medical care and strong advocacy is not in place to support a full recovery and return to meaningful work (Crook & Moldofsky, 1994; Kisner & Pratt, 1999; Bailer et al., 2003). The development of an illness or injury that is related to work puts in motion a cascade of financial, personal, and work-related stressors. These concerns are especially burdensome because workers' compensation systems are extremely difficult to navigate (Lax & Klein, 2008; Kilgour et al., 2015). Studies entertaining all aspects of health—social, psychological, behavioral, and ecological—give reason for caution. Working longer may negatively impact short- and long-term health when there is risk of injury or work-related illnesses (Mulatu & Schooler, 1999; Kenny et al., 2008).

The case of arthritis highlights the necessity for occupational health professionals to engage in problem solving around chronic diseases common in old age. The prevalence of arthritis reaches 50 percent for persons aged 65 and older (Caban-Martinez et al., 2011). Arthritis is marked by progressively worsening pain and inflammation of the joints, deleteriously affecting employment rates (Allaire, Al Heresh, & Keysor, 2013). Many musculoskeletal problems in older workers are work-related, while most arthritis cases are probably not caused by work but may be exacerbated by working conditions. Assessing the impact of work on health in older workers requires careful attention to working conditions and accurate assessment of work-relatedness of common conditions like arthritis. Arthritis is related to increased job strain, increased job instability, and negative workplace experiences that may affect men differently than women (Gignac et al., 2013). Workers sometimes work long after it would have been in their best interests to stop working.

Old age is not considered a disability covered under the Americans with Disabilities Act (ADA), but older workers would benefit from attention to accommodation (Head et al., 2006; Vickerstaff, Phillipson, & Wilkie, 2013). In 1967, the Age Discrimination in Employment Act was signed into law, protecting workers aged 40–65. The ADEA protects certain applicants and employees 40 years of age and older from discrimination on the basis of age in hiring, promotion, discharge, compensation, or terms, conditions, or privileges of employment. Prior to the enactment of ADEA, it was legal to discriminate against workers on the basis of age. Many companies had mandatory retirement ages and workers were forced to retire regardless of their abilities. The 1986 amendment to the ADEA eliminated the upper age limit, effectively halting mandatory retirement except for a few select occupations. The ADEA does not require accommodations for age-related needs in the same way that the ADA does for disabilities, but it does prohibit employer policies that may appear to be age neutral but which may have a disparate impact on older workers. For example, older workers tend to have lower tolerance for heat and may therefore require more breaks than younger workers in a hot working environment. However, the protection afforded by the ADEA is difficult to obtain, since a complaint would need to be filed with the EEOC, and the process for obtaining relief is likely to be complex and prolonged. ADEA cases have generally involved hiring or firing and the case law on workplace accommodations is not well developed.

Accommodation includes attention to a wide range of factors influencing the quality of work life such as work arrangements, job attributes, organizational climate, safety culture, job security, and work-life balance. Adjustments can lead to the retention of older workers and improve the health by reducing long-term health and disability (Sauter, Streit, & Hanseman, 2009; Reinhardt, Wahrendorf, & Siegrist, 2013). Realizing that older people may be readily accommodated, researchers assess work design and redesign (Sauter, Streit, & Hanseman, 2009; Sharit & Czaja, 2012). Significant gaps in our understanding of the physiological, biomechanical, and psychosocial elements affecting older workers (Wegman & McGee, 2004) must be addressed.

Redefining the Process of Retirement

Retirement is constantly being redefined. The earliest conceptions were more focused on retirement as a status, while modern expectations for retirement evoke a protracted stage of life with good health enjoyed in the absence of work-related responsibilities. Over time, the concept of retirement has changed in many other ways as well. Notably, it has evolved from a milestone event to a bridging process that takes place over a period of time. Retirement decisions are characterized by pushes and pulls usually centered on fairly obvious financial trade-offs. These factors have been shaped and reshaped by social, economic, and political contexts over the last several decades. Retirees' decisions about retirement continue to be impacted by a changing employment landscape and increasingly diverse types of living arrangements.

In, "Rethinking Retirement," Melissa Hardy (2011) describes how retirement has been conceptualized over several decades. In 1935, the United States created the Social Security system that actively encouraged older covered workers to retire. For the next few decades, various pro-retirement policies shaped a layer of protection around vulnerable elders to ensure a federal system of economic security and supportive health benefits into old age. In the 1970s, industries were providing early exit strategies through pensions. Retirement as a life event eventually became an accepted norm, especially for those who had built substantial financial security. Then in the 1980s, problems with the Social Security program began to emerge especially over the way the dependency ratio was affecting funding (Polivka & Luo, 2015; DuBoff, 1997). As more retirees took benefits, the program's fiscal challenges grew. At the same time, private pensions offered by companies began to face serious fiscal shortfalls. The United States faced a period of deindustrialization, growing service economies, and growing legions of retirees drawing benefits. As public and private pensions retrenched, retirement became less of an event and more of a process. Some older workers took retirement packages rather than face unemployment while others were simply displaced or laid off. As the U.S. economy shifted, so did the process of retiring.

Since the 1990s, prowork policies have dominated policy shifts and are of major importance to organized labor, employers, and the government especially because they have been "transferring risks from employers and government to workers" (McNamara, Sano, & Williamson, 2012). The elimination of mandatory retirement ages served as a prowork strategy. Examples of other prowork policies that shifted risks during the 1990s include the relaxation of the Social Security earnings test, which encourages income even among beneficiaries, and the trend away from defined-benefit pensions and toward defined-contribution pensions, which shifts investment risks from companies to individuals making them less financially secure as they approach old age (McNamara, Sano, & Williamson, 2012).

Most retirees now face complex retirement decisions highly dependent on financial literacy. Transitions to retirement now included bridge employment and returning to work after retirement. For some, these blurred lines may have provided a kind of weaning from satisfying work roles by responding to desires for flexible employment arrangements; however, for others these transitions were driven by narrowing opportunities. Aging workers make retirement decisions in the face of skill obsolescence and corporate downsizing. Some employers strive to retain older workers through accommodation, but others rely on job insecurity in the labor market to pressure workers to remain in stressful jobs (Phillipson, 2013).

The process of retirement is clearly influenced by economic contexts, but it is far from being unidimensional. Ideas about retirement form over the entire working lifetime and are embedded in family circumstances, institutional factors, and more general social norms (Clark & Mitchell, 2005; Ekerdt, Kosloski, & DeViney, 2000). Expected retirement age shifted later with the concern over the economic downturn, but also was influenced by other factors such as individual debt, work conditions, work arrangements, ADL limitations, and spouse's work status (Dew & Yorgason, 2010; Szinovacz, Davey, & Martin, 2014). For some, remaining in the workforce longer creates positive gains from multiple social attachments and roles that provide opportunities for mastery and work/family enhancement. Often work simply becomes too physically demanding, other caregiving responsibilities take precedence over working, or the older worker is marginalized at the workplace and feels pressured to leave. Retirement planning involves an array of decisions driven by balancing financial needs, social opportunities, and institutional constraints.

The experience of retirement is highly gendered (Moen, 1996, 2005). Retirement timing often takes into account partner's retirement and care work responsibilities. Indeed, marital status influences retirement as spouses attempt to synchronize their work and family life (Svinovacz & DeViney, 2000; Szinovacz & Davey, 2005). Whether married or single, older men and women make decisions within the context of financial obligations, care needs of the family, traditional social roles, and great disparities in health and income.

Women have been consistently more involved with care work and domestic responsibilities and frequently occupy lower-paying positions relative to men. Since they have not been able to garner strong enough financial security due to less labor-force participation over their life course, many are working after age 65 to catch up. Intentions to continue working beyond retirement age are rooted in circumstances emerging from the midlife years (Shacklock, Brunetto, & Nelson, 2009; Damman, Henkens, & Kalmijn, 2011, 2013). Retirement takes on different meanings and levels of satisfaction based on domestic contexts (Loretto & Vickerstaff, 2013; Smith & Moen, 2004).

The average retirement age has been stable for the last decade at age 64 for men and 62 for women (Munnell, 2015). Over 41 million retired workers are drawing Social Security Retirement benefits. Today's preretirees have a different landscape in which to make their retirement decisions. Women are less financially prepared for retirement than men (Wang & Scultz, 2010). Blacks and Latinos also retire with fewer savings than whites (Rhee, 2013). Poor health strongly motivates people to leave the workforce (McGarry, 2002); however, some work longer because they enjoy their work or desire to engage in a new type of career or entrepreneurial pursuit. Others report that they plan to retire later due to immediate financial constraint, persistent debts, or concerns about the inadequacy of Social Security benefits (Greenhouse, 2013). Often disability in one spouse prompts retirement, but for those in good health, longevity provides a stage for a period of reevaluation of personal and financial goals. There is evidence that voluntary transitions over time promote enhanced self-efficacy and life satisfaction over involuntary and fixed retirement schemes (Dingemans & Henkens, 2015). As expected, those with greater economic resources and better health tend to report greater satisfaction during retirement; those with fewer economic resources and poorer health face greater challenges.

Discussion

Americans are working longer than ever before, and the health and economic impacts of these trends, vary significantly by age, gender, race, ethnicity, and nativity. The relationship between work and health over the life course continues to be challenging as aging individuals make decisions in an ever-changing employment landscape. Working into the later decades of life may have numerous positive benefits on health and well-being for those with good enough health and good enough employment options. But for those for whom health is already compromised, and for whom jobs are physically or emotionally demanding, the impact on health may indeed be negative. More work is needed by researchers and employers alike to understand the needs of older workers and the best ways to accommodate them. Moreover, as key economic and political factors have changed, so has the practice and meaning of retirement. More changes are expected in the decades ahead.

Retirement has been redesigned. It has achieved a fluidity that blurs traditional career stages. This reworking of a historic work status raises significant policy questions with relevance to many disciplines at the intersection of aging, work, and health. Examining the current economic contexts with the accompanying proliferation of low-wage work and noting strong concerns about the occupational health of older workers, this chapter considered how the aging workforce is redefining work and retirement. Attention was paid to critical gerontology, the life-course paradigm, and public health lenses.

As political and economic pressures mount to keep people working longer, it will be increasingly important to keep in mind that the United States has never kept an aging workforce engaged under current economic and social conditions. On the one hand, for many, cumulative disadvantages in the form of chronic comorbidities, decreased wealth attainment, and poor occupational choices may prove highly burdensome. On the other hand, with good accommodation practices, working longer may be an attractive option leading to increased health and meaning in later life, greater social integration, and maximized financial security. If we value elders intrinsically, then more meaningful futures in both work and retirement arenas could be crafted by identifying and rectifying significant gaps that exist in the knowledge about workplace accommodation, about how aging workers acquire skills, and how to engage the older workers' voice in the formation of retirement options.

References

Abraham, J. D., & Hansson, R. O. (1995). Successful aging at work: An applied study of selection, optimization, and compensation through impression management. *Journals of Gerontology, Series B: Psychological Sciences and Social Sciences*, *50*(2), 94–103.

Algarni, F. S., Gross, D. P., Senthilselvan, A., & Battie, M. C. (2015). Ageing workers with work-related musculoskeletal injuries. *Occupational Medicine (London)*, 65(3), 229–237. doi:10.1093/occmed/kqu213

Allaire, S. J., AlHeresh, R., & Keysor, J. J. (2013). Effect of arthritis and other rheumatic conditions on employment. *Work: A Journal of Prevention Assessment & Rehabilitation*, *45*(3), 417–420. doi:10.3233/wor-131629

Andel, R., Kareholt, I., Parker, M. G., Thorslund, M., & Gatz, M. (2007). Complexity of primary lifetime occupation and cognition in advanced old age. *Journal of Aging and Health*, *19*(3), 397–415. doi:10.1177/0898264307300171

Arcury, T. A., Grzywacz, J. G., Chen, H., Mora, D. C., & Quandt, S. A. (2014). Work organization and health among immigrant women: Latina manual workers in North Carolina. *American Journal of Public Health*, *104*(12), 2445–2452. doi:10.2105/ajph.2013.301587

Bailer, A. J., Bena, J. F., Stayner, L. T., Halperin, W. E., & Park, R. M. (2003). External cause-specific summaries of occupational fatal injuries. Part II: An analysis of years of potential life lost. *American Journal of Industrial Medicine*, *43*(3), 251–261. doi:10.1002/ajim.10190

Baltes, P. B., & Smith, J. (2003). New frontiers in the future of aging: From successful aging of the young old to the dilemmas of the fourth age. *Gerontology*, *49*(2), 123–135. doi:10.1159/000067946

Baron, S. L., Beard, S., Davis, L. K., Delp, L., Forst, L., Kidd-Taylor, A., . . . Welch, L. S. (2014). Promoting integrated approaches to reducing health inequities among low-income workers: Applying a social ecological framework. *American Journal of Industrial Medicine*. doi:0.1002/ajim.22174

Behncke, S. (2012). Does retirement trigger ill health? *Health Economics*, *21*(3), 282–300. doi:10.1002/hec.1712

Bohle, P., Di Milia, L., Fletcher, A., & Rajaratnam, S. (2008). Introduction: Aging and the multifaceted influences on adaptation to working time. *Chronobiology International*, *25*, 155–164.

Bohle, P., Pitts, C., & Quinlan, M. (2010). Time to call it quits? The safety and health of older workers. *International Journal of Health Services*, *40*(1), 23–41.

Brooke, L., & Taylor, P. (2005). Older workers and employment: Managing age relations. *Ageing and Society*, *25*, 415–429. doi:10.1017/s0144686x05003466

Brooke, E., Taylor, P., McLoughlin, C., & Di Biase, T. I. A. (2013). Managing the working body: Active ageing and limits to the "flexible" firm. *Ageing and Society*, *33*(8), 1295–1314. doi:http://dx.doi.org/10.1017/S0144686X12000426

Bureau of Labor Statistics. (2013). Foreign-born workers: Labor force characteristics 2013. http://www.bls.gov/news.release/pdf/forbrn.pdf

Bureau of Labor Statistics. (2014a). Displaced workers summary. http://www.bls.gov/news.release/disp.nr0.htm

Bureau of Labor Statistics. (2014b). Foreign-born workers: Labor force characteristics 2014. http://www.bls.gov/news.release/pdf/forbrn.pdf

Bureau of Labor Statistics (2014c). Highlights of women's earnings in 2013. Report 1051. http://www.bls.gov/opub/reports/cps/highlights-of-womens-earnings-in-2013.pdf

Bureau of Labor Statistics. (2014d). Labor force statistics from the Current Population Survey. http://www.bls.gov/cps/cpsaat37.htm

Bureau of Labor Statistics (2014e). U.S. Census Bureau, Current Population Survey. Annual Social and Economic Supplement.

Butrica, B. (2011). Making a case for working longer at older ages. *Public Policy & Aging Report*, *21*(2), 22–26. doi:10.1093/ppar/21.2.22

Caban-Martinez, A.J., Lee, D.J., Fleming, L.E., Tancredi, D.J., Arheart, K.L., LeBlanc, W.G., . . . Muennig, P.A. (2011). Arthritis, occupational class, and the aging US workforce. *American Journal of Public Health*, *101*(9), 1729–1734. doi:10.2105/AJPH.2011.300173

Cahill, K.E., Giandrea, M.D., & Quinn, J.F. (2006). Retirement patterns from career employment. *Gerontologist*, *46*(4), 514–523.

Cahill, K.E., Giandrea, M.D., & Quinn, J.F. (2012). Older workers and short-term jobs: Patterns and determinants. *Monthly Labor Review*, *135*(5), 19–32.

Cahill, K.E., Pitt-Catsouphes, M., McNamara, T.K., & Valcour, M. (2012). Employment experiences of older workers in the context of shifts in the national economy. *Gerontologist*, *52*, 676.

Calasanti, T.P. (2002). Work and retirement in the 21st century: Integrating issues of diversity and globalization. *Ageing International*, *27*(3), 3–20. doi:10.1007/s12126-003-1000-1

Calvo, E., Haverstick, K., & Sass, S.A. (2009). Gradual retirement, sense of control, and retirees' happiness. *Research on Aging*, *31*(1), 112–135. doi:10.1177/0164027508324704

Cappelli, P. (1995). Rethinking employment. *British Journal of Industrial Relations*, *33*(4), 563–602.

Choi, S.D. (2009). Safety and ergonomic considerations for an aging workforce in the US construction industry. *Work*, *33*(3), 307–315. doi:10.3233/wor-2009-0878

Christ, S.L., Lee, D.J., Fleming, L.E., LeBlanc, W.G., Arheart, K.L., Chung-Bridges, K., . . . McCollister, K.E. (2007). Employment and occupation effects on depressive symptoms in older Americans: Does working past age 65 protect against depression? *The Journals of Gerontology, Series B: Psychological Sciences and Social Sciences*, *62*(6), S399–S403.

Clark, R.L., & Mitchell, O.S. (2005). *Reinventing the retirement paradigm*. New York; Oxford, UK: Oxford University Press.

Clarke, M., Lewchuk, W., de Wolff, A., & King, A. (2007). 'This just isn't sustainable': Precarious employment, stress and workers' health. *International Journal of Law and Psychiatry*, *30*(4–5), 311–326. doi:10.1016/j.ijlp.2007.06.005

Costa, G., & Di Milia, L. (2008). Aging and shift work: A complex problem to face. *Chronobiology International: The Journal of Biological & Medical Rhythm Research*, *25*(2/3), 165–181.

Crook, J., & Moldofsky, H. (1994). The probability of recovery and return to work from work disability as a function of time. *Quality of Life Research*, *3*(Suppl. 1), S97–S109.

Damman, M., Henkens, K., & Kalmijn, M. (2011). The impact of midlife educational, work, health, and family experiences on men's early retirement. *The Journals of Gerontology, Series B: Psychological Sciences and Social Sciences*, *66B*(5), 617–627. doi:10.1093/geronb/gbr092

Damman, M., Henkens, K., & Kalmijn, M. (2013). Late-career work disengagement: The role of proximity to retirement and career experiences. *The Journals* of Gerontology Series B: Psychological Sciences and Social Sciences, 68(3), 455–463. doi:10.1093/geronb/gbt001

Dannefer, D. (2003). Cumulative advantage/disadvantage and the life course: Cross-fertilizing age and social science theory. *Journals of Gerontology, Series B: Psychological Sciences and Social Sciences, 58*(6), S327–S337.

Dave, D., Rashad, I., & Spasojevic, J. (2008). The effects of retirement on physical and mental health outcomes. *Southern Economic Journal, 75*(2), 497–523.

Dew, J., & Yorgason, J. (2010). Economic pressure and marital conflict in retirement-aged couples. *Journal of Family Issues, 31*(2), 164–188. doi:10.1177/0192513x09344168

Dingemans, E., & Henkens, K. (2015). How do retirement dynamics influence mental well-being in later life? A 10-year panel study. *Scandinavian Journal of Work, Environment & Health, 41*(1): 16–23.

Downs, M., Phillipson, C., Vincent, J.A., & British Society of, G. (2006). *The Futures of Old Age*. London: SAGE Publications Ltd.

DuBoff, R.B. (1997). A slippery slope: Economist and social insurance in the United States. *International Journal of Health Services, 27*(3), 297–408. doi:10.2190/1UF9-T8QC-3G3X-9KU0

Elder, G.H., Johnson, M.K., & Crosnoe, R. (2003). The emergence and development of life course theory. In J. T. Mortimer & M. J. Shanahan (Eds.), *Handbook of the life course* (pp. 3–19). New York: Kluwer Academic/Plenum Publishers.

Ekerdt, D.J., Kosloski, K., & DeViney, S. (2000). The normative anticipation of retirement by older workers. *Research on Aging, 22*(1), 3–22. doi:10.1177/0164027500221001

Estes, C.L. (2001). *Social policy & aging: A critical perspective*. Thousand Oaks, CA: Sage Publications.

Estes, C.L., & Phillipson, C. (2002). The globalization of capital, the welfare state, and old age policy. *International Journal of Health Services, 32*(2), 279–297.

Freedman, M. (2006). The social purpose encore career: Baby boomers, civic engagement, and the next stage of work. *Generations—Journal of the American Society on Aging, 30*(4), 43–46.

Freund, A.M., & Baltes, P.B. (1998). Selection, optimization, and compensation as strategies of life management: Correlations with subjective indicators of successful aging. *Psychology and Aging, 13*(4), 531–543. doi:10.1037//0882-7974.13.4.531

Frisoni, G.B., Rozzini, R., Bianchetti, A., & Trabucchi, M. (1993). Principal lifetime occupation and MMSE score in elderly persons. *Journal of Gerontology, 48*(6), S310–S314. doi:10.1093/geronj/48.6.S310

Gallo, W., Bradley, E., Dubin, J., Jones, R., Falba, T., Cramer, L., & Kasl, S. (2003). The persistence of depressive symptoms in older workers who experience involuntary job loss. *Gerontologist, 43*, 329.

Gallo, W.T., Bradley, E.H., Siegel, M., & Kasl, S.V. (2001). The impact of involuntary job loss on subsequent alcohol consumption by older workers: Findings from the health and retirement survey. *Journals of Gerontology, Series B: Psychological Sciences and Social Sciences, 56*(1), S3–S9.

Gallo, W.T., Teng, H.M., Falba, T.A., Kasl, S.V., Krumholz, H.M., & Bradley, E.H. (2006). The impact of late career job loss on myocardial infarction and stroke: A 10 year follow up using the health and retirement survey. *Occupational and Environmental Medicine, 63*(10), 683–687. doi:10.1136/oem.2006.026823

George, L.K. (1993). Sociological perspectives on life transitions. *Annual Review of Sociology, 19*, 353–373.

Gignac, M.A., Badley, E.M., Moore, L., Bowring, J., & Cao, X. (2013). The employment experience of people with arthritis: Findings from an on-line survey. *Arthritis and Rheumatism, 65*, S1221–S1221.

Greenhouse, Steven. Pushing back retirement, and not always for money. *New York Times*. March 12, 2013.

Hallqvist, J., Lynch, J., Bartley, M., Lang, T., & Blane, D. (2004). Can we disentangle life course processes of accumulation, critical period and social mobility? An analysis of disadvantaged socio-economic positions and myocardial infarction in the Stockholm Heart Epidemiology Program. *Social Science and Medicine, 58*(8), 1555–1562. doi:10.1016/s0277-9536(03)00344-7

Hao, Y. (2008). Productive activities and psychological well-being among older adults. *Journals of Gerontology, Series B: Psychological Sciences and Social Sciences, 63*(2), S64–S72.

Hardy, M. (2011). Rethinking retirement. In R. A. Settersten & J. L. Angel (Eds.) *Handbook of Sociology of Aging*. New York: Springer.

Harrington Meyer, M. (2013). Changing social security in the US: Rising insecurity? *Social Policy and Society, 12*(01), 135–146. doi:10.1017/S1474746412000486

Harrington Meyer, M., & Herd, P. (2007). *Market friendly or family friendly? The state and gender inequality in old age*. New York: Russell Sage Foundation.

Harrington Meyer, M., & Parker, W.M. (2012). The changing worlds of family and work. In R. A. Settersten & J. L. Angel (Eds.), *Handbook of sociology and aging*. New York: Springer.

Hartmann, H., Rose, S., & Lovell, V. (2006). How much progress in closing the long-term earnings gap? In Blau, F.D., Brington, M.C., & Grusky, D.B. (Eds.), *The declining significance of gender?* New York: Russell Sage Foundation.

Hayutin, A., Beals, M., & Borges, E. (2013). *The aging US workforce: A chartbook of demographic shifts*. Stanford, CA: Stanford Center on Longevity.

Hayutin, A., Beals, M., & Borges, E. (April 9, 2013). Demographics of the aging workforce—summary. Paper presented at the Stanford Center on Longevity Conference: Adapting to an Aging Workforce. Conference Proceedings, Stanford, CA.

Head, L., Baker, P.M.A., Bagwell, B., & Moon, N.W. (2006). Barriers to evidence based practice in accommodations for an aging workforce. *Work (Reading, Mass.), 27*(4), 391–396.

Hegewich, A., Ellis, E. (2015). The gender gap by occupation 2014 and by race and ethnicity. Institute for Women's Policy Research. Washington, DC.

Hill, E.J., Grzywacz, J.G., Allen, S., Blanchard, V.L., Matz-Costa, C., Shulkin, S., & Pitt-Catsouphes. (2008). Defining and conceptualizing workplace flexibility. *Community, Work and Family, 11*(2), 149–163. doi:10.1080/13668800802024678

Kalleberg, A. L. (2013). Good jobs, bad jobs: The rise of polarized and precarious employment systems in the United States, 1970s to 2000s. *Work Employment and Society, 27*(5), 896–898. doi:10.1177/0950017013480403

Kenny, G. P., Yardley, J. E., Martineau, L., & Jay, O. (2008). Physical work capacity in older adults: Implications for the aging worker. *American Journal of Industrial Medicine, 51*(8), 610–625. doi:10.1002/ajim.20600

Kilgour, E., Kosny, A., McKenzie, D., & Collie, A. (2015). Healing or harming? Healthcare provider interactions with injured workers and insurers in workers'compensation systems. *Journal of Occupational Rehabilitation, 25*(1), 220–39. doi:10.1007/s10926-014-9521-x

Kim, J., & Durden, E. (2007). Socioeconomic status and age trajectories of health. *Social Science & Medicine, 65*(12), 2489–2502. doi:10.1016/j.socscimed.2007.07.022

Kisner, S. M., & Pratt, S. G. (1999). Occupational injury fatalities among older workers in the United States, 1980–1994. *American Journal of Industrial Medicine, Supplement 1*, 24–25.

Kiss, P., De Meester, M., & Braeckman, L. (2008). Differences between younger and older workers in the need for recovery after work. *International Archives of Occupational and Environmental Health, 81*(3), 311–320. doi:10.1007/s00420-007-0215-y

Krause, N., Scherzer, T., & Rugulies, R. (2005). Physical workload, work intensification, and prevalence of pain in low wage workers: Results from a participatory research project with hotel room cleaners in Las Vegas. *American Journal of Industrial Medicine, 48*(5), 326–337.

Kuh, D., Ben-Shlomo, Y., Lynch, J., Hallqvist, J., & Power, C. (2003). Life course epidemiology. *Journal of Epidemiology and Community Health, 57*(10), 778–783.

Lacey, R. J., Belcher, J., & Croft, P. R. (2013). Does life course socio-economic position influence chronic disabling pain in older adults? A general population study. *European Journal of Public Health, 23*(4), 534–540. doi:10.1093/eurpub/cks056

Lax, M. B., & Klein, R. (2008). More than meets the eye: Social, economic, and emotional impacts of work-related injury and illness. *New Solutions: A Journal of Environmental and Occupational Health Policy, 18*(3), 343–360. doi:10.2190/NS.18.3.i

Lazazzara, A., Karpinska, K., & Henkens, K. (2013). What factors influence training opportunities for older workers? Three factorial surveys exploring the attitudes of HR professionals. *International Journal of Human Resource Management, 24*(11), 2154–2172. doi:10.1080/09585192.2012.725077

Lee, J., & Smith, J. P. (2009). Work, retirement, and depression. *Journal of Population Ageing, 2*(1–2), 57–71. doi:http://dx.doi.org/10.1007/s12062-010-9018-0

Leigh, J. P. (2012). Numbers and costs of occupational injury and illness in low-wage occupations. Center for Poverty Research and Center for Health Care Policy Research, University of California Davis.

Loretto, W., & Vickerstaff, S. (2013). The domestic and gendered context for retirement. *Human Relations, 66*(1), 65–86. doi:10.1177/0018726712455832

Loucks, E.B., Lynch, J.W., Pilote, L., Fuhrer, R., Almeida, N.D., Richard, H., . . . Benjamin, E.J. (2009). Life-course socioeconomic position and incidence of coronary heart disease. *American Journal of Epidemiology, 169*(7), 829–836. doi:10.1093/aje/kwn403

Lynch, C. (2012). *Retirement on the line: Age, work, and value in an American factory*. Ithaca, NY: Cornell University Press.

McDonough, P., & Berglund, P. (2003). Histories of poverty and self-rated health trajectories. *Journal of Health and Social Behavior, 44*(2), 198–214.

McGarry, K. (2002). Health and retirement: Do changes in health affect retirement expectations? *National Bureau of Economic Research Working Paper 9317*, Cambridge, MA.

McMullin, J.A., & Bereger, E.D. (2006). Gendered ageism/age(ed) sexism: The case of unemployed older workers. In Calasanti, T.M. & Slevin, K.F. (Eds.), *Age matters*. New York: Routledge.

McNamara, T.K., Sano, J.M., & Williamson, J.B. (2012). The pros and cons of pro-work policies and programs for older workers. In Hedge, J.W. & Borman, W.C. (Eds.), *The Oxford handbook of work and aging*. New York: Oxford University Press, Publishers.

McNamara, T.K., Brown, M., Aumann, K., Pitt-Catsouphes, M., Galinsky, E., & Bond, J.T. (2013). Working in retirement: A brief report. *Journal of Applied Gerontology, 32*(1), 120–132. doi:10.1177/0733464811408085

McNamara, T.K., Pitt-Catsouphes, M., Brown, M., & Matz-Costa, C. (2012). Access to and utilization of flexible work options. *Industrial Relations, 51*(4), 936–965. doi:10.1111/j.1468-232X.2012.00703.x

Mein, G., Martikainen, P., Hemingway, H., Stansfeld, S., & Marmot, M. (2003). Is retirement good or bad for mental and physical health functioning? Whitehall II longitudinal study of civil servants. *Journal of Epidemiology and Community Health, 57*(1), 46–49.

Mirowsky, J., & Ross, C.E. (1999). Economic hardship across the life course. *American Sociological Review, 64*(4), 548–569. doi:10.2307/2657255

Moen, P. (1996). A life course perspective on retirement, gender, and well-being. *Journal of Occupational Health Psychology, 1*(2), 131–144. doi:10.1037/1076-8998.1.2.131

Moen, P. (2005). Beyond the career mystique: "Time in," "Time out," and "Second Acts." *Sociological Forum, 20*(2), 189–208. doi:10.2307/4540892

Moen, P., Flood, S., & Louis, V. (2011). A third age of the life course? Gendered time working and volunteering, ages 50 to 75. *Gerontologist, 51*, 19–20.

Moen, P., Robison, J., & Fields, V. (1994). Women's work and caregiving roles: A life course approach. *Journals of Gerontology, 49*(4), S176–S186.

MorBarak, M.E. (1995). The meaning of work for older adults seeking employment: The generativity factor. *International Journal of Aging & Human Development, 41*(4), 325–344. doi:10.2190/vgtg-epk6-q4bh-q67q

Morrow, I.J. (2011). Managing the older worker: How to prepare for the new organizational order. *Personnel Psychology, 64*(4), 1053–1056. doi:10.1111/j.1744-6570.2011.01228_2.x

Mulatu, M.S., & Schooler, C. (1999). Longitudinal effects of occupational, psychological, and social background characteristics on health of older workers.

In N. E. Adler, Marmot, M., McEwen, B. & Stewart, J. (Eds.), *Socioeconomic status and health in industrial nations: Social, psychological, and biological pathways* (Vol. 896, pp. 406–408).

Munnell, A.J. (2015). *The average retirement age—An update.* (Report No. 15–4). Chestnut Hill, MA: Center for Retirement Research at Boston College. http://crr.bc.edu/wp-content/uploads/2015/03/IB_15–4.pdf

Mutchler, J.E., Burr, J.A., Massagli, M.P., & Pienta, A. (1999). Work transitions and health in later life. *The Journals of Gerontology, Series B: Psychological Sciences and Social Sciences, 54B*(5), S252–S261. doi:10.1093/geronb/54B.5.S252

Nair, S.N., Czaja, S.J., & Sharit, J. (2007). A multilevel modeling approach to examining individual differences in skill acquisition for a computer-based task. *Journals of Gerontology, Series B: Psychological Sciences and Social Sciences, 62*, 85–96.

Passel, Jeffrey S., Cohn, D'Vera, Krogstad, Jens Manuel, & Gonzalez-Barrera, Ana (2014). As growth stalls, unauthorized immigrant population becomes more settled. Washington, DC: Pew Research Center's Hispanic Trends Project.

Peeters, M.C.W., & van Emmerik, H. (2008). An introduction to the work and well-being of older workers—From managing threats to creating opportunities. *Journal of Managerial Psychology, 23*(4), 353–363. doi:10.1108/02693940810869006

Phillipson, C. (2004a). Older workers and retirement: Critical perspectives on the research literature and policy implications. *Social Policy and Society, 3*(02), 189–195. doi:doi:10.1017/S1474746403001659

Phillipson, C. (2004b). Work and retirement transitions: Changing sociological and social policy contexts. *Social Policy and Society, 3*(02), 155–162. doi:doi:10.1017/S1474746403001611

Phillipson, C. (2013). Commentary: The future of work and retirement. *Human Relations, 66*(1), 143–153. doi:10.1177/0018726712465453

Platman, K. (2004). 'Portfolio careers' and the search for flexibility in later life. *Work Employment and Society, 18*(3), 573–599. doi:10.1177/0950017004045551

Polivka, L., & Luo, B.Z. (2015). The neoliberal political economy and erosion of retirement security. *Gerontologist, 55*(2), 183–190.

Posthuma, R.A., & Campion, M.A. (2009). Age stereotypes in the workplace: Common stereotypes, moderators, and future research directions. *Journal of Management, 35*(1), 158–188. doi:10.1177/0149206308318617

Pransky, G.S., Benjamin, K.L., & Savageau, J.A. (2005). Early retirement due to occupational injury: Who is at risk? *American Journal of Industrial Medicine, 47*(4), 285–295. doi:10.1002/ajim.20149

Pransky, G.S., Benjamin, K.L., Savageau, J.A., Currivan, D., & Fletcher, K. (2005). Outcomes in work-related injuries: A comparison of older and younger workers. *American Journal of Industrial Medicine, 47*(2), 104–112. doi:10.1002/ajim.20122

Quadagno, J. (2004). Why the United States has no national health insurance: Stakeholder mobilization against the welfare state, 1945–1996. *Journal of Health and Social Behavior, 45 Supplement*, 25–44.

Quinlan, M., Mayhew, C., & Bohle, P. (2001). The global expansion of precarious employment, work disorganization, and consequences for occupational health: A review of recent research. *International Journal of Health Services, 31*(2), 335–414.

Reinhardt, J. D., Wahrendorf, M., & Siegrist, J. (2013). Socioeconomic position, psychosocial work environment and disability in an ageing workforce: A longitudinal analysis of SHARE data from 11 European countries. *Occupational and Environmental Medicine, 70*(3), 156–163. doi:10.1136/oemed-2012-100924

Rhee, N. (2013). Race and Retirement Insecurity in the United States. National Institute on Retirement Security. Washington, DC.

Robson, S. M., & Hansson, R. O. (2007). Strategic self development for successful aging at work. *International Journal of Aging & Human Development, 64*(4), 331–359. doi:10.2190/q303-171u-7686-8517

Rogers, E., & Wiatrowski, W. J. (2005). Injuries, illnesses, and fatalities among older workers. *Monthly Labor Review, 128*(10), 24–30.

Roscigno, V. J., Mong, S., Byron, R., & Tester, G. (2007). Age discrimination, social closure and employment. *Social Forces, 86*(1), 313–334. doi:10.1353/sof.2007.0109

Rose, S. J., & Hartmann, H. (2008). Still a man's labor market: The long-term earnings gap. Institute for Women's Policy Research, Washington, DC.

Ross, C. E., & Wu, C. L. (1996). Education, age, and the cumulative advantage in health. *Journal of Health and Social Behavior, 37*(1), 104–120. doi:10.2307/2137234

Sauter, S., Brightwell, S., Colligan, M., Hurrell, J., Katz, T., LeGrande, D., . . . Tetrick, L. (2002). The changing organization of work and the safety and health of working people: Knowledge gaps and research directions. Cincinnati, OH: National Institute for Occupational Safety and Health, Washington, DC.

Sauter, S., Streit, J., & Hanseman, D. (2009). Work organization and health in an aging workforce. In S. J. Czaja & J. Sharit (Eds.), *Aging and work: Issues and implications in a changing landscape*. Baltimore, MD: Johns Hopkins University Press.

Schooler, C., Mulatu, M. S., & Oates, G. (1999). The continuing effects of substantively complex work on the intellectual functioning of older workers. *Psychology and Aging, 14*(3), 483–506. doi:10.1037/0882-7974.14.3.483

Seghal, E. (1985). Foreign born in the U.S. labor market: The results of a special survey. *Monthly Labor Review, 108*(7):18–24.

Shacklock, K., Brunetto, Y., & Nelson, S. (2009). The different variables that affect older males' and females' intentions to continue working. *Asia Pacific Journal of Human Resources, 47*(1), 79–101. doi:10.1177/1038411108099291

Shaefer, L. (2009). Part-time workers: Some key differences between primary and secondary earners. *Monthly Labor Review, 132*(10). http://www.bls.gov/opub/mlr/2009/10/art1full.pdf.

Sharit, J., & Czaja, S. J. (2012). Job design and redesign for older workers. In J. W. Hedge & W. C. Borman (Eds.), *The Oxford handbook of work and aging*. Oxford: Oxford University Press.

Sharit, J., Hernandez, M. A., Czaja, S. J., & Pirolli, P. (2008). Investigating the roles of knowledge and cognitive abilities in older adult information seeking on the Web. *ACM Transactions on Computer-Human Interaction, 15*(1). doi:10.1145/1352782.1352785

Silverstein, M. (2008). Meeting the challenges of an aging workforce. *American Journal of Industrial Medicine, 51*(4), 269–280. doi:10.1002/ajim.20569

Smith, D. B., & Moen, P. (2004). Retirement satisfaction for retirees and their spouses—Do gender and the retirement decision-making process matter? *Journal of Family Issues, 25*(2), 262–285. doi:10.1177/0192513x03257366

Smith, P., Bielecky, A., & Mustard, C. (2012). The relationship between chronic conditions and work-related injuries and repetitive strain injuries in Canada. *Journal of Occupational and Environmental Medicine, 54*(7), 841–846. doi:10.1097/JOM.0b013e31824e11f7

Soumerai, S. B., & Avorn, J. (1983). Perceived health, life satisfaction, and activity in urban elderly: A controlled study of the impact of part-time work. *Journal of Gerontology, 38*(3), 356–362. doi:10.1093/geronj/38.3.356

Steege, A. L., Baron, S. L., Marsh, S. M., Menéndez, C. C., & Myers, J. R. (2014). Examining occupational health and safety disparities using national data: A cause for continuing concern. *American Journal of Industrial Medicine, 57*(5), 527–38. doi:10.1002/ajim.22297

Strangleman, T. (2012). Work identity in crisis? Rethinking the problem of attachment and loss at work. *Sociology, 46*(3), 411–425. doi:10.1177/0038038511422585

Szinovacz, M. E., & Davey, A., (2005). Retirement and marital decision making: Effects on retirement satisfaction. *Journal of Marriage and Family, 67*(2), 387–398. doi:10.1111/j.0022-2445.2005.00123.x

Svinovacz, M. E., & DeViney, S. (2000). Marital characteristics and retirement decisions. *Research on Aging, 22*, 479–489.

Szinovacz, M. E., Davey, A., & Martin, L. (2014). Did the Great Recession influence retirement plans? *Research on Aging*. doi:10.1177/0164027514530171

Szinovacz, M. E., Martin, L., & Davey, A. (2014). Recession and expected retirement age: Another look at the evidence. *The Gerontologist, 54*(2), 245–257. doi:10.1093/geront/gnt010

Taylor, P., Brooke, L., McLoughlin, C., & Di Biase, T. (2010). Older workers and organizational change: Corporate memory versus potentiality. *International Journal of Manpower, 31*(3), 374–386. doi:10.1108/01437721011050639

Toossi, M. (2013). Labor force projections to 2022: The labor force participation rate continues to fall. *Monthly Labor Review 28.*

Toossi, M. (2015a). Labor force projections to 2014: Retiring boomers. *Monthly Labor Review, 128*(11), 25–44.

Toossi, M. (2015b). United States Census. Labor force statistics from the current population survey. 2015, http://data.bls.gov/timeseries/LNS14000000

Unson, C., & Richardson, M. (2013). Insights into the experiences of older workers and change: Through the lens of selection, optimization, and compensation. *The Gerontologist, 53*(3), 484–494. doi:10.1093/geront/gns095

Vickerstaff, S., Phillipson, C., & Wilkie, R. (Eds.) (2013). *Work, health and well-being: The challenges of managing health at work*. Bristol: Policy Press.

Voelpel, S. C., & Dous, M. (2006). Lost knowledge: Confronting the threat of an aging workforce. *Academy of Management Perspectives, 20*(4), 125–126.

Wang, M, & Shultz, K. (2010). Employee retirement: A review and recommendations for future investigation. *Journal of Management, 36*(1): 172–206.

Wegman, D. H. (1999). Older workers. *Occupational Medicine, 14*(3), 537–557.

Wegman, D. H., & McGee, J. P. (2004). In D. H. Wegman & J. P. McGee (Eds.), *Health and safety needs of older workers*. National Research, Council Institute of Medicine Committee on the Health & Safety Needs of Older Workers, Washington, DC.

Wickrama, K. A. S., Lorenz, F. O., Conger, R. D., Matthews, L., & Elder, G. H. (1997). Linking occupational conditions to physical health through marital, social, and intrapersonal processes. *Journal of Health and Social Behavior, 38*(4), 363–375. doi:10.2307/2955431

Wickrama, K. K., O'Neal, C. W., Kwag, K. H., & Lee, T. K. (2013). Is working later in life good or bad for health? An investigation of multiple health outcomes. *The Journals of Gerontology, Series B: Psychological Sciences and Social Sciences, 68*(5), 807–815. doi:10.1093/geronb/gbt069

Zajacova, A., Montez, J. K., & Herd, P. (2014). Socioeconomic disparities in health among older adults and the implications for the retirement age debate: A brief report. *Journals of Gerontology, Series B: Psychological and Social Sciences, 69*(6), 973–978. doi:10.1093/geronb/gbu041

Zwerling, C., Sprince, N. L., Wallace, R. B., Davis, C. S., Whitten, P. S., & Heeringa, S. G. (1996). Risk factors of occupational injuries among older workers: An analysis of the health and retirement study. *American Journal of Public Health, 86*(9), 1306–1309.

CHAPTER EIGHT

Veterans and the Life Course

Andrew S. London

In the last decade, a range of scholars of aging and the life course have produced a set of critical evaluations of the extant research literature on the consequences of military service (Carlson & Andress, 2009; London & Wilmoth, 2008, 2016; MacLean & Elder, 2007; Settersten, 2006; Wilmoth & London 2013, 2016). These synthetic overviews build on prior reviews (Modell & Haggerty, 1991) and draw from a body of literature that dates back several decades to the seminal work of Glen H. Elder, Jr. (1986, 1987), and even earlier (Browning, Lopreato, & Poston, 1973; Card, 1983; Hogan, 1981). The vast majority of the research reviewed in these overviews focuses on entry into the military, the transition to civilian life, the transition to adulthood, and/or follows veterans through midlife. Mostly, researchers have focused on educational and socioeconomic attainment, and marriage and family. Less research focuses on the more-distal, later-life consequences of military service (Settersten, 2006; Spiro, Schnurr, & Aldwin, 1997; Wilmoth & London, 2016). While several decades of scholarship have yielded important conceptual models, empirical results, and policy-relevant insights, Teachman (2013: 275) recently began his evaluation of the existing literature by stating: "Research on military service has a long and rich history. . . . Yet despite this research heritage, fifty years after the publication of *The American Soldier*, we know surprisingly little about the ways military service is linked to the lives of the men and women who have served their country." It is unfortunate that the existing body of research does not yield a more-comprehensive understanding of the life-course consequences of military service. It is also imperative that we learn from the past and take steps now to put in place firm foundations for future research on military service, aging, and the life course.

In this chapter, I use the life-course perspective to focus attention on the lives of veterans who served prior to the advent of the All-Volunteer Force (AVF) at the end of the Vietnam-era draft in 1973, and, more specifically, on veterans who served during the Vietnam era. Those who entered the military in the period prior to 1973 were born in 1955 or earlier. Thus, surviving veterans of the pre-AVF era will for the next several decades constitute the majority of the population of older adult veterans who live in our families and communities, participate in research studies, seek care in healthcare facilities, and need family, community-based, and institutional care. In the first section of the chapter, I provide a brief overview of how and why we expect military service to affect aging and the life course, and introduce the cumulative exposure model of the life course as a framework for thinking about the life-course consequences of military service. I then provide a brief description of the size and composition of the pre-AVF veteran population in 2013, and how it will change over the next several decades. Next, I turn to a critical evaluation of what we know about selection into military service during the Vietnam era, and how Vietnam-era service affected the transition to adulthood and the midlife socioeconomic attainment, marriage/family, and health outcomes of veterans relative to nonveterans. At present, we know relatively little about how military service will shape the later-life trajectories and outcomes of Vietnam-era veterans because they are just entering older adulthood. Thus, in addition to reviewing emergent research that is beginning to examine later-life outcomes, I present findings from an original analysis of data from the 2009 American Community Survey (ACS). Specifically, I describe differences between late-midlife nonveterans, Vietnam-era veterans with no service-connected disability, and Vietnam-era veterans with service-connected disability, separately for men and women. I chose 2009 for these analyses because it is the most-recent year that service-connected disability is measured in the ACS (prior to the recent release of the 2013 ACS data), and because analysis of these data provides a relatively contemporary, albeit selective, profile of the Vietnam-era cohort as they enter older adulthood. Finally, I conclude with a discussion of the opportunities that an intensified effort to comparatively study the later lives of Vietnam-era veterans and nonveterans provides, some changes we need to make so that we don't miss the chance, and the challenges that must be overcome if we are going to be successful.

Life-Course Perspectives on Military Service

The life-course perspective generally encompasses five principles—lifelong development, location in time and place, timing and sequencing, human agency, and linked lives (Elder, Johnson, & Crosnoe, 2003; Settersten, 2003; Mortimer & Shanahan, 2003). Each of these is important for understanding the consequences of military service. Human development and aging are processes that unfold over time and in particular historical, geographical, social, and economic contexts. What happens earlier conditions, but does not determine absolutely, what happens in subsequent life stages because individuals make choices and institutions—such as the military—exert influences that change the trajectory of development. The life-course perspective highlights the critical importance of having comprehensive data on military service experiences, as well as longitudinal, comparative data that enable researchers to address selection, disentangle aging from period and cohort effects, and understand the variable or disproportionate effects of early-life military service on different outcomes in different stages of the life course (Teachman, 2013).

The military is a complex, hierarchical, and potentially transformative social institution (Kelty & Segal, 2013). For those who serve, the military can have long-term effects on identity, life satisfaction, and well-being (Aldwin, Levenson, & Spiro, 1994; Card, 1983; Smith & True, 2014), as well as subsequent choices, trajectories, and outcomes (Wilmoth & London, 2013). Historically, less than 1 percent of the U.S. population has served in the armed forces at any given time, with the exception of brief periods when the country has been at war (Segal & Segal, 2004, Figure 1). There are five branches of the U.S. armed forces—Air Force, Army, Coast Guard, Marine Corps, and Navy—as well as Reserve and National Guard components that are variably associated with them. Within each branch, enlisted personnel and officers are distinguished, with more-fine-grained, hierarchal distinctions drawn within each category. Most active-duty personnel serve during young adulthood for periods of four to eight years, although reenlistment, particularly during periods of war, can lead to longer durations of service. The relatively small percentage of service members who seek careers in the military generally retire after 20 years of active-duty service and are eligible for benefits that may enhance their later-life financial and health security (Street & Hoffman, 2013). Veteran status indicates prior active-duty service with a better-than-dishonorable discharge. Exposure to combat is not required for active-duty or veteran status, or benefits eligibility. The availability of specific veterans' benefits varies by historical period, duration of service, rank, and disability status, and the take-up of benefits varies across the life course (Bennett & McDonald, 2013; Street & Hoffman, 2013; Wilmoth & London, 2011; Wilmoth, London, & Heflin, 2015). In specific circumstances, family members may also receive benefits as a result of a spouse or parent's active-duty service or service-related death.

Understanding the consequences of military service over the life course is complicated because the effects of military service may be mixed and countervailing. Military service unevenly exposes young adults to an array of risks and benefits; for any particular life-course outcome, the extent to which military service is beneficial, has negative consequences, or has no consequences depends on the particularities of historical circumstance, the prevailing organization and policies of the armed forces, individual characteristics, service experiences, and access to benefits.

Wilmoth and London (2013, Figure 1.1) advocate using a cumulative exposure model of the life course as a conceptual framework for studying the consequences of military service. This conceptual model focuses attention on various mechanisms by which military service influences aging and variation in later-life trajectories and outcomes, as well as the historical embeddedness of aging and development. The cumulative exposure model proposes three key domains of mechanisms that might drive variation in life-course trajectories and outcomes in relation to military service. These include: the range of early-life individual and contextual factors that affect selection into military service—the preservice period of the military life course; military service experiences, including but not limited to exposure to combat—the active-duty period of the military life course; and the effects of variable military service experiences on postservice outcomes—the veteran period of the military life course. They propose that early-life factors influence selection into military service, and that military service experiences, in turn, can mediate, moderate, or have no effect on the associations between such factors and later-life outcomes. The possibility that military service might produce positive or negative turning points—discontinuities—in the life course is a central tenet of this conceptual model (Browning et al., 1973; Elder 1986, 1987; Laub & Sampson, 2003; Sampson & Laub, 1996). This conceptual model also posits that military service has the potential to directly shape or reshape mid- and later-life educational, employment, marriage/family, and health trajectories and outcomes. Ultimately, this conceptual model suggests that the consequences of military are neither automatic nor uniform. Rather, they are individually, socially, and historically contingent, and can best be evaluated with longitudinal studies that compare those with and without military service histories, controlling for selection and taking variation in military service experiences into account.

The Pre-AVF and Vietnam-Era Veteran Population

Older adult veterans are a large and policy-relevant population (Wilmoth & London, 2011). From 2013 to 2043, the population of male veterans aged 50 and over is projected to decline by 43 percent from 15,113,268 to 8,564,570, while the population of female veterans aged 50 and over is projected to increase by 64 percent from 972,048 to 1,594,593 (National Center for Veterans Analysis and Statistics, 2014a).[1] Several decades ago, 100 percent of the older-adult veterans who researchers observed in their data sets, clinicians treated in health-care facilities, and individuals encountered in institutions and community-based settings had served in the military prior to the advent of the AVF at the end of the poorly implemented and controversial Vietnam-era draft (Kelty & Segal, 2013). Among men transitioning to adulthood in the mid-twentieth century, military service was a normative part of the life course. From 1915 to 1935, rates of participation in the military were over 50 percent for each single-year birth cohort, with rates over 70 percent for those born between 1919 and 1927 (Hogan, 1981). Some served voluntarily during this period, but many others were drafted—and may even have felt coerced—into service during World War II, the Korean War, and the Vietnam War. A substantial number of Vietnam-era men, especially those with higher academic aptitude in high school, enlisted in order to avoid being drafted (Card, 1983). They enlisted unwillingly in order to try to improve the terms of their service.

As of 2013, pre-AVF-era veterans constituted approximately 56 percent of the estimated 22,299,350 living veterans—59 percent of the 20,298,098 male veterans and 23 percent of the 2,001,252 female veterans. By 2023, the percentage of living veterans who served prior to the advent of the AVF is projected to decline sharply to 40 percent as the estimated 3.2 million old-old veterans who served during or between World War II and the Korean War and were alive in 2013 pass away, and as veterans of Operation Enduring Freedom, Operation Iraqi Freedom, and Operation New Dawn enter the population. By 2043, it is projected that about 7 percent of living veterans will have entered military service during the pre-AVF era.

Although the percentage of pre-AVF-era veterans will decline over the next several decades, the percentage of surviving pre-AVF-era veterans who served during a war is projected to increase from 82 percent in 2013 to 96 percent in 2043. As seen in Figure 8.1, this shift is driven by the fact that Vietnam-era veterans are projected to constitute an increasingly large proportion of surviving pre-AVF-era veterans over the course of the next three decades. Overall, nearly 9 million Americans served during the Vietnam War. In 2013, it is estimated that there were 7,387,059 living Vietnam-era veterans, which constituted 33 percent of all living veterans and 44 percent of all living wartime veterans. In 2043, it is projected that there will be 965,845 surviving pre-AFV-era veterans, of whom 95 percent will be Vietnam-era veterans. Thus, in 2043, it is projected that there will still be nearly 1 million surviving old-old wartime veterans almost all whom served during the Vietnam War.

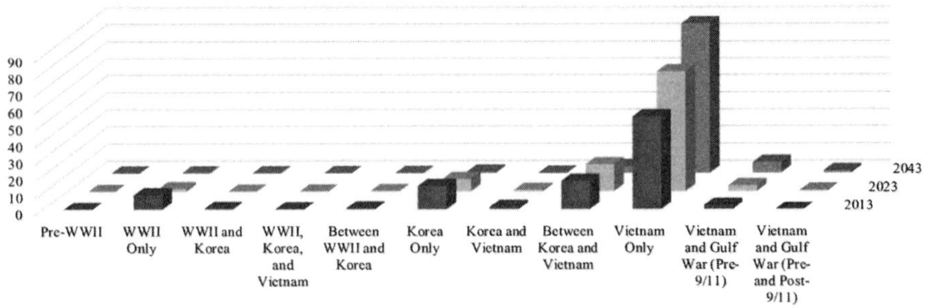

Figure 8.1 Projected trends in the percent distribution of pre-AVF-era veterans by period of service from 2013 to 2043. (Data for this Figure were obtained from VetPop2014, Table 2L [National Center for Veterans Analysis and Statistics.] [2014])

Given these trends that will unfold over the next three decades, it is critically important that we assess the extant research related to Vietnam-era veterans. Just as the last few decades of research on and care for older adult and old-old veterans has focused primarily on veterans of World War II and the Korean War, the next few decades will primarily focus on the lives of Vietnam-era veterans. How these veterans fare as older adults will depend on their early-life experiences, military service experiences, and experiences over the life course, as well as the policies and programs that are in place to meet their needs (Wilmoth & London, 2011). Such policies and programs, which contribute to later-life health and financial security, and family well-being, include: veterans administration health care; service-connected disability, specific war-service, and career-service pensions; life insurance; and support services for family caregivers (National Center for Veterans Analysis and Statistics, 2014b; Nichols et al., 2011; Street & Hoffman, 2013). Vietnam-era veterans are part of the large, post–World War II baby boom cohort, born between 1946 and 1964, which will put substantial demands on family, social service, and health-care systems as they age. Older adult Vietnam-era veterans will benefit from existing and emergent policies and programs available to all older adults, such as Medicare and Social Security, but they may also have specific needs that will require more-focused policies and programs both within and outside of the Veterans Administration.

Vietnam-Era Military Service and the Life Course

The cumulative exposure model of the life course, discussed above, sensitizes us to the need to consider selection and military service experiences when assessing the life-course consequences of military service. Thus, before turning to a review of what is known about the consequences of Vietnam-era military service for socioeconomic attainment, marriage/family, and health outcomes, it is important to consider the factors that affected selection into military service in this era and, briefly, some of the military-institutional factors that may have shaped later-life outcomes.

Selection

The military is a selective institution. From 1941 to 1973, American men were subject to a draft, and during World War II, the Korean War, and the Vietnam War, many men were in fact conscripted into service (Fligstein, 1980; Flynn, 1993). However, even during the draft era, some men, and all women, voluntarily enlisted or sought to join the military academies in order to be commissioned as officers. While some factors, such as having a family history of military service and socioeconomic disadvantage, increased the likelihood of volunteering for military service, demographic characteristics, such as age, race/ethnicity, nativity status, gender, and sexual orientation, have variably constrained entry into the military in various historical periods (Brown, 2013; Kelty & Segal, 2013; Lutz, 2013).

In the context of a draft or voluntary enlistment, entry into the military is not guaranteed. Recruiters may dissuade some would-be service men, and increasingly women, from applying. Individuals who apply must take the Armed Forces Qualifying Test (AFQT) and score high enough to ensure that they have the aptitudes necessary to successfully complete basic training programs and the duties required by particular military occupational specialties (Sackett & Mavor, 2006). Individuals must also pass preinduction exams that are designed to identify a range of disqualifying physical and mental health conditions, impairments, abnormalities, and behaviors. Rejection rates vary by year depending on the personnel needs of the armed forces and the characteristics of applicants, but, from 1950 to 1971, they were above 30 percent in every year and over 40 percent for much of the period (Wolf, Wing, & Lopoo, 2013, Figure 13.1).

Although differential rejection due to differential failure of preinduction exams and screenings will remain an aspect of selection that must be considered in life-course studies, a well-implemented draft has the potential to reduce the influence of voluntary factors on selection into the military because selection is random. A draft has the potential to level the playing field in the sense that the selective force of economic need, family culture, and individual choice do not drive entry. However, it is important to note that the Vietnam-era draft was notorious for not being well-implemented, which contributed to social and racial strife, as well as to efforts to reform military personnel policy and the shift to the AVF (Kelty & Segal, 2013). The deferment system in place during the Vietnam War allowed college students to avoid service, which provided a means for primarily white, middle- and upper-class men to avoid the draft. Middle-class and white men may also have been more able to obtain exemptions for other reasons or enroll in the Reserves to avoid the risk of deployment to the war zone. Presidential decisions to keep the Reserve/Guard at home made them a relatively safe haven (Kelty & Segal, 2013). Given that lower-class men and blacks made up a large portion of the troops who served in Vietnam during the Vietnam War, allegations were made that "blacks and the poor were serving as cannon fodder" (Armor, 1996: 9).

Despite the poor implementation of the draft, there is some evidence that differences between those who did and did not serve may be limited. In her extensive analysis of preservice, baseline Project Talent data, which were collected when the men she studied were 14 or 15 years old, Card (1983) found that men from upper-class backgrounds were significantly less likely to have served than men from other socioeconomic class backgrounds, and lower-class and black men were more likely to serve in the Army and Marine Corps, where combat exposure was more common. However, she did not find an overall race difference in participation. Moreover, she found very few other differences between those who did not serve, those who served but not in the Vietnam theater of operations, and those who served in Vietnam across a very broad range of demographic characteristics, cognitive tests, and measured aptitudes and aspirations. Compared to those who did not serve, those who served were less calm, received less guidance outside of high school, participated less in extracurricular activities, and were less interested in selected vocations. But, differences were small. She concluded that the combination of the draft and the differential rejection of both draftees and enlistees may have helped level the playing field to some extent. For example, with respect to race, countervailing forces may have worked to equalize participation. Blacks were more likely than whites to be drafted because they were less able to obtain deferments, but they were four times more likely to be rejected because they failed preinduction physical and mental health exams. Card (1983: 24) summarized her findings related to selection into service by stating: "The groups of veterans and nonveterans are not as different from one another as popular belief might suggest."

Accounting for such selective forces, by one means or another, is important in life-course studies of the consequences of military service. To the extent possible, analysts want to be sure that they are identifying a causal relationship between military service and some outcome, which can only be done if selection is adequately addressed. This may be done by controlling for observed preservice characteristics, using sibling fixed effects models (London et al., *in review*), or using the draft-era lottery or something else as an instrumental variable to control for unobserved heterogeneity (Angrist, 1990, 1991; Angrist, Imbens, & Rubin, 1996). The extent to which this can be done, of course, depends on the availability of adequate data.

Active-Duty

Analysts interested in the life-course consequences of military service are often limited to investigating simple veteran status differences because of data constraints. As valuable as such analyses are, they represent a limited starting point. In such analyses, the specific aspect of service that matters is masked. Moreover, because the undocumented influences of different aspects of military service may be countervailing and cancel each other out, we may sometimes incorrectly conclude that the effect is small or nonexistent. Entering the military exposes young adults to a range of opportunities and risks, which are historically, geographically, and institutionally contingent. If military service, per se, has consequences for understanding variation in the life course, then something about active-duty military service must matter for some aging-related process or outcome. However, our capacity to empirically delineate dimensions of military service in relation to the range of outcomes that are of interest to scholars of aging and the life course is severely limited. Most longitudinal data sets that include important life-course outcomes do not include measures of draft status, branch of service, rank, military occupational specialty, duration of service, location of service, exposure to combat, or service-connected disability.

Theoretically, there are good reasons to expect different aspects of military service to matter for different life-course outcomes. With respect to employment outcomes, each branch and rank initially selects individuals with particular characteristics with the goal of staffing specific military occupational specialties. Military occupational specialties provide different kinds of educational and training opportunities, risks, and rewards, which variably translate into the civilian labor market (Kleykamp, 2013). The training and education service members receive in their military occupational specialty may be one of the factors that produces variation in employment outcomes during the veteran period of the life course. It may do so because it is the only education and training the individual receives beyond high school and before entering the labor force, or because it sets the individual on a postservice trajectory toward additional education in a particular field via access to GI Bill benefits. It may also be one of the factors that contributes to positive turning points in the lives of men and women from disadvantaged backgrounds. While these processes operate across time periods of service, their effects likely vary in response to changing institutional and historical conditions. Thus, the effects of training and educational opportunities during the Vietnam-era active-duty period may be very different than those that prevailed in other periods. Moreover, some evidence from the Vietnam era suggests that veteran status served as a negative screening device in the labor market (Berger & Hirsch, 1985; Hogan, 1981).

With respect to marriage and family formation, Lundquist and Smith (2005) found that organizational and economic incentives in the family-friendly AVF promoted early marriage and family formation among military women. However, this mechanism is unlikely to have operated in the less family-friendly Vietnam-era military. In part because of the draft and the implementation of deferments for those with dependents, men who served in the Vietnam era tended to be very young and childless. Some married rapidly in advance of induction, while others waited until after they completed their service (Hogan, 1981). Thus, for the Vietnam-era cohort of service members, marriage and/or family formation tended to happen during the veteran period rather than before it (Burland & Lundquist, 2013). Combat exposure and service-connected physical and mental health problems that are rooted in the active-duty period may exert a negative influence on marital and family outcomes in this era. Such negative influences may have been exacerbated by the unpopularity of the war and the stigma many Vietnam-era service members experienced upon their return home (Frey-Wouters & Laufer, 1986; Kulka et al., 1990).

Another set of service-connected factors might shape health outcomes, for better or worse. Those who serve in the military are initially selected on the basis of healthiness. Some aspects of military service might enhance service members' health and well-being, such as rank (MacLean & Edwards, 2010). During the active-duty period, service members engage in a substantial amount of regular exercise and achieve relatively high levels of physical fitness. In some circumstances, socialization into the military role and unit cohesion may foster a sense of mastery, social support, and self-esteem that provide psychosocial resources that can be beneficial for well-being.

However, there are a broad range of factors related to the mission and culture of the institution that potentially threaten health and well-being. Wartime service is not randomly assigned or equally distributed. In the context of the Vietnam War, characteristics that indicated the ability to perform noncombat functions reduced combat assignments and service in the Vietnam theater of operations, although indicators of aggression and stress management also played a role in predicting combat exposure

(Gimbel & Booth, 1996). Wartime service often involves combat exposure, which increases the risk of short-term injury and long-term disability (Elder, Shanahan, & Clipp, 1994, 1997; MacLean, 2010), physical and mental health problems (MacLean, 2013; Wilmoth, London, & Parker, 2010), sleep problems (London, Burgard, & Wilmoth, 2014), and later-life mortality (Elder et al., 2009). More-mundane overtraining injuries and accidents also contribute to long-term health problems and disabilities. In the context of service in the Vietnam theater of operations, exposure to Agent Orange is a critical issue, although in other contexts, such as World War II and the Gulf War, environmental exposures may also have mattered for long-term health. Health outcomes are also negatively affected by the culture of the institution regarding tobacco, alcohol, and drugs. For example, the military has been described as "pro-tobacco" (Jahnke et al., 2011: 1382), and "highly hospitable to smoking" (Smith & Malone, 2012: 1202). It is an institution that has a long history of having a culture that supports and encourages tobacco use by its members (Nelson & Pederson, 2008), "institutional norms that promote smoking" (Conway, 1998: 291), and, from a policy perspective, "a culture of tobacco 'exceptionalism'" (Smith & Malone, 2012: 1202). Policy changes in the mid-1980s appear to have reduced some types of drug use (Miech et al., 2013), but less progress has been made with respect to reducing alcohol consumption and smoking. For women, and to a lesser extent men, the experience of military sexual trauma during the active-duty period may be a factor that affects long-term health and well-being (Kimmerling et al., 2007; Suris & Lind, 2008).

With some exceptions, such as combat exposure, theoretical conceptualizations of what it is about military service that explains variation in life-course outcomes among older adults have outstripped empirical examinations of them (Wilmoth & London, 2013). For the Vietnam-era cohort, we are just at the beginning of the window of opportunity to examine whether and how their military service experiences influence their later-life trajectories and outcomes relative to their nonveteran older-adult peers. Although there are challenges, moving forward, it is critically important that we continue to expand our capacity to conduct theoretically informed, comparative, empirical analyses that aim to elucidate the mechanisms by which participation in the Vietnam-era military affected later-life trajectories and outcomes.

Veteran Period

We know less than we should about the impact of Vietnam-era military service on the lives of the men and women who served, as well as those whose lives are linked to them. However, the extant research literature does provide a set of empirical studies about the effects of Vietnam-era service on the transition to adulthood and socioeconomic attainment, marriage/family, and health outcomes through midlife. This body of research can serve as a foundation for the further study of the long-term, later-life consequences of Vietnam-era service.

Socioeconomic Attainment. In contrast to World War II and Korean War veterans, who achieved higher educational attainment than their nonveteran peers, Vietnam-era veterans achieved lower levels of educational attainment than their peers at the time of discharge (Cohen, Segal, & Temme, 1986; Cohen & Temme, 1986; Stanley, 2003). This may have been due to selection, as well as the fact that during the Vietnam era some nonveterans achieved that status by receiving deferments because they were in college, and because of changes in federal policies that made financial aid that was not tied to military service more available and changes in the GI Bill benefits that were available to veterans (Bennett & McDonald, 2013, Table 6.1). For example, in 1975, Vietnam-era GI Bill benefits represented 34 percent of monthly wages in manufacturing, in contrast to 54 percent at the peak of World War II-era GI Bill use (Mattila, 1978). The lower value of Vietnam-era GI Bill educational benefits relative to manufacturing wages may have increased the opportunity costs of pursuing additional schooling for some veterans.

Yet, there is evidence that use of GI Bill benefits did influence the educational attainment of Vietnam-era veterans. Focusing on the transition to adulthood and early midlife—ages 36–37 years—Card (1983) found that male Vietnam-era veterans finished school at significantly older ages than their nonveteran classmates. Angrist (1993) used data from the 1987 Survey of Veterans and found that veterans' benefits increased years of schooling by one and a half years for men aged 35–44 years, 95 percent of whom served during the Vietnam era. The majority of the veterans in the sample had volunteered for service and had served for three to five years, and they had twelve and a half years of education at the time they were discharged from service. Overall, 63 percent received some sort of financial aid, 78 percent acquired some additional education or training after discharge, and 52 percent attended college or graduate school. Taken together, the available evidence suggests that Vietnam-era veterans were able to catch up to their nonveteran peers to some extent and close the educational attainment gap over time (Teachman, 2005; Teachman & Call, 1996). This conclusion is bolstered by recent research that has followed the Vietnam-era cohort over a longer period of time. Angrist and Chen (2011) used 2000 Census data to obtain draft-lottery estimates of the causal effect of Vietnam-era military service on educational attainment.

They found large gains for veterans, which they attribute to use of the GI Bill rather than draft avoidance behavior. Elman and O'Rand (2004) find that military service significantly increased school reentry in midlife among men, which might partly account for the narrowing of the gap.

The employment and earnings prospects of veterans and nonveterans are tied to some extent to macroeconomic and labor-market circumstances, as well as their educational attainment. Vietnam-era veterans are part of the large baby boom cohort, whose members have had to compete for jobs and weather the economic recessions of the 1970s and 1980s relatively early in their careers (Wilmoth and London, 2016, Figure 1). The unpopularity of the Vietnam War may also have affected their initial reception in the labor market. Compared to World War II–era veterans, the unemployment rates for Vietnam War veterans were much higher. Browning et al. (1973) report that the unemployment rate for Vietnam-era veterans was 11 percent overall—11 percent for whites and 15 percent for nonwhites—compared to 5 percent for World War II–era veterans. This circumstance certainly influenced their labor-market opportunities and may have contributed to their overrepresentation in public-sector employment in midlife (Angrist & Chen, 2011).

The available literature indicates that Vietnam-era veterans, overall, have not done as well as their nonveteran peers with respect to income and earnings (Berger & Hirsch, 1983; Bryant, Samaranayake, & Wilhite, 1993; Hirsch & Mehay, 2003; Martindale & Poston, 1979; Savoca & Rosenheck, 2000; Teachman, 2004). Hogan (1981) attributes this to intercohort change in the occupational and income returns of being a veteran, and disadvantages associated with a service-connected disorderliness in the transition to adulthood in this era. Using Social Security administrative records through the early 1980s, Angrist (1990) employed the draft lottery to estimate the causal effect of veteran status on civilian earnings. He found a 15 percent earnings penalty for white male veterans relative to white male nonveterans. However, there is some indication that veterans earnings have caught up to those of nonveterans over time. Angrist and Chen (2011) found no Vietnam-era veteran status difference in draft-lottery estimates of earnings in 2000, which they in part attributed to a modest economic return to GI Bill-subsidized educational attainment.

Although the overall profile of earnings and income relative to Vietnam-era service is negative, there is some indication that military service produced positive and negative turning points for economically disadvantaged and advantaged men, respectively. Kleykamp (2013: 148) notes: "One of the most consistent findings across generations of veterans is the fact that the effect of military service appears to be more positive—or at least less negative—among racial and ethnic minorities." Consistent with this view, a range of studies indicate an earnings advantage among African American Vietnam-era veterans, and an earnings penalty among whites (Berger & Hirsch, 1983; Browning et al., 1973; Lopreato & Poston, 1977; Martindale & Poston, 1979; Rosen & Taubman, 1982; Teachman, 2004). The earnings advantage among blacks is consistent with the positive turning point hypothesis, which posits that military service may knife off individuals from early-life disadvantage and place them in a bridging environment, where education and training in young adulthood, prior to the adoption of adult roles, can redirect the life course in positive ways. The earnings penalty among white men may be indicative of a negative turning point, or an undermining of early-life advantage. This is consistent with findings from a study based on a convenience sample of elite, Ivy League college-educated men who served in Vietnam (Bookwala, Frieze, & Grote, 1994). These men were less satisfied in midlife with their careers, finances, and life in general, and more likely to have changed careers, moved, used alcohol, experienced depression, and questioned their values than nonveterans. Some of these consequences were specific to those who served in the Vietnam theater of operations and thus may be associated with combat exposure.

Marriage/Family. The literature on the consequences of Vietnam-era service on marriage and family outcomes is somewhat smaller than that on socioeconomic outcomes, and the evidence is more mixed. Card (1983) found that male Vietnam-era veterans got married and became fathers at significantly older ages than their nonveteran classmates. Others have also reported that the effect of military service on marriage, especially early age at marriage, was negative during the Vietnam era (Cooney & Hogan, 1991; Goldscheider & Waite, 1986), which is different than the effect in other historical eras (Hogan, 1981). However, Call and Teachman (1996) examined marital stability in relation to the timing of first marriage and Vietnam-era military service. They found that Vietnam combat and noncombat veterans married at the same rate as nonveterans, and marriages contracted before or during service were not negatively impacted with respect to marital stability. Laufer and Gallops (1985) studied a probability sample of nonveterans, Vietnam-era veterans who did not serve in the theater of operations, and Vietnam veterans who did serve in the theater of operations. Vietnam veterans were more likely to enter marriage than nonveterans, but combat exposure contributed to higher rates of divorce. Other research finds that Vietnam-era military service had little effect on the risk of divorce in well-controlled models (Cohen & Segal, 2009; Ruger, Wilson, & Waddoups, 2002), although there is some evidence that combat exposure increased the odds of marital dissolution among all cohorts (Ruger et al., 2002). Heerwig and Conley (2013) used an instrumental variable approach to studying family dynamics and found that Vietnam-era service actually reduced the likelihood of divorce among white men. In general, the extent to which variation in Vietnam-era military service experiences, combat exposure, and service-connected disability affect marriage and family outcomes is underexplored in the available literature.

Health. Later-life measurements of the health and well-being of those who served in the Vietnam era will be based on those who survive to the point of observation, and selective mortality is an issue with which life-course scholars interested in older adults and later-life outcomes must grapple (Wolf et al., 2013). MacLean (2013, Table 10.1) estimates that 58,000 U.S. service members were killed during the Vietnam War. Many others survived, but were wounded in combat. The odds of being wounded relative to being killed were much better in the Vietnam War than they were for either World War II or the Korean War, which perhaps reflects improvements in technology and in-theater medical and surgical care (MacLean, 2013). Suicide rates were also higher among military personnel than civilians during the Vietnam War (Ritchey, 2009), and there is some evidence that Vietnam-era veterans were more likely to die from accidents, suicide, and homicide in the period immediately following separation from service (Boehmer et al., 2004; Boscarino, 2006). Other evidence suggests that Vietnam veterans are more likely to attempt suicide if they have a psychiatric disorder (Fontana & Rosenheck, 1995).

Among wartime veterans of all eras, combat exposure is one of the key drivers of veteran status differences in physical and mental health over the life course (MacLean, 2010, 2013; Vogt et al., 2004). Card (1983) documents that veterans who served in the Vietnam theater of operations had significantly more symptoms of post-traumatic stress disorder—nightmares, loss of control over behavior, emotional numbing, withdrawal, hyperalertness, anxiety, depression—than veterans who did not serve in the Vietnam theater of operations and nonveterans, respectively. Research that directly compares veterans to nonveterans consistently indicates that Vietnam veterans are in worse health than nonveterans. Some evidence suggests that physical health disparities increase with age (Dobkin & Shabani, 2009). Vietnam veterans also have worse psychological outcomes (Dohrenwend et al., 2006; Laufer et al., 1981), including late-onset stress symptomology among older-adult combat veterans (Davison et al., 2006).

Several longitudinal, life-course studies have begun to investigate the later-life health and health behaviors of Vietnam-era veterans to the extent possible given that this cohort is currently entering early older adulthood. In later life, veterans who served during the Vietnam War have more chronic health conditions and poorer self-rated health around retirement age than veterans who served during World War II (Wilmoth et al., 2010).

Using cohorts defined on the basis of the year individuals turned 18 and became eligible for military service during particular historical periods, which facilitates comparisons of veterans and nonveterans, Wilmoth, London, and Himes (2015) examined inter- and intra-cohort variation in body mass index (BMI). They observed the Vietnam-era cohort over the 36–64 age range and found that members of this cohort were significantly heavier than members of earlier cohorts at the same ages. Across cohorts, they found that BMI followed the same trajectory over age, and that within each cohort, veterans were significantly heavier than nonveterans. For the older cohorts, BMI declined substantially and faster at older ages. Whether the same will be true for the Vietnam-era cohort remains to be seen. London et al. (*in review*) conducted an age-period-cohort analysis of smoking that included the cohorts in which men would have been eligible to serve in Vietnam. They found that veterans were significantly more likely to smoke than nonveterans in the 30–64 age range. Moreover, for both relevant cohorts, the intercohort change for veterans was positive, while it was negative for nonveterans. These results suggest that service in the military may have been a driver of population-level changes in smoking behavior in this era.

Another factor that appears to be affecting the later-life health of Vietnam-era veterans is Agent Orange exposure. Vietnam veterans have attributed some of their later-life illnesses to exposure to Agent Orange during their active-duty wartime service (Scott, 1992). In 2001, veterans with Type 2 diabetes associated with exposure to Agent Orange in Vietnam became eligible for Disability Compensation. Duggan, Rosenheck, and Singleton (2010) estimate that this policy change increased enrollment in the Disability Compensation program by 6 percentage points, and increased the amount of benefits received by enrollees by almost 2 percent. These estimated impacts related to this one disease suggest that a substantial number of individuals were exposed to and harmed by Agent Orange.

In addition to the available life-course literature, there is an extensive body of research on Vietnam-era veterans' health that is based on users of Veterans Administration health-care services, which is a highly selected and disadvantaged segment of the veteran population. The National Center for Veterans Analysis and Statistics (2014b) estimates that 40 percent of living veterans used at least one Veterans Administration service in 2012 and that users tend to have lower household incomes than non-users. As important as this research is for policy and program management, it does not allow for assessment of the impact of military service on health because it is not directly comparative. It also does not allow for examinations of change over age and across the life course because it is generally based on cross-sectional samples. Like the life-course literature on health, it tends to focus on health problems. Often left unexplored in both of these literatures is the question of whether and how military service in this era might have engendered resilience, stress-related growth, and positive outcomes, which it sometimes does (Aldwin et al., 1994; Card, 1983).

The Vietnam-Era Cohort in Late-Midlife

The Vietnam-era cohort is entering the retirement and older adult years, yet we know relatively little about how their contemporary circumstances vary by veteran status or how service-connected disability has shaped how they have fared to this point. With the foregoing review as context, I turn now to a description of selected demographic, socioeconomic, marriage/family, and health outcomes using data from the 2009 ACS. The sample includes all men and women, regardless of veteran or service-connected disability status, who were aged 52–63 years in 2009. This age range is consistent with the start, August 5, 1964, and stop, May 7, 1975, dates for Vietnam War service recorded in the U.S. Code of Federal Regulations (2014) and was selected because it is the age range of the Vietnam-era veterans identified in the 2009 ACS. The total sample includes 507,219 individuals, of whom about 48 percent are male. As seen in Table 8.1, weighted descriptive statistics are presented separately for men and women, and focus on comparisons of nonveterans, veterans with no service-connected disability, and veterans with service-connected disability, all severities combined. Overall, among men, 74 percent are nonveterans, 21 percent are veterans with no service-connected disability—nondisabled veterans, and 5 percent are veterans with a service-connected disability—disabled veterans, while among women, 99 percent are nonveterans, 1 percent are nondisabled veterans, and less than 1 percent are disabled veterans. Self-reported service-connected disability is likely to be underreported (Griffin & Stein, 2015). To the extent that veteran status is accurately reported, such underreporting likely results in some disabled veterans reporting themselves to be nondisabled veterans. There is also likely to be considerable heterogeneity in the consequences of more- and less-severe service-connected disabilities, which is masked by combining all severities together. Although it would be desirable to differentiate veterans along a broad range of service-related dimensions, such as by branch, rank, duration of service, such distinctions are not possible with the ACS.

In late-midlife, veteran status differences in demographic characteristics are broadly similar for men and women. For both men and women,

Table 8.1 Percentage of 52–63-Year-Old Vietnam-Era Nonveterans, Veterans with No Service-Connected Disability, and Veterans with Service-Connected Disability, by Gender, 2009 American Community Survey

	Men			Women		
	Non-veteran %	Veteran, no service-connected disability %	Veteran, service-connected disability %	Non-veteran %	Veteran, no service-connected disability %	Veteran, service-connected disability %
Demographic						
Race:						
White	80.4	86.0	77.8	79.7	79.1	68.2
African American	9.7	9.7	15.5	11.3	15.7	24.1
Other	10.0	4.2	6.7	9.0	5.2	7.7
Hispanic	10.6	4.7	6.4	9.0	4.4	5.4
U.S.-born	83.2	97.4	97.1	86.5	97.0	96.5
Living in South	34.5	38.0	44.7	36.4	43.3	54.6
Non-metro	16.5	19.3	20.3	16.9	17.6	18.6
Socioeconomic						
>High school	53.2	55.2	58.3	50.9	70.2	80.1
Employed	71.2	66.0	47.3	61.0	64.9	48.7
>Median Personal Income	59.6	62.2	64.8	38.0	47.5	62.7
In poverty	9.1	7.1	6.9	9.9	8.1	6.9
Owns home	79.1	81.6	80.0	79.9	77.5	75.7
Marriage/Family						
Marital status:						
Never-married	11.4	6.7	6.1	8.5	11.1	14.5
Married	69.5	71.0	68.4	62.4	54.0	43.3
Previously married	19.1	22.3	25.5	29.0	34.9	42.2
Married 2+ times	27.5	38.8	42.7	30.4	43.2	46.1
Percentage 1+ coresident children	32.9	23.8	24.4	29.2	25.6	21.8

	Men			Women		
	Non-veteran %	Veteran, no service-connected disability %	Veteran, service-connected disability %	Non-veteran %	Veteran, no service-connected disability %	Veteran, service-connected disability %
Health						
Any limitation/ disability	16.6	17.9	43.1	17.4	19.3	38.7
Any health insurance	84.8	91.5	97.5	87.3	92.3	99.5

Source: Author's calculations.

nondisabled veterans are as or more likely than nonveterans to be white and less likely to be coded other race or of Hispanic ethnicity. Disabled veterans are more likely than nonveterans and nondisabled veterans to be African American (16% vs. 10% for men and 24% vs. 11–16% among women). Disabled veterans are also somewhat more likely than nondisabled veterans to be coded other race or of Hispanic ethnicity. Since service-connected disability ratings are generally assigned early in the life course, close to service members' transitions to civilian life, these racial differences likely reflect the often-noted racial stratification in military and combat roles during the war. Both veteran groups are overwhelmingly U.S.-born. Veterans, especially disabled veterans, are more likely than nonveterans to reside in the South and in nonmetro areas, which has implications for health-care and service delivery.

The late-midlife socioeconomic profiles of Vietnam-era men and women differ somewhat in relation to veteran status. Among men, both nondisabled and disabled veterans are more likely than nonveterans to have more than high school education, but the rate is highest among disabled veterans. The same pattern is observed among women, but there is a much larger difference between disabled veterans and the other two groups. Approximately 80 percent of disabled female veterans have more than high school education, compared to 51 percent of female nonveterans; the difference for men is about 5 percentage points and only 58 percent of disabled male veterans have more than high school educational attainment. Among both men and women, less than half of disabled veterans are employed; employment rates among the other groups range from 61 to 71 percent, with nondisabled male veterans working less than male nonveterans and nondisabled female veterans working more than female nonveterans. Perhaps reflecting the importance of Veterans Administration Disability Compensation and/or Social Security Disability Insurance (Wilmoth, London, & Heflin, 2015), the percentage with personal income above the median for both men and women is highest among disabled veterans. As was the case with education, veteran status differences are much smaller among men than among women. Among both men and women, the rate of poverty is highest among nonveterans and lowest among disabled veterans. Home ownership varies slightly more among women than men. It is also lower among both groups of female veterans than among nonveterans, but, for all groups of men and women, home ownership exceeds 75 percent.

Outcomes in the marriage and family domain also vary by veteran status and gender. Among men, nonveterans have the highest rate of never marrying and disabled veterans the lowest. Among women, the pattern is the mirror image. Among all three groups of men, the rates of being currently married are about the same. Disabled male veterans have the highest rate of being previously married, but differences are relatively small. Among women, the rate of being currently married is highest among nonveterans and lowest among disabled veterans; female veterans in general, and disabled female veterans in particular, have low rates of current marriage. Disabled female veterans are the most likely to be previously married—42 percent. Both male and female disabled veterans have high rates of two or more marriages—43 and 46 percent, respectively. The rate of multiple marriages is more similar among the two veteran groups than between the veteran and nonveteran groups for both men and women. Nonveteran men are more likely than either of the veteran groups to have one or more children in the household. Among women, nonveterans are the most likely to have one or more children in the household.

The ACS does not include many health variables. However, six measures of functional limitation/disability are included. These indicate difficulty with cognition, ambulation, independent living, self care, vision, and hearing (see also, Wilmoth, London, & Parker, 2011). The any disability measure used for the analysis presented in Table 8.1 equals 1 if the respondent has any one of these six functional limitations/disabilities, and 0 otherwise. For both men and women, there is relatively little difference in the rate of any limitation/disability between nonveterans and nondisabled veterans. However, high rates are observed for both male and female disabled veterans—43 and 39 percent, respectively. It is likely they would be even higher if other forms of disability were measured, such as that associated with psychiatric and substance abuse disorders. Among both men and women, veterans, particularly disabled veterans, have higher rates of any health insurance coverage than nonveterans.

Discussion

Almost a decade ago, in the lead article to a special issue of *Research on Aging* on Military Service, the Life Course, and Aging, which he guest-edited, Richard A. Settersten, Jr. (2006: 12) wrote: "Most scholarship on aging is based on cohorts born early in the 20th century, and these cohorts have had significant experience with war. Wartime experiences may therefore be critical but largely hidden variables underlying current scientific knowledge about aging." Wilmoth and London (2013: 2) expanded this claim by noting that the "institutional influence of military service on lives has more generally been under-acknowledged among life-course scholars, and more broadly within Sociology and other disciplines that study human lives." Their recent content analysis of papers published between January 1980 and December 2013 in the five Gerontology Society of America-sponsored journals, *Research on Aging*, and *Journal of Aging and Health* lends credence to these notions (Wilmoth & London, 2016). In total, over the 34-year period, these seven mainstream aging journals published a total of 101 military-related articles, or three per year, on average. The vast majority were cross-sectional, nonrepresentative, and focused exclusively on veterans or Veterans Administration health-care facilities and programs that serve older veterans. Although these studies address important, policy-relevant questions, they do not contribute substantially to our understanding of how military service affects variation in long-term life-course outcomes because almost none of these studies directly compares veterans to nonveterans over time in carefully controlled models.

The Vietnam-era cohort of veterans is now entering the retirement and older adult years. While the extant literature provides some indications of how their lives have unfolded to this point, the knowledge base is thin on most topics. The descriptive results from analysis of the 2009 ACS that are presented in this chapter raise more questions than they answer. Perhaps, they will stimulate further research. Further research is needed because, even where our knowledge base is deepest, such as with respect to the effects of combat and consequences of military service for socioeconomic attainment, there are important gaps or uncertainties. It is critically important that researchers use available data sources to fill in the gaps in our knowledge to the extent possible. It is also important that we develop new opportunities to study the later lives of Vietnam-era veterans and nonveterans. Questions about military service experiences can be added to ongoing longitudinal data collection efforts. There is much to be learned about how different aspects of military service experiences affect a range of outcomes among older adult baby boomers in general and the Vietnam-era veterans among them in particular. As we follow surviving cohort members forward, we will need to make efforts to better understand the sources of, and adjust for, differential attrition and mortality by veteran status. There are challenges, but they can be overcome.

At the same time that efforts are being made to follow Vietnam-era veterans and nonveterans through older adulthood, we must also expand our capacity to prospectively follow younger cohorts as they age. Teachman (2013) has provided a set of recommendations to help address the data limitations that currently exist with regard to studying military service and the life course. For starters, he recommends that data: be longitudinal; contain information about nonveterans, active-duty personnel, Reserve/Guard members, and veterans so that comparative analyses can be undertaken; begin prior to the age of eligibility for military service; and comprehensively measure heterogeneity in military service experiences. He further recommends that we consider selection dynamically since the confounding factors that distinguish veterans and nonveterans may not be stable over time; continue to follow individuals when they enter service; measure contextual information to capture the effects of time and place; consider to whom veterans lives are linked and collect data about them as well; and undertake qualitative investigations as well as quantitative studies. These are sound recommendations, but finding the funds to implement them is a challenge.

Failure to act now to enhance the capacity of the social science research community to study military service, aging, and the life course will represent a missed opportunity. Not only will we perpetuate the notion that military service is a hidden variable in research on aging and the life course, we will also miss the opportunity to study how the transition to the AVF and military experiences during the late twentieth and early twenty-first centuries shaped aging and life-course processes and outcomes among those entering older adulthood in the mid-twenty-first century. As more women serve in the military, and as lesbian-, gay-, and bisexual-identified individuals serve openly for the first time in U.S. history, there are new opportunities to expand the reach of research on military service and the life course. Additionally, important questions related to spouses, children, and the lives of those who are linked to service members are emerging as key issues for future data collection and research. Of the 2 million individuals who have served in the active-duty military since September 11, 2001, nearly 45 percent had children (Cozza & Lerner, 2013). In 2011, the ratio of spouses and children to active-duty service members was 1.4 to 1 (Clever & Segal, 2013). Further investigation of military service in the United States, as well as carefully constructed international and cross-national comparative research, can elucidate the mechanisms by which military service affects lives, and how that varies by individual characteristics and historical circumstances. There is important work to be done that has the potential to significantly impact policies and programs that aim to support those who volunteered and, potentially, sacrificed for us all, as well as those whose lives are linked to them.

Arguably, military service is now an emergent variable in life-course research (London & Wilmoth, 2016). However, the continued emergence of military service in life-course studies is not guaranteed. If the availability of data and knowledge related to military service and the life course does continue to expand and deepen, this research initiative has the potential to provide important insights about how early-life institutions shape later-life outcomes. Hopefully, several decades from now, researchers will not look back and lament that we know very little about how military service affects the lives of those who served and the lives of those who are linked to them as Teachman (2013) recently did.

Note

1. VetPop2014, Tables 1L and 2L (National Center for Veterans Analysis and Statistics 2014a) are the sources for all of the population size estimates presented in this section. VetPop2014 is the latest official projection model of the veteran population provided by the Office of the Actuary. Original calculations based on data from VetPop2014 were completed by the author.

References

Aldwin, C. M., Levenson, M. R., & Spiro, A. (1994). Vulnerability and resilience to combat exposure: Can stress have lifelong effects? *Psychology and Aging, 9*(1), 34–44.

Angrist, J. D. (1990). Lifetime earnings and the Vietnam era draft lottery—Evidence from social security administrative records. *American Economic Review, 80*(3), 313–336.

Angrist, J. D. (1991). The draft lottery and voluntary enlistment in the Vietnam era. *Journal of the American Statistical Association, 86*(415), 584–595.

Angrist, J. D. (1993). The effect of veterans benefits on education and earnings. *Industrial & Labor Relations Review, 46*(4), 637–652.

Angrist, J. D., & Chen, S. H. (2011). Schooling and the Vietnam-era GI Bill: Evidence from the draft lottery. *American Economic Journal: Applied Economics, 3*, 96–118.

Angrist, J. D., Imbens, G. W., & Rubin, D. B. (1996). Identification of causal effects using instrumental variables. *Journal of the American Statistical Association, 91*(434), 444–455.

Armor, D. J. (1996). Race and gender in the US military. *Armed Forces & Society, 23*(1), 7–27.

Bennett, P.R., & McDonald, K.B. (2013). Military service as a pathway to early socioeconomic achievement for disadvantaged groups. In J.M. Wilmoth & A.S. London (Eds.), *Life-course perspectives on military service* (pp. 119–143). New York: Routledge.

Berger, M.C., & Hirsch, B.T. (1983). The civilian earnings experience of Vietnam-era veterans. *Journal of Human Resources, 18*(4), 455–479.

Berger, M.C., & Hirsch, B.T. (1985). Veteran status as a screening device during the Vietnam era. *Social Science Quarterly, 66*(1), 79–89.

Boehmer, T.K.C., Flanders, D., McGeehin, M.A., Boyle, C., & Barrett, D.H. (2004). Postservice mortality in Vietnam Veterans—30 year follow-up. *Archives of Internal Medicine, 164*(17), 1908–1916.

Bookwala, J., Frieze, I., & Grote, N. (1994). The long-term effects of military service on quality of life—the veteran experience. *Journal of Applied Social Psychology, 24*(6), 529–545.

Boscarino, J.A. (2006). Posttraumatic stress disorder and mortality among US Army veterans 30 years after military service. *Annals of Epidemiology, 16*(4), 248–256.

Brown, M.T. (2013). Military service and lesbian, gay, bisexual, and transgender lives. In J.M. Wilmoth & A.S. London (Eds.), *Life-course perspectives on military service* (pp. 97–118). New York: Routledge.

Browning, H.L., Lopreato, S.C., & Poston, D.L. (1973). Income and veteran status—Variations among Mexican Americans, blacks and Anglos. *American Sociological Review, 38*(1), 74–85.

Bryant, R.R., Samaranayake, V.A., & Wilhite, A.L. (1993). The effect of military service on the subsequent civilian wage of the post-Vietnam veteran. *Quarterly Review of Economics and Finance, 33*(1), 15–31.

Burland, D., & Lundquist, J.H. (2013). The best years of our lives: Military service and family relationships—A life-course perspective. In J.M. Wilmoth & A.S. London (Eds.), *Life course perspectives on military service* (pp. 165–184). New York: Routledge.

Call, V.R.A., & Teachman, J.D. (1996). Life-course timing and sequencing of marriage and military service and their effects on marital stability. *Journal of Marriage and the Family, 58*(1), 219–226.

Card, J.J. (1983). *Lives after Vietnam: The personal impact of military service.* Lexington, MA: Lexington Books.

Carlson, E., & Andress, J. (2009). Military service by twentieth-century generations of American men. *Armed Forces & Society, 35*(2), 385–400.

Clever, M., & Segal, D.R. (2013). The demographics of military children and families. *The Future of Children, 23*(2), 13–39.

Cohen, J., & Temme, L.V. (1986). Military service was an educational disadvantage to Vietnam-era personnel. *Sociology and Social Research, 70*(3), 206–208.

Cohen, J., & Segal, M.W. (2009). Veterans, the Vietnam era, and marital dissolution: An event history analysis. *Armed Forces & Society, 36*(1), 19–37.

Cohen, J., Segal, D.R., & Temme, L.V. (1986). The educational cost of military service in the 1960s. *Journal of Political & Military Sociology, 14*(2), 303–319.

Conway, T.L. (1998). Tobacco use and the United States military: A longstanding problem. *Tobacco Control*, 7(3), 219–221.

Cooney, T. M., & Hogan, D. P. (1991). Marriage in an institutionalized life course: First marriage among American men in the twentieth century. *Journal of Marriage and the Family, 53*(1), 178–190.

Cozza, S. J., & Lerner, R. M. (2013). Military children and families: Introducing the issue. *The Future of Children, 23*(2), 3–11.

Davison, E. H., Pless, A. P., Gugliucci, M. R., King, L. A., King, D. W., Salgado, D. M., Spiro, A., & Bachrach, P. (2006). Late-life emergence of early-life trauma—The phenomenon of late-onset stress symptomology among aging combat veterans. *Research on Aging, 28*(1), 84–114.

Dobkin, C., & Shabani, R. (2009). The health effects of military service: Evidence from the Vietnam draft. *Economic Inquiry, 47*(1), 69–80.

Dohrenwend, B. P., Turner, B., Turse, N. A., Adams, B. G., Koenen, K. C., & Marshall, R. (2006). The psychological risks of Vietnam for US veterans: A revisit with new data and methods. *Science, 313*(5789), 979–982.

Duggan, M., Rosenheck, R., & Singleton, P. (2010). Federal policy and the rise in disability enrollment: Evidence for the Veterans' Affairs Disability Compensation Program. *Journal of Law and Economics, 53*(2), 379–398.

Elder Jr., G. H. (1986). Military times and turning points in men's lives. *Developmental Psychology, 22*(2), 233–245.

Elder Jr., G. H. (1987). War mobilization and the life course: A cohort of World War II veterans. *Sociological Forum, 2*(3), 449–472.

Elder Jr., G. H, Clipp, E. C., Brown, J. S., Martin, L. R., & Friedman, H. W. (2009). The life-long mortality risks of World War II experiences. *Research on Aging, 31*(4), 391–412.

Elder Jr., G. H., Johnson, M. K., & Crosnoe, R. (2003). The emergence and development of life course theory. In J. T. Mortimer & M. J. Shanahan (Eds.), *Handbook of the life course*, (pp. 3–19). New York: Kluwer Academic/Plenum.

Elder Jr., G. H., Shanahan, M. J., & Clipp, E. C. (1994). When war comes to men's lives: Life-course patterns in family, work, and health. *Psychology and Aging, 9*(1), 5–16.

Elder Jr., G. H., Shanahan, M. J., Clipp, E. C. (1997). Linking combat and physical health: The legacy of World War II in men's lives. *American Journal of Psychiatry, 154*(3), 330–336.

Elman, C., & O'Rand, A. (2004). The race is to the swift: Socioeconomic origins, adult education, and wage attainment. *American Journal of Sociology, 10*(1), 123–160.

Fligstein, N. D. (1980). Who served in the military, 1940–73. *Armed Forces & Society, 6*(2), 297–312.

Flynn, G. Q. (1993). *The draft 1940–1973*. Lawrence: University Press of Kansas.

Fontana, A., & Rosenheck, R. (1995). Attempted suicide among Vietnam veterans—A model of etiology in a community sample. *American Journal of Psychiatry, 152*(1), 102–109.

Frey-Wouters, E., & Laufer, R. S. (1986). *Legacy of a war: The American soldier in Vietnam*. New York: Routledge.

Gimbel, C., & Booth, A. (1996). Who fought in Vietnam? *Social Forces, 74*(4), 1137–1157.

Goldscheider, F. K., & Waite, L. J. (1986). Sex differences in the entry into marriage. *American Journal of Sociology*, *92*(1), 91–109.

Griffin Jr., C.L., & Stein, M.A. (2015). Self-perception of disability and prospects for employment among U.S. veterans. *Work, 50*, 49–58.

Heerwig, J.A., & Conley, D. (2013). The causal effects of Vietnam-era military service on post-war family dynamics. *Social Science Research, 42*, 299–310.

Hirsch, B.T., & Mehay, S.L. (2003). Evaluating the labor market performance of veterans using a matched comparison group design. *Journal of Human Resources, 38*(3), 673–700.

Hogan, D.P. (1981). *Transitions and social change: The early lives of American man.* New York: Academic.

Jahnke, S.A., Hoffman, K.M., Haddock, K., Long, M.A.D., Williams, L.N., Landon, H.A., & Poston, W.S.C. (2011). Military tobacco policies: The good, the bad, and the ugly. *Military Medicine, 176*(12), 1382–1387.

Kelty, R., & Segal, D.R. (2013). The military as a transforming influence: Integration into or isolation from normal adult roles? In J.M. Wilmoth and A.S. London (Eds.), *Life-course perspectives on military service* (pp. 19–47). New York: Routledge.

Kimmerling, R., Gima, K., Smith, M.W., Street, A, & Frayne, S. (2007). The veterans health administration and military sexual trauma. *American Journal of Public Health, 97*(12), 2160–2166.

Kleykamp, M. (2013). Labor market outcomes among veterans and military spouses. In J.M. Wilmoth & A.S. London (Eds.), *Life-course perspectives on military service* (pp. 144–164). New York: Routledge.

Kulka, R.A., Schlenger, W.E., Fairbank, J.A., Hough, B.K.J., Marmar, C.R., Weiss, D.S., Grady, D.A., & Cranston, A. (1990). *Trauma and the Vietnam War generation: Report of findings from the National Vietnam Veterans Readjustment Study*. New York: Brunner/Mazel.

Laub, J.H., & Sampson, R.J. (2003). *Shared beginnings, divergent lives: Delinquent boys to age 70.* Cambridge, MA: Harvard University Press.

Laufer, R.S., & Gallops, M.S. (1985). Life-course effects of Vietnam combat and abusive violence—marital patterns. *Journal of Marriage and the Family, 47*(4), 839–853.

Laufer, R.S., Yager, T. Frey-Wouters, E., & Donnellan, J. (1981). Postwar trauma: Social and psychological problems of Vietnam veterans in the aftermath of the war. In A. Egendorf, C. Kadushin, R.S. Laufer, G. Rothbart, & L. Sloan (Eds.), *Legacies of Vietnam: Comparative adjustment of veterans and their peers* (pp. 19–44). New York: Center for Policy Research.

London, A.S., Burgard, S.A., & Wilmoth, J.M. (2014). The influence of veteran status, psychiatric diagnosis, and traumatic brain injury on inadequate sleep. *Journal of Sociology & Social Welfare,* XLI(4), 49–67.

London, A. S., Herd, P., Miech, R. A., & Wilmoth, J.M. (*in review*). The influence of men's military service on smoking across the life course.

London, A.S., & Wilmoth, J.M. (2008). Military service. In D. Carr, R. Crosnoe, M.E. Hughes, & A. Pienta (Eds.), *Encyclopedia of the life course and human development* (pp. 292–299). Farmington Hills, MI: Gale.

London, A. S., & Wilmoth, J. M. (2016). Military service in lives: Where do we go from here? In M. J. Shanahan, J. T. Mortimer, & M. Kirkpatrick Johnson

(Eds.), *Handbook of the life course (Volume II)* (pp. 277–300). Switzerland: Springer International Publishing.

Lopreato, S. C., & Poston, D. L. (1977). Differences in earnings and earnings ability between black veterans and non-veterans in the United States. *Social Science Quarterly, 57*(4), 750–766.

Lundquist, J. H., & Smith, H. L. (2005). Family formation among women in the US Military: Evidence from the NLSY. *Journal of Marriage and Family, 67*(1), 1–13.

Lutz, A. C. (2013). Race–ethnicity and immigration in the U.S. military. In J. M. Wilmoth & A. S. London (Eds.), *Life-course perspectives on military service* (pp. 68–96). New York: Routledge.

MacLean, A. (2010). The things they carry: Combat, disability, and unemployment among U.S. men. *American Sociological Review, 75*(4), 563–585.

MacLean, A. (2013). A matter of life and death: Military service and health. In J. M. Wilmoth & A. S. London (Eds.) *Life course perspectives on military service* (pp. 200–220). New York: Routledge.

MacLean, A., & Edwards, R. D. (2010). The pervasive role of rank in the health of U.S. veterans. *Armed Forces & Society, 36*(5), 765–785.

MacLean, A., & Elder Jr., G. H. (2007). Military service in the life course. *Annual Review of Sociology, 33,* 175–196.

Martindale, M., & Poston, D. L. (1979). Variations in veteran-non-veteran earnings patterns among World War II, Korea, and Vietnam War cohorts. *Armed Forces & Society, 5*(2), 219–243.

Mattila, J. P. (1978). GI Bill benefits and enrollments—How did veterans fare? *Social Science Quarterly, 59*(3), 535–545.

Miech, R. A., London, A. S., Wilmoth, J. M., & Koester, S. (2013). The effects of the military's antidrug policies over the life course: The case of past-year hallucinogen use. *Substance Use & Misuse, 48,* 837–853.

Modell, J., & Haggerty, T. (1991). The social impact of war. *Annual Review of Sociology, 17,* 205–224.

Mortimer, J. T., & Shanahan, M. J. (2003). *Handbook of the life course.* New York: Kluwer Academic/Plenum Publishers.

National Center for Veterans Analysis and Statistics. (2014a). Office of the Actuary, Veteran Population Projections Model (VetPop2014), Tables 1L and 2L. Last retrieved July 1, 2015, http://www.va.gov/vetdata/Veteran_Population.asp

National Center for Veterans Analysis and Statistics (2014b). Unique veteran users report FY 2012. Last retrieved July 1, 2015, https://catalog.data.gov/dataset/fy-2012-profile-of-unique-veteran-users

Nelson, J. P., & Pederson, L. L. (2008). Military tobacco use: A synthesis of the literature on prevalence, factors related to use, and cessation interventions. *Nicotine & Tobacco Research, 10*(5), 775–790.

Nichols, L. O., Martindale-Adams, J., Burns, R., Graney, M. J., & Zuber, J. (2011). Translation of a dementia caregiver support program in a health care system—REACH VA. *Archives of Internal Medicine, 171*(4), 353–359.

Ritchey, J. (2009). US Army, mental health experts team up to fight rising suicide rate. Last retrieved July 1, 2015, http://www.voanews.com/content/a-13-2009-01-30-voa59-68626972/407478.html

Rosen, S., & Taubman, P. (1982). Changes in life-cycle earnings—What do social security data show? *Journal of Human Resources, 17*(3), 321–338.

Ruger, W., Wilson, S. E., & Waddoups, S. L. (2002). Warfare and welfare: Military service, combat, and marital dissolution. *Armed Forces & Society, 29*(1), 85–107.

Sackett, P. R., & Mavor, A. S. (2006). *Assessing fitness for military enlistment: Physical, medical, and mental health standards*. Washington, DC: National Academies Press.

Sampson, R. J., & Laub, J. H. (1996). Socioeconomic achievement in the life course of disadvantaged men: Military service as a turning point, circa 1940–1965. *American Sociological Review, 61*(3), 347–367.

Savoca, E., & Rosenheck, R. (2000). The civilian labor market experiences of Vietnam-era veterans. *Journal of Mental Health Policy and Economics, 3*(4), 199–207.

Scott, W. J. (1992). PTSD and Agent Orange—Implications for a sociology of veterans issues. *Armed Forces & Society, 18*(4), 592–612.

Segal, D. R., & Segal, M. W. (2004). America's military population. *Population Bulletin, 59*(4), 1–40.

Settersten Jr., R. A. (2003). *Invitation to the life course: Toward new understandings of later life*. Amityville, NY: Baywood.

Settersten Jr., R. A. (2006). When nations call: How wartime military service matters for the life course and aging. *Research on Aging, 28*(1), 12–36.

Smith, E. A., & Malone, R. A. (2012). Why strong tobacco control measures "can't" be implemented in the U.S. military: A qualitative analysis. *Military Medicine, 177*(10), 1202–1207.

Smith, R. T., & True, G. (2014). Warring identities: Identity conflict and the mental distress of American veterans of the wars in Iraq and Afghanistan. *Society and Mental Health, 4*(2), 147–161.

Spiro, A., Schnurr, P. P., & Aldwin, C. M. (1997). A life-span perspective on the effects of military service. *Journal of Geriatric Psychiatry, 30*(1), 91–128.

Stanley, M. (2003). College education and the midcentury GI Bills. *Quarterly Journal of Economics,* 118(2), 671–708.

Street, D, &, Hoffman, J. (2013). Military service, social policy, and later-life financial and health security. In J. M. Wilmoth & A. S. London (Eds.), *Life-course perspectives on military service* (pp. 221–242). New York: Routledge.

Suris, A., & Lind, L. (2008). Military sexual trauma—A review of prevalence and associated health consequences in veterans. *Trauma, Violence, and Abuse, 9*(4), 250–269.

Teachman, J. D. (2004). Military service during the Vietnam era: Were there consequences for subsequent civilian earnings? *Social Forces, 83*(2), 709–730.

Teachman, J. D. (2005). Military service in the Vietnam era and educational attainment. *Sociology of Education, 78*(1), 50–68.

Teachman, J. D. (2013). Setting an agenda for future research on military service and the life course. In J. M. Wilmoth & A. S. London (Eds.), *Life course perspectives on military service* (pp. 254–274). New York: Routledge.

Teachman, J. D., & Call, V. R. A. (1996). The effect of military service on educational, occupational, and income attainment. *Social Science Research, 25*(1), 1–31.

U.S. Code of Federal Regulations. (2014). 38 §3.2, periods of war. Last retrieved July 1, 2015, http://www.ecfr.gov/cgi-bin/text-idx?rgn=div5&node=38:1.0.1.1.4#se38.1.3_12

Vogt, D. S., King, D. W., King, L. A., Savarese, V. W., & Suvak, M. K. (2004). War-zone exposure and long-term general life adjustment among Vietnam veterans: Findings from two perspectives. *Journal of Applied Social Psychology, 34*(9), 1797–1824.

Wilmoth, J. M., & London, A. S. (2011). Aging veterans: Needs and provisions. In J. L. Angel & R. Settersten (Eds.), *Handbook of the sociology of aging* (pp. 445–461). New York: Springer.

Wilmoth, J. M., & London, A. S. (2013). *Life-course perspectives on military service.* New York: Routledge.

Wilmoth, J. M., & London, A. S. (2016). The influence of military service on aging. In K. F. Ferraro, L. K. George, & D. Carr (Eds.), *Handbook of aging and the social sciences* (8th ed., pp. 227–250). New York: Springer.

Wilmoth, J. M., London, A. S., & Heflin, C. M. (2015). The use of VA disability benefits and social security disability insurance among veterans. *Disability and Health Journal, 8*, 388–396.

Wilmoth, J. M., London, A. S., & Himes, C. L. (2015). Inter-cohort variation in the consequences of U.S. military service on men's body mass index trajectories in mid- to late-life. In C. Burton-Jeangros, S. Cullati, A. Sacker, & D. Blane (Eds.), *A life course perspective on health trajectories and transitions* (pp. 133–154). London: Springer.

Wilmoth, J. M., London, A. S., & Parker, W. M. (2010). Military service and men's health trajectories in later life. *Journal of Gerontology: Social Science, 56*(6), 744–755.

Wolf, D. A., Wing, C., & Lopoo, L. M. (2013). Methodological problems in determining the consequences of military service. In J. M. Wilmoth & A. S. London (Eds.), *Life-course perspectives on military service* (pp. 254–274). New York: Routledge.

CHAPTER NINE

Immigration, Life Course, and Aging

Ynesse Abdul-Malak and Rebecca Wang

The number of immigrants arriving in the United States and the number of older immigrants are both expected to grow in the coming two decades. How are immigrants faring particularly as they approach older ages? Life-course-based theoretical frameworks such as segmented assimilation and cumulative inequality aid in contextualizing the various economic and physical well-being of immigrants. In this chapter, we review the literature on the economic and health impacts of immigration in the United States. We begin with a broad demographic look at who immigrates to the United States and highlight several different contexts in which migration occurs. Then, we review various ways in which immigrants fare economically and in health, placing special emphasis on where immigrants are advantageous and where they are most vulnerable.

Demographic Trends

According to the 2013 American Community Survey, there are roughly 41 million foreign-born immigrants in the United States (Zong & Batalova, 2015). Together, immigrants comprise approximately 13 percent of the total U.S. population. While the proportion of immigrants has been steadily increasing since the 1970s, the peak share of immigrants occurred in 1890, with immigrants accounting for almost 15 percent of the total U.S. population (Zong and Batalova, 2015). Within this immigrant population, foreign-born older immigrants in the United States aged 60 and older represent approximately 7 percent of all admitted immigrants each year with numbers ranging from 50,398 in 1998 to 100,554 in 2006 (Wilmoth,

2012). Overall, the foreign-born older population increased from 2.7 to 4.6 million people between 1990 and 2010, an increase of nearly 70 percent (Population Reference Bureau, 2013). The greatest increase has been among Asian and Latino foreign-born older immigrants who accounted for roughly 38 percent and 29 percent, respectively, aged 65 years and older in 2010 (Wilmoth, 2012). This section will highlight key demographic trends of the immigrant population in the United States, including country of origin, age, gender, intergenerational households, and geography of immigrant settlement.

Early to late twentieth century brought immigrants from a variety of countries of origin to the United States and was largely shaped by sociohistorical time and policy. Immigrants arriving at the turn of the twentieth century largely came from southern, central, and eastern Europe and in particular, Italians, Polish, and eastern European Jewish (Perlmann, 2005). However, this time was also characterized by great feelings of xenophobia, prompting restrictionist policies such as quotas on all immigrant groups as well as bans on specific immigrant groups such as the Chinese. The passage of the 1965 Immigration Act lifted quotas and bans on immigration and saw a surge in immigrants from Asia and Latin America. The top sending countries in 2013 were Mexico, China, India, Philippines, and Vietnam and account for about 45 percent of the total U.S. immigrant population (Zong & Batalova, 2015). Figure 9.1 illustrates the shift in birth countries of immigrants. In 1960, approximately three-quarters of the immigrants were from Europe (Zong & Batalova, 2015). Countries such as Germany, Italy, Poland, and the former Soviet Union accounted for a large share of immigrants. In contrast, European originating immigrants in 2013 comprised 12 percent of the immigrant population (Zong & Batalova, 2015). Asian and Latin American-born immigrants experienced the opposite trend. In 2013, Asian and Latin American countries accounted for 68 percent of the immigrant population in the United States, compared to just 14 percent in 1960 (Zong & Batalova, 2015).

Although the average age of the immigrant population is higher than that of the U.S.-born population, the difference fluctuates across time. In 2013, the average age of the U.S.-born population was approximately 36 years compared to approximately 43 years for the foreign-born population (Zong & Batalova, 2015). The large majority of the foreign-born population is of working age, with about 80 percent of the foreign-born population between the ages of 18 and 64 years (Zong & Batalova, 2015). While the 65 years and older group is similar across foreign-born and U.S.-born, at about 14 percent, there has been an increase in immigrants arriving in later life (Zong & Batalova, 2015). Researchers distinguish between two distinct groups of older immigrants in the United States: Those who migrated earlier

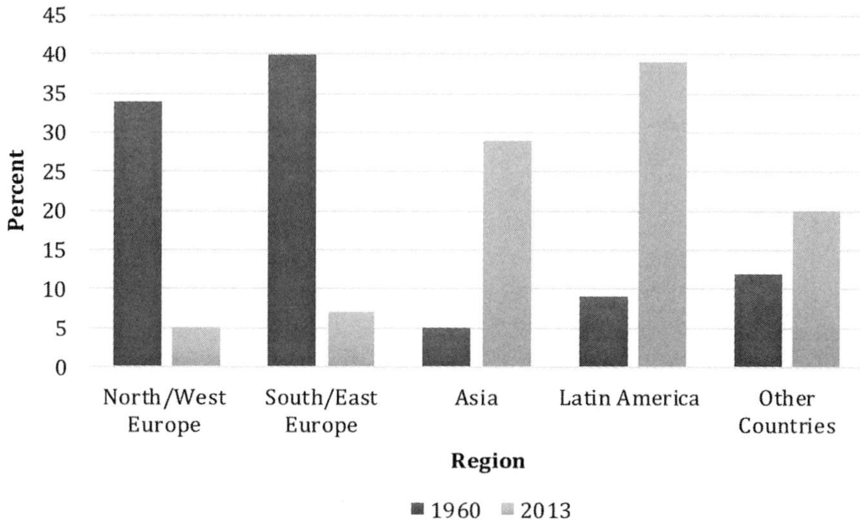

Figure 9.1 Immigrant population by geographic region, 1960 and 2013. (Migration Policy Institute tabulation of data from the 2013 American Community Surveys. Data for 1960 are from Campbell J. Gibson and Emily Lennon, "Historical Census Statistics on the Foreign-Born Population of the United States: 1850 to 1990" [Working Paper No. 29, U.S. Census Bureau, Washington, DC, 1999].)

in life and those who migrated later in life. The 2010 American Community Survey estimates that 10 percent of immigrants over the age of 65 had been living in the United States for fewer than 10 years (Population Reference Bureau, 2013). Demographers have found that the aging experiences of early-arriving immigrants who migrated at a younger age and have aged in the United States generally reflect their U.S.-born counterparts in terms of health and health-care utilization in later life (Choi, 2011). In comparison, immigrants who arrive later in life, particularly after 65 years, face unique challenges.

Compared to the early twentieth century, the gender composition of the U.S. immigrant population has shifted due to increased numbers of female immigrants. From 1870 to 1950, there were more men than women immigrants in the United States, with the highest sex ratio in 1910 of 131 immigrant men to every 100 immigrant women (Zong & Batalova, 2015). In 2013, the sex ratio was 95 immigrant men to every 100 immigrant women, meaning that there are fewer immigrant men than women in the United States (Zong & Batalova, 2015). Because women live longer than men, on average, consequently, many of the problems of aging are disproportionately experienced by women whose life course experiences shape their later-life outcomes, including health conditions, economic status, and social relationships. The variability in intergenerational family experiences of older immigrants is directly and indirectly influenced by sociohistorical and sociopolitical contexts. Sociohistorical time not only provides the context to society's warm or hostile welcome, it also provides the context in which immigrants develop key cultural values and norms that are transferred across generations. For example, Chinese family formations were directly shaped by historical policies such as the Chinese Exclusion Act of 1882. Xenophobic attitudes towards Chinese immigrants forced families into close living quarters, known as Chinatowns. Most Chinatowns consisted of tight knit ethnic enclaves featuring strong social and economic support systems. As a result, it was not uncommon to have large, extended families, many not biological (Rumbaut, 2005). This greatly shaped the experiences of Chinese older immigrants as they were not only much more likely to be independent, but these immigrant grandparents had the "respect of an entire community" (Zhou, 2009, p. 25). These grandpas often times kept watch over the children in Chinatowns. In stark contrast, the family and intergenerational experiences of contemporary immigrant generations are typically characterized as dissonant and filled with struggles (Foner & Dreby, 2011; Treas, 2008b). Values of familism and filial piety are not always found consistently across generations. This is perhaps best seen in multigenerational households. Some scholars have found that in multigenerational homes, some intergenerational relationships are privileged over other relationships (Silverstein & Attias-Donfut, 2010; Treas, 2008b; Usita & Shakya, 2012). For example, a strong degree of familism may be present in the parent-child relationship, but not in the grandparent-grandchild relationship. This relationship is further moderated by the degree of acculturation experienced by the younger generation (Foner & Dreby, 2011). Silverstein and Attias-Donfut (2010) suggest that acculturation among the later-generation children is negatively associated with feelings of emotional solidarity with their grandparents. That is, as the immigrant children become more acculturated into American mainstream culture, they feel less close to their grandparents.

A distinctive hallmark of the post-1965 wave of migration has been the decreasing geographic concentration of immigrant settlement. One of the significant demographic changes has been geographic disbursement of immigrants away from the Big Five states: California, New York, Texas, Florida, and Illinois. This trend has been particularly well documented by researchers for the Mexican immigrant population, as the Mexican migration patterns have experienced the most diversity (Donato et al., 2008; Leach & Bean, 2008; Lichter et al., 2010). Before 1990, 86 percent of Mexican immigrants settled in the Big Five states. This number decreased to 61 percent in 2000 according to the PUMS data. For example, the increase of Mexican immigrants in the same time period settling in new destinations states rose from 10 percent to 30 percent (Massey & Capoferro, 2008). While this is largely driven by Latino immigration, in a comparison of Asian immigrant groups, the trend is similar, but was more modest than Latino immigrant trends (Bump, Lowell, & Pettersen, 2005; Massey & Capoferro, 2008). The passage of Immigration Reform and Control Act of 1986 (IRCA) coupled with growing economies, particularly in service and construction, played a large role in the new geography of immigrant settlements. As a provision of IRCA, undocumented migrants who have been living in the United States since January of 1982 were granted amnesty. Essentially, this allowed for immigrants to relocate without the fear of deportation. Moreover, traditional immigrant destinations such as California were experiencing saturation of local markets, pushing immigrants to look elsewhere for work. The top three states experiencing the largest percent growth of immigrants in the past decade are Tennessee, North Carolina, and Kentucky (Zong & Batalova, 2015). Many of these nontraditional places share a similar story, such as Dalton, Georgia, where growing industrial economies generated labor shortages that immigrants quickly filled.

As immigration to the United States steadily increases, the demographic trends of immigrants reveal several noteworthy shifts. While the bulk of immigrants are still migrating during working-age years, there has been a substantial growth of immigrants arriving in later life. Immigrant sex ratio trends indicate a shift to more immigrant women to men, placing them in a more vulnerable position to later-life hardships. Contemporary intergenerational household dynamics challenge the traditional immigrant assumptions of filial piety and familism. Finally, the geographic settlement of immigrants has expanded far beyond the traditional destinations of immigrants.

Contextualizing Migration Patterns

Why do immigrants migrate to the United States? Immigrants arrive in the United States under very different contexts. Understanding the reasons for international migration helps to contextualize the experiences across the life course of immigrants. For immigrants, the different details of why people migrate are critical to contextualizing the experiences across the life course. This section highlights push-pull influences of migration, chained migration, and rolling migration.

Factors that push people to immigrate vary depending on the economic climate of a particular period of time. In the 1980s and 1990s, scholars focused on the pressures to migrate as a result of global capitalism (Portes & Walton, 2013; Sassen, 1990). World systems theory emphasizes the effect of globalization. Globalization is marked by the growth of multinational capitalists with branches and factories in the global south and has a direct effect of immigration because it dislocates groups of people, many of whom are forced to move elsewhere. This nonvoluntary immigration is an inevitable consequence of the growth of profit-driven capitalists in search of land, raw materials, and labor (Massey et al., 1993). For example, despite high unemployment rates in the United States during the 1970s, Asian and Caribbean immigration remained steady because of the increased expansion of global corporations and industries into Southeast Asian and Caribbean countries and displacing physical homes, jobs, and means for survival (Sassen, 1990). As a result, immigrants who are pushed into a new country often face more difficulties because of the absence of migration incentives such as better wages. Today, the appendages of global capitalism still create constrained opportunities to thrive in less-developed countries, pressuring families and individuals to immigrate to an unfamiliar place.

On the other end of the spectrum, international migration occurs as a result of many sources of incentive, or pull factors. At the most elementary level, incentives can be seen as a basic cost-benefit calculation and maximizing income with minimal risk for individuals and families. Federal programs, such as the Bracero Program during the 1940s, created large-scale incentives for international migration. At its peak, the U.S. government brought in almost half a million contracted Mexican laborers to meet the labor demand (Portes & Rumbaut, 2014). The Bracero Program stipulations included set wages, housing, and some medical care (Massey, Durand, & Malone, 2002). To cut costs, rural farmers began to hire undocumented immigrants who were willing to work and farmers did not have to provide the same standards of pay and living as contracted braceros. Moreover, when the Bracero Program ended in the 1965, farmers were reluctant to hire back native workers, which would ultimately increase wages and decrease profit. So, while the official incentives of labor migrants may have disappeared, the incentive for labor migrants, particularly undocumented immigrants remained strong. Contemporary pull factors for immigrants include postsecondary education, family reunification, and opportunities for both skilled and unskilled labor.

As immigration increases, so does the possibility for chained migration. That is, changing norms in the sending and receiving country create an embedded incentive for migration. For example, a consequence of the Bracero Program was that the social definition of a farm laborer became strongly associated with foreign or immigrant work, essentially creating an institutionalized demand for immigrant laborers. In the sending countries, increased migration and remittances made households with family members working abroad become more common (Massey, 1999). The greater visibility of international migration then becomes ingrained into their values changing norms and cultural values (Massey, 1999). These factors produce an increasing incentive for others to follow in the footsteps of their fellow, former community members and migrate. Moreover, with each wave of migration, a foundation of knowledge and social capital is developed; thus, the risks of future waves decrease (Massey, 1999).

The flow of migration is not always permanent, as in the case of rolling migrants. Rolling migration refers to immigrants who strategically divide their time between the United States and their country of origin. Policy changes, along with more restrictionist laws, have resulted in the use of more innovative strategies. Contemporary immigrants are becoming increasingly transnational, through strategies of using tourist visas or dual citizenship. Transnational, or global, families refers to families that are split with part of the family in the United States and part of the family in their respective home country (Silverstein & Attias-Donfut, 2010). These groups of migrants differ from the traditional younger, working-age labor migrants and are often the older parents of adult immigrant children. Transnational older adults mainly come to help their adult children and grandchildren. For many older immigrants, this is achieved through "strategic use of immigration policies that presume a desire for permanent U.S. settlement and constrain international travel patterns" (Treas, 2008a, p. 471). Some strategies include using tourist visas to stay in the United States for six months, then returning to their home country in order to apply for a new travel visa (Treas, 2008a). Though technically considered temporary, some older immigrants continue this cycle for many years. For some immigrants, the transnational life may be ideal as some immigrants value the preservation of ties to their home country. However, as some qualitative research suggest, for older immigrants who have the resources to live a transnational life, commuting between two countries and the back-and-forth nature of the visits disrupts the lives of older immigrants' adult children and grandchildren who have come to depend on the different types of support provided by their elder parents (Gilberson, 2009). Nevertheless, this circulatory transnational migration pattern is increasingly becoming the reality for contemporary immigrants.

Theories for Assessing Impacts of Immigration on Economic Well-Being and Health

The body of research studying the impacts of immigration on economic well-being and health often draws from the rich theoretical developments in both the sociology of immigration as well as social gerontology. Encouraging the use of diverse theories from multiple disciplines provides the best framework for better capturing the diversity in immigrant lives. This section pays special attention to how these conceptual frameworks inform our understanding of immigrants' socioeconomic circumstances and health. We explore how segmented assimilation theory contributes to our understanding of immigrants' socioeconomic status and health; then, we discuss how cumulative inequality theory adds to our understanding of the social location of new wave immigrants and its association with their economic well-being and health.

Segmented Assimilation Theory

Segmented assimilation theory emerged as an alternative to classical assimilation theory to explain the process of assimilation of various immigrant groups. Classical assimilation theory was more relevant to describe the experiences of European immigrants, while segmented assimilation theory is used to elucidate the adaptation and experiences of the new wave of immigrants, specifically the second generation (Portes & Zhou, 1993; Zhou, 1997). It recognizes that contextual differences are what accounted for the new immigrants' assimilation. Successful assimilation is shaped by a wide range of factors such as skin color, geographic location, and access to economic opportunities (Portes & Zhou, 1993). The new immigrants are so diverse, ranging from laborers to professionals, who are received in various sectors of American society, from impoverished urban settings to affluent suburbs (Zhou, 1997). Consequently, these contextual differences shape their paths of social mobility. Those who start from the bottom echelon might be trapped there and the ones who are on top have more opportunities to move upward. For example, professional migrants are more likely to assimilate to mainstream U.S. culture (Finch et al., 2007). In the United States, structural forces that are inherent due to the prevalence of spatial segregation can explain some of the differences in the social mobility of different immigrant groups. Rumbaut (1997) conjectures that these structural forces could hinder healthy behaviors of the new wave second-generation immigrants. That is, some immigrants, specifically those who are blacks, are more likely to live in urban settings and are more likely to adapt to the American way of life, poor dietary habits and lack of exercise.

Cumulative Inequality Theory

Cumulative inequality theory provides insights into economic and health disparities that exist in different immigrant groups across the life course. It is a middle-range theory that integrates elements from the life course perspective with cumulative advantage/disadvantage theory to study health and aging and the accumulation of inequality (Ferraro & Shippee, 2009). Cumulative inequality theory posits that life course trajectories are shaped by disparities in resources, accumulation of risk, and human agency (Ferraro, Shippee, & Schafer, 2009). It looks at the interaction of the individuals with their environments. Specifically, it highlights how with demographic changes, social systems might generate inequality over the life course and that "personal trajectories are shaped by the accumulation of risk, available resources, perceived trajectories, and human agency" (Ferraro, Shippee, & Schafer, 2009: 334). Looking at the accumulation of inequality highlights more than later-life outcomes; it also places emphasis on the aging process as a whole. Moreover, cumulative inequality theory recognizes that social forces generate inequality and that individual choices are structurally constructed. Social antecedents are correlated with current- and future-life conditions. In other words, immigrants' early-life conditions and events can impact their later-life outcomes. Indeed, immigrants who achieve early socioeconomic accomplishments such as higher education might have better later-life outcomes, such as economic success and better health in the United States. Furthermore, cumulative inequality theory underscores how disadvantages generate more exposure to risk while advantages facilitate opportunities. This is not merely a linear relationship. Multiple domains could interact to generate inequality. This can be illustrated with the case of highly educated immigrants who are more likely to capitalize in their human capital when they migrated to the United States. Finally, cumulative inequality theory focuses on how life course trajectories are not deterministic and that risk accumulation, available resources, and human agency are constantly interacting to shape later-life outcomes. The concept of human agency is very salient when it comes to how different individuals respond to a risk or an opportunity. Immigrants can overcome adversities and prosper.

In sum, cumulative inequality theory highlights how minority immigrant health is linked to early-life trajectories, such as lack of resources in their native countries and current economic inequalities in the United States. It provides insights on how country of origin and time of migration are important factors in determining health status. Cumulative life course exposure to low socioeconomic conditions can lead to chronic diseases (Pollitt, Rose, & Kaufman, 2005; Wakabayashi, 2010). For example, immigrants with fewer resources early in life in their home countries often continue to have fewer resources in the United States, and as a result they struggle with more adverse health effects through their life trajectories.

We find this theory to be the most plausible at explaining minorities' economic disparities and health.

Economic Impacts of Immigration

What are the economic impacts of immigration on the receiving country? What are the economic impacts of immigration on immigrants across the life course? How do older immigrants fare economically? Economic impacts of immigration are usually measured in terms of labor market and utilization of social programs. This section assesses the economic impacts of immigration on the U.S. economy and on various immigrant groups by looking at its effects on labor market, poverty and employment rates, wage differentials, wealth as in savings and home ownership, and immigrant usage of social assurance programs.

Scholarly works on the impacts of immigration on the U.S. labor market are mixed and inconclusive. Immigrant inflows can provide mixed economic effects to the United States because of the heterogeneity of immigrant groups and structural/institutional factors. For example, high-skilled immigration might be conducive to economic growth by increasing productivity and innovation (Orrenius & Zavodny, 2012; Peri, 2012), while low-skilled workers might have a negative impact on natives' wages (Borjas, 2003; Hanson, 2008). Using national data, Borjas (2003) found that between the years 1960 and 2000, immigration negatively impacted labor wages and low-skilled labor supply, specifically for young high school dropouts, who experienced slower wage growth. Conversely, looking at data from 1960 to 2008, Peri (2010) found that the effect of immigration had not been deleterious to the U.S. economy. In fact, immigration increased the wages of U.S-born Americans.

Economic impacts of immigration on immigrants can be assessed by looking at poverty rates across immigrants from different region/country of origin, age, and generational cohorts. In general, immigrants are more likely to live in poverty than native-born Americans, at 19 percent and 15 percent, respectively (Grieco et al., 2012). Specifically, immigrants from Latin America are more likely to live below the poverty line compared to those from African, European, and Asian countries. Based on the American Community Survey, for immigrant families that poverty is determined, Figure 9.2 illustrates that about 23 percent of Latin American immigrants live below 100 percent of the poverty level compared to 10 percent of European immigrants (U.S. Census Bureau, 2015). When region of origin is disaggregated into countries, the disparity in poverty level is even more apparent with Mexican immigrants having the highest rates at 29 percent, followed by Guatemalans at 27 percent, and

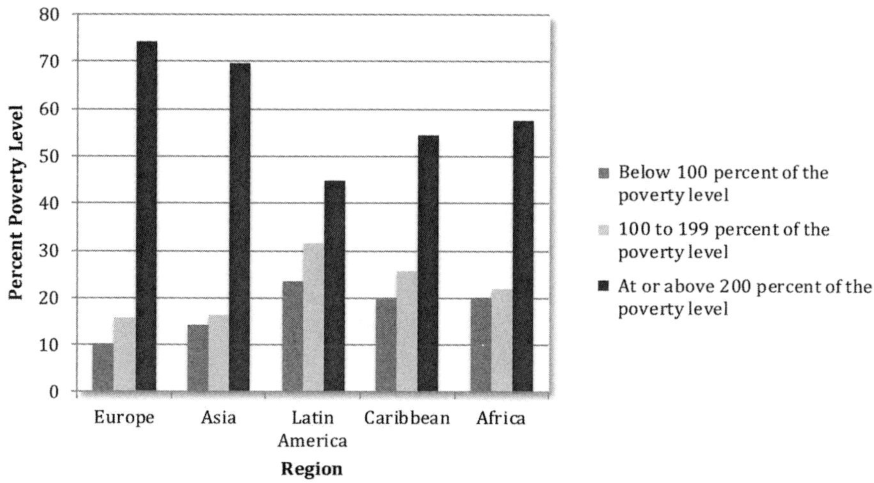

Figure 9.2 Immigrant poverty level for past 12 months by region of origin. (U.S. Census Bureau, 2009–2013, 5-Year American Community Survey)

Dominicans at 26 percent (Portes & Rumbaut, 2014, p. 34). Poverty varies across different age groups, about 31 percent of foreign-born children of 18 years or younger live below the poverty line compared to 21 percent of U.S.-born children (Grieco et al., 2012). In 2009, while 40 percent of children from Mexico and the Dominican Republic lived below the poverty line, only 6 or 7 percent of those from India and the Philippines did (Borjas, 2011). For older adults, despite working in the labor market for more years, on average, older immigrants are more susceptible to poverty than U.S.-born older adults. The poverty rate for immigrants, 65 years and older, is 16 percent compared to 8 percent of the native-born (Grieco et al., 2012). About 20 percent of Hispanic older immigrants and 14 percent of Asian older immigrants live under the federal poverty line, compared to 9 percent of the U.S.-born older adult population (Gerst & Burr, 2012). In 1970, the relative wage of immigrants 65 years and older compared to native-born was 5 percent and has widened to 30 percent in 2007 (Borjas, 2009). This widening gap is partially explained by country of origin, limited acculturation, and lack of opportunities for paid employment. Late-life-arriving immigrants and those who reside in the United States for less than 10 years have lower income, and they are less likely to receive retirement benefits and pensions (Borjas, 2009).

How do rates and types of employment differ among immigrants according to region/country of origin, generational cohorts, and gender? Employment is one major reason why people migrate. While the current employment profile of U.S. immigrants has diversified in comparison to that of the early twentieth-century immigrants, immigrants are still disproportionately represented in labor-intensive, low-skilled, often dangerous work. Immigrants in the early twentieth century were generally poor and took jobs in low-skill industries. Southern and central European immigrants were concentrated in construction, mining, and factory jobs. In comparison, in 2013, approximately 30 percent of the employed immigrant population worked in "management, professional, and related occupations," or white-collar occupations (Zong & Batalova, 2015). However, many contemporary labor immigrants occupy jobs at the lower end of the occupation spectrum. The difference is that these jobs are no longer held by European immigrants, but rather by Hispanic immigrants, especially Mexicans (Perlmann, 2005). Immigrants comprise 16 percent of the U.S. labor force that is overwhelmingly represented by Hispanic and Asian immigrants, 48 percent and 24 percent, respectively (Bureau of Labor Statistics, 2014). The unemployment rate in 2013 for immigrants was slightly lower than U.S.-born Americans, 6.9 percent and 7.5 percent, respectively (Bureau of Labor Statistics, 2014). However, the rates for black immigrants' unemployment is 11 percent compared to 5 percent of Asian immigrants (Bureau of Labor Statistics, 2014). By gender, in 2013, immigrant men comprised about 58 percent of the labor force compared to 52 percent of their U.S.-born counterparts and among various immigrant groups, 66 percent are men (Bureau of Labor Statistics, 2014).

The geographic proximity of Latin America to the United States renders the migration of low-skilled migrants more feasible, while it creates education selectivity among other groups such as Asians and Africans. Immigrants with less education tend to hold manual jobs that many natives would not hold, such as in factories, farmlands, construction, and service industries. Latin American immigrants are more likely to work in service occupations, 31 percent, while only about 11 percent of European and Asian immigrants are likely to (Grieco et al., 2012). This explains the large numbers of immigrants who are overrepresented in these industries. Immigrants from Latin America including Mexico are more likely to come to the United States and occupy these positions because the journey is not as expensive. On the other hand, immigrants from Asia, Africa, and Europe tend to be more educated, thus they can afford to make the long journey to the United States and they occupy more managerial and professional positions. By gender, in 2013, immigrant women were more likely to be in service occupations compared to U.S.-born women, 33 percent and 20 percent, respectively (Bureau of Labor Statistics, 2014).

To measure immigrant wealth, we can look at wage differentials, home ownership, and savings by region/country of origin, gender, and education level. In general, immigrant earnings are less than native-born Americans, with its relative wages declining. In 2010, the median income for families of U.S.-born householders was $62,358 compared to $49,785 for families of immigrant householders (Grieco et al., 2012). However, there was great income disparity in immigrants' income depending on region of origin, with Asians' 2013 weekly earning to be at $951, followed by blacks at $649 and Hispanics at $509 (Bureau of Labor Statistics, 2014).

Wealth among immigrants is different according to gender. In 2013, immigrant women earned 15 percent less than their U.S.-born counterparts (Bureau of Labor Statistics, 2014) and 13 percent less than immigrant men (Immigration Policy Center, 2010). Mexican immigrant women earned less than any other immigrant group with a median annual income of $21,489, while Indian women had the highest median annual income at $61,767 (Immigration Policy Center, 2010). About 75 percent of married immigrants of 51 or older are homeowners compared to 88 percent U.S.-born Americans (Sevak & Schmidt, 2014). Looking at immigrant wealth by educational level reveals a positive association. The most educated immigrants are those from Asian countries, while those from Latin America have the lowest level of educational attainment. About 49 percent of Asian immigrants have a Bachelor's degree or higher while only 11 percent of those from Latin America do (Grieco et al., 2012). At the country of origin level, about 75 percent of Indians and only 5 percent of Mexicans are college graduates (Portes & Rumbaut, 2014). Therefore, immigrants with higher level of education tend to be better off economically. Even when accounting for variables such as country of origin, education, and gender, in general, immigrants fare worse when it comes to wealth accumulation. Using the Survey of Income and Program Participation (SIPP) from 2001 to 2003, Seto and Bogan (2013) showed that immigrants are 4.41 percent and 3.38 percent less likely to own stocks and mutual funds, respectively. Immigrants have a family net worth of $100,000 less than U.S-born (Sevak & Schmidt, 2014).

Immigrant use of social programs such as Temporary Assistance to Needy Families (TANF), Supplemental Security Income (SSI), Supplemental Nutrition Assistance Program (SNAP), Women, Infants, and Children nutrition program (WIC), and housing assistance is mostly determined by immigration status, country of origin, and age. Before the Personal Responsibility and Work Opportunity Reconciliation Act of 1996 (PRWORA), immigrants with legal status were allowed to participate in means-tested federal benefit programs, albeit their usage of such programs was considered low. With the implementation of PRWORA, participation of immigrants in social programs dropped significantly because citizenship status is one of the qualifications for eligibility for some of these programs.

Under the provisions of PRWORA, immigrants must reside in the United States for longer than five years to be eligible for certain assistance programs. Using data from the Current Population Survey (CPS) Annual Social and Economic Supplement (ASEC), controlling for legal status and low incomes, Capps, Fix, and Henderson (2009) found that usage of TANF, SSI, and food stamps remained low among legal permanent residents compared to native families. From 1994 to 2002, TANF and food stamps usage among legal permanent residents decreased by 18 percent and 14 percent, respectively. Together, this represented a 50 percent greater decrease compared to U.S.-born families (Capps, Fix, & Henderson, 2009). Based on 2011 CPS data, the use of any type of social programs was higher among immigrants from Latin American countries such as Mexico (57%) and Guatemala (55%) and lower in European countries such as Germany (10%) and UK (6%) (Camarota, 2012). Moreover, legal barriers to accessing social assurance programs often make the later-life immigrant population not only vulnerable, but also place strain on their adult children and extended family who typically absorb the consequences of these structural barriers (Choi, 2011; Gerst & Burr, 2012).

How do older immigrants fare economically? Late-life immigrants are vulnerable to economic hardship, despite their sponsors' affidavit to provide economic support until older immigrants "are naturalized citizens or they work for 40 quarters" (Gerst & Burr, 2012, p. 15). Older immigrants may become naturalized and share the same access to social benefits as United States citizens. However, many late-life immigrants are much less likely to become naturalized because they are more likely to arrive to the United States with limited human capital, making it difficult to successfully pass the English proficiency and literacy tests associated with the naturalization process (Gerst & Burr, 2012). For these late-life immigrants, they are much less likely to work for the 40 quarters needed to gain eligibility for Social Security because of their age and their limited English proficiency. Additionally, policy changes from the PRWORA changed eligibility requirements for federal programs such as Temporary Aid to Needy Families, making some older immigrant populations even more vulnerable. For the late-arriving older immigrants who do not have access to these state resources, many are much more reliant on their adult children. This shift of "responsibility for support of the most vulnerable from government to family members" places a heavy burden on the families of the newly arrived older immigrants (Gerst & Burr, 2012, p. 15). Ineligibility not only negatively affects older immigrants, it also disproportionately affects the lower-income adult children and grandchildren who may have existing financial strains.

Health Impacts of Immigration

What are the health impacts of immigration? With the rising number of older immigrants to the United States, specifically the new wave of immigrants from Latin America and Asia, there has been a lot of focus on the health status of these immigrants and how they impact the U.S. health-care system. In general, immigrants experience a health advantage and have lower adult mortality than their U.S.-born counterparts (Abraído-Lanza et al., 2006; Derose, Escarce, & Lurie, 2007; Heron, Schoeni, & Morales, 2003; Kim et al., 2006; Read, Emerson, & Tarlov, 2005; Singh & Miller, 2004; Singh & Siahpush, 2001; Singh & Yu, 1996). Explanations for this immigrant health advantage have focused on many factors such as selective migration and culturally relevant healthy behaviors (Abraido-Lanza, Chao, & Florez, 2005; Akresh & Frank, 2008; Antecol & Bedard, 2006; Cho et al., 2004; Jasso et al., 2004). However, many scholarly works have shown that with age and time, this health advantage dissipates and immigrant health converges with the native-born levels (Abraido-Lanza, Chao, & Florez, 2005; Antecol & Bedard, 2006; Wakabayashi, 2010). This section focuses on major health impacts of immigration in terms of infant mortality, health behaviors, and chronic conditions on various immigrant groups and its impact on the U.S. health-care system.

Generally, immigrants' infant mortality rate (IMR) is lower than of U.S.-born women. However, most scholarly works on this topic have focused on Hispanics, mostly Mexicans, and non-Hispanic white immigrants (Frisbie et al., 2010; Henry-Sanchez & Geronimus, 2013; Mathews & MacDorman, 2010). Using data from the National Center for Health Statistics (NCHS) of three time periods, 1989–1991, 1995–1998, and 1999–2001 and tracing trends over time in IMR due to specific leading causes, Frisbie et al. (2010) showed that there are great disparities in IMR among various American mothers. Comparing immigrants' IMR to U.S.-born non-Hispanic white women, the odds ratios of infant mortality from all-causes are 1.56 for non-Hispanic black immigrants, 0.85 for Mexican immigrant, and 0.73 for non-Hispanic white immigrants. The IMR for black immigrants is much higher than any other immigrant group. That is, black immigrant infants are less likely to see their first birthdays compared to other immigrant groups. To our knowledge, there are no studies that disaggregate the pan-ethnic grouping of black immigrant women to country of origin, in order to fully capture and understand the disparity of IMR among that group.

There are stark differences in patterns and distribution of chronic health conditions among various immigrant groups in the United States by generational cohorts, country of origin, and gender. First-generation, or foreign-born, immigrants are generally healthier and have fewer chronic health conditions than the second generation, born in the United States. Data from the nationally representative, Second Longitudinal Survey of Aging (LSOAII) show that second-generation immigrants are over six times more likely to have cancer than their late-arriving, first-generation counterparts (Choi, 2011). Second-generation older immigrants have, on average, 1.2 percent more reported chronic conditions compared to the late-arriving, first-generation immigrants (Choi, 2011). Using data from 1997 to 2005 of the National Health Interview Survey (NHIS), Oza-Frank and Narayan (2008) showed that immigrants from Mexico, Central America, and the Caribbean have higher prevalence of diabetes compared to European immigrants, 7 percent and 3 percent, respectively. With the National Survey of American Life (NSAL) data, Erving (2011) found that after controlling for SES and social roles, Caribbean black immigrant women are 43 percent more likely to report greater chronic illness (including cancer, hypertension, diabetes, stroke, blood circulation problems, and heart trouble) relative to men. Incidence of chronic health conditions seem to increase with increased length of stay in the United States. Difference in chronic health conditions between different immigrant women is understudied and not well understood. Very few studies disaggregate immigrant groups into country of origin and different demographic factors.

How do health behaviors explain health differentials among U.S. immigrants? Health behaviors such as smoking, exercise, and dietary habits are important determinants of overall health. Understanding how health behaviors operate or change with migration might provide insights on immigrants' health disparity. Over time, immigrants adopt traditional American health behaviors and their health status begins to converge with that of the general U.S. population. Singh and Siahpush (2001) analyzed a longitudinal data set from the National Longitudinal Mortality Study (NLMS) and Behavioral and health status data, originating from the 1993 and 1994 NHIS to examine several factors associated with all-cause and cause-specific mortality in the United States, specifically whether health status and behaviors vary among immigrant groups and by length of stay in the United States. After adjusting for the effects of several socioeconomic and demographic factors, immigrants who reside in the United States for less than a year are 52 percent less likely to smoke cigarettes than the U.S.-born; those who are in the United States for 10–15 years and those who are residing in the country longer than 15 years are less likely to smoke than their U.S.-born counterparts, 32 percent and 18 percent, respectively (Singh & Siahpush, 2001). Additionally, immigrants residing in the United States for more than 15 years are

13 percent less likely to be overweight compared to newly arrived immigrants, who are 61 percent less likely to be overweight. Pérez-Escamilla (2011) conducted a systematic review of nationally representative surveys related to Hispanics' health behaviors and concluded that higher acculturation among Hispanics is associated with poor dietary habits such as lower consumption of fruits and vegetables and higher consumption of sugar and added fats. Among immigrant women, Roshania, Narayan, and Oza-Frank (2008) found that longer stay in the United States for early-arriving immigrants, those who arrived at 20 years old or younger, was related to a change in dietary habits and they were more likely to be overweight/obese compared to those who came at 50 years old or older, odds ratios of 0.46 and 0.38, respectively. Using similar data, Choi (2012) found that immigrants from all regions, except the Middle East/north Africa, are more likely to be obese/overweight with longer stay in the United States. The longer immigrants stay in the United States, the more likely their health behaviors including smoking status and dietary habits, and risk factors for cardiovascular diseases, converge to the lifestyles of Americans.

Immigrants have lower rates of health insurance coverage than U.S.-born populations, and there is disparity of coverage along country of origin, SES, gender, and age. Immigrants from Latin America, the Caribbean, Vietnam, and Korea are least likely to have health-care coverage, while immigrants from Europe and Canada have the highest insurance coverage rates (Carrasquillo, Carrasquillo, & Shea, 2000). Indeed, immigrants from Central America or the Caribbean are least likely to be covered by some form of health insurance and only 63 percent of those from the Caribbean with health insurance are covered by a private insurer (Grieco et al., 2012). One explanation for lower coverage is that immigrants are more likely to work for employers who do not offer health benefits or are self-employed (Buchmueller et al., 2007). Moreover, access to jobs with access to health benefits is positively associated with education.

Immigrant groups such as Indians, who enjoy an 89 percent high school graduation rate, also enjoy a high percentage of health-care coverage (Derose, Escarce, & Lurie, 2007). Disparities in health insurance coverage among immigrants are even greater across gender and age. Using the National Health Interview Surveys from 1992–2002, Kaushal and Kaestner (2007) found that single immigrant women are less likely to have coverage, about 19 percent lack insurance. Among immigrant families, children of immigrants are much more susceptible to not having health insurance than children of nonimmigrants, controlling for income. That is, among lower-income families, children of immigrants are three times as likely to lack health insurance than children of nonimmigrants (Huang, Stella, & Ledsky, 2006). Among older immigrants, country of origin, marital status, gender, and work quarters are strong predictors of health-care coverage. Overall, older immigrants are less likely to have health insurance. Further, Latino immigrants are 22 times as likely than European immigrants to be without health insurance (Choi, 2006). The 1996 PRWORA significantly restricted immigrants' eligibility for federally funded services such as Medicaid for noncitizens, especially unmarried women (Derose et al., 2009; Kaushal & Kaestner, 2007). Additionally, many older immigrants might not be qualified for Medicare because they have not worked in the United States long enough or were self-employed. Approximately one-quarter of older immigrants qualify for Medicare, because most older immigrants have less than 40 quarters of work experience (Carr & Tienda, 2013).

The U.S. safety net, such as Medicaid and Medicare, does not negate the health disparities by providing equal health-care access. Country of origin, SES, gender, and age are variables that are associated with healthcare access. Overall, noncitizen immigrants made up less than 5 percent of the population receiving Medicare or Medicaid (Carrasquillo, Carrasquillo, & Shea, 2000). U.S. policies advantage certain immigrant groups over others. For example, those who are considered refugees or asylum seekers for political reasons are automatically eligible for government-funded health-care coverage. This creates a disparity regarding health-care access based on country of origin. Cuban and Russian immigrants are considered refugees and thus enjoy government-funded health-care coverage. Whereas, 60 percent of migrant farm workers, mostly from Mexico, Guatemala, El Salvador, and Haiti, do not meet the basic eligibility criteria for government assistance (Carrasquillo, Carrasquillo, & Shea, 2000). The situation is even more precarious for undocumented immigrants. Immigrant children, who entered the United States after the implementation of PRWORA, are ineligible for insurance coverage under SCHIP programs. Kaushal & Kaestner (2007) found that welfare reform was associated with a 28 to 40 percent increase in the proportion of lack health-care coverage among low-educated, immigrant single mothers. Older immigrants, especially those who have not paid into the system, are not qualified to receive Medicare. According to New York City Department of Health and Mental Hygiene, immigrant adults living in NYC with low incomes are less likely to have Medicaid than the U.S.-born, 29 percent and 42 percent, respectively (Kim et al., 2006). The newly implemented Affordable Care Act (ACA) aims to address the unequal health-care access; however, its coverage is not as comprehensive as Medicaid and Medicare (Pandey, Cantor, & Lloyd, 2014). Scholarly works need to evaluate the effectiveness of the ACA at providing health-care coverage for many uninsured and whether it has an effect at decreasing health disparities among various immigrant groups.

Discussion

Contemporary waves of immigration vary greatly in demographics, economic well-being, and physical health. Political and social histories not only shape the demographic compositions of immigrants, but also the contextual climate for migration and reception. The motivations, strategies, and paths on which immigrants arrive to the United States can range from simple cost-benefit calculations of voluntary migrants to the dislocating structural forces of global capitalist expansion.

Drawing directly and indirectly from life course perspectives, theoretical frameworks such as cumulative inequality and segmented assimilation aid in contextualizing the various economic and physical well-being of immigrants. The economic and health impacts of immigration vary not only by cultural origins, but also by a diverse set of factors such as generational cohort, age, and gender. Disparities such as greater rates of poverty and lower median incomes have long-lasting effects across the life course for immigrants, such as having much more limited financial savings in retirement. Moreover, much of low-skilled labor positions in the United States are occupied by immigrants. The physical demands associated with these occupations will no doubt carry long-lasting effects into later life. Finally, policy influences such as the restrictions from the 1996 Welfare Reform Act have only produced negative effects on immigrants and their families, who must absorb the additional weight.

Regarding physical health, immigrants in the United States enjoy some advantages but are much more vulnerable in other health-related areas. With the exception of late-life immigrants, first-generation immigrants experience better health. Infant mortality rates are lower for immigrant women than non-Hispanic and U.S.-born white women, but higher for black immigrants. In addition, immigrants enjoy fewer chronic conditions than their U.S.-born counterparts. However, immigrants are much more vulnerable when it comes to health-care access. Lack of health-care coverage is detrimental to long-term health. Moreover, health-care access and coverage are subject to federal program regulations and restrictions that often disproportionately affect immigrants.

The intricate nexus of immigration, life course, and aging allows much room for additional research. For example, with increasing numbers of immigrants moving and settling in nontraditional destinations, so does the need to better understand processes of incorporation. While scholarship on the demography of these populations has been well documented, additional quantitative research on the experiences of incorporation in these new destinations is much more limited. Researchers in the future are tasked with creating innovative methodology to access this population, especially the need to disaggregate the pan-ethnic grouping into country of origin. Furthermore, research on aging has not yet been included in this area. For now, the numbers of older immigrant are still small. However, it is quite likely that these numbers will be increasing in the coming years, especially for the late-life immigrants because of the more relaxed restrictions of family reunification policy. Older immigrants already face higher risk of isolation and loneliness. A lack of established immigrant coethnic communities, especially in nonmetropolitan new destinations, may be the most detrimental to the well-being and health of older immigrants. Though perhaps small in absolute number, the growth rates of immigrants in new destinations represent an overlooked, yet emergent population.

References

Abraído-Lanza, A. F., Armbrister, A. N., Flórez, K. R., & Aguirre, A. N. (2006). Toward a theory-driven model of acculturation in public health research. *American Journal of Public Health, 96*(8), 1342–1346.

Abraido-Lanza, A. F., Chao, M. T., & Florez, K. R. (2005). Do healthy behaviors decline with greater acculturation? Implications for the Latino mortality paradox. *Social Science & Medicine (1982), 61*(6), 1243.

Akresh, I. R., & Frank, R. (2008). Health selection among new immigrants. *American Journal of Public Health, 98*(11), 2058–2064. doi:10.2105/AJPH.2006.100974

Antecol, H., & Bedard, K. (2006). Unhealthy assimilation: Why do immigrants converge to American health status levels? *Demography, 43*(2), 337–360.

Borjas, G. (2003). The labor demand curve is downward sloping: Reexamining the impact of immigration on the labor market. *Quarterly Journal of Economics, 118*(4), 1335–1374. doi:10.3386/w9755

Borjas, G. (2009). *Economic well-being of the elderly immigrant population.* (No. orrc09–02). National Bureau of Economic Research.

Borjas, G. (2011). Poverty and program participation among immigrant children. *The Future of Children, 21*(1), 247–266.

Buchmueller, T. C., Lo Sasso, A. T., Lurie, I., & Dolfin, S. (2007). Immigrants and employers-sponsored health insurance. *Health Services Research, 42*(1p1), 286–310.

Bump, M. N., Lowell, B. L., & Pettersen, S. (2005). The growth and population characteristics of immigrants and minorities in America's new settlement areas. In E. Gozdziak, & S. Martin (Eds.), *Beyond the gateway: Immigrants in a changing America* (pp. 19–37). Lanham, MD: Lexington Books.

Bureau of Labor Statistics. (2014). *Foreign-born workers: Labor force characteristics—2013.* U.S. Department of Labor. Retrieved March 1, 2015, from http://www.bls.gov/news.release/forbrn.nr0.htm

Camarota, S. A. (2012). *Immigrants in the United States, 2010: A profile of America's foreign-born population.* Center for Immigration Studies Washington, DC.

Retrieved March 1, 2015 from http://cis.org/2012-profile-of-americas-foreign-born-population

Capps, R., Fix, M., & Henderson, E. (2009). Trends in immigrants' use of public assistance after welfare reform. In M. Fix (Ed.), *Immigrants and welfare* (pp. 93–122). New York: Russell Sage Foundation.

Carr, S., & Tienda, M. (2013). Family sponsorship and late-age immigration in aging America: Revised and expanded estimates of chained migration. *Population Research and Policy Review, 32*(6), 825–849.

Carrasquillo, O., Carrasquillo, A. I., & Shea, S. (2000). Health insurance coverage of immigrants living in the United States: Differences by citizenship status and country of origin. *American Journal of Public Health, 90*(6), 917–923.

Cho, Y., Frisbie, W.P., Hummer, R.A., & Rogers, R.G. (2004). Nativity, duration of residence, and the health of Hispanic adults in the United States. *International Migration Review, 38*(1), 184–211. doi:10.1111/j.1747–7379.2004.tb00193.x

Choi, J.Y. (2012). Prevalence of overweight and obesity among US immigrants: Results of the 2003 new immigrant survey. *Journal of Immigrant and Minority Health, 14*(6), 1112–1118.

Choi, S. (2006). Insurance status and health service utilization among newly-arrived older immigrants. *Journal of Immigrant and Minority Health, 8*(2), 149–161.

Choi, S. (2011). Longitudinal changes in access to health care by immigrant status among older adults: The importance of health insurance as a mediator. *The Gerontologist, 51*(2), 156–169. doi:10.1093/geront/gnq064

Derose, K.P., Bahney, B.W., Lurie, N., & Escarce, J.J. (2009). Review: Immigrants and health care access, quality, and cost. *Medical Care Research and Review, 66*(4), 355–408.

Derose, K.P., Escarce, J.J., & Lurie, N. (2007). Immigrants and health care: Sources of vulnerability. *Health Affairs, 26*(5), 1258–1268.

Donato, K.M., Tolbert, C., Nucci, A., & Kawano, Y. (2008). Changing faces, changing places: The emergence of new nonmetropolitan immigrant gateways. In D.S. Massey (Ed.), *New faces in new places: The changing demography of American immigration* (pp. 75–98). New York: Russell Sage Foundation.

Erving, C.L. (2011). Gender and physical health: A study of African American and Caribbean black adults. *Journal of Health and Social Behavior, 52*(3), 383–399. doi:10.1177/0022146511415857

Ferraro, K.F., & Shippee, T.P. (2009). Aging and cumulative inequality: How does inequality get under the skin? *The Gerontologist, 49*(3), 333–343. doi:10.1093/geront/gnp034

Ferraro, K.F., Shippee, T.P., & Schafer, M.H. (2009). Cumulative inequality theory for research on aging and the life course. In V.L. Bengtson, D. Gans, N.M. Putney & M. Silverstein (Eds.), *Handbook of theories of aging* (2nd ed., pp. 413–433). New York: Springer New York.

Finch, B.K., Lim, N., Perez, W., & Phuong, D., Do. (2007). Toward a population health model of segmented assimilation: The case of low birth weight in Los Angeles. *Sociological Perspectives, 50*(3), 445–468.

Foner, N., & Dreby, J. (2011). Relations between the generations in immigrant families. *Annual Review of Sociology, 37*, 545–564.

Frisbie, W. P., Hummer, R. A., Powers, D. A., Song, S., & Pullum, S. G. (2010). Race/ethnicity/nativity differentials and changes in cause-specific infant deaths in the context of declining infant mortality in the US: 1989–2001. *Population Research and Policy Review, 29*(3), 395–422.

Gerst, K., & Burr, J. A. (2012). Welfare program participation among older immigrants. *Public Policy and Aging Report, 22*(2), 12–16.

Gilberson, G. (2009). Caregiving across generations: Aging, state assistance, and multigenerational ties among immigrants from the Dominican Republic. In N. Foner (Ed.), *Across generations: Immigrant families in America* (pp. 135–159). New York: New York University Press.

Grieco, E. M., Acosta, Y. D., de la Cruz, G Patricia, Gambino, C., Gryn, T., Larsen, L. J., Walters, N. P. (2012). The foreign-born population in the United States: 2010. *American Community Survey Reports,* Retrieved September 1, 2014, from https://www.census.gov/prod/2012pubs/acs-19.pdf

Hanson, G. H. (2008). The economic consequences of the international migration of labor. *National Bureau of Economic Research Working Paper Series, No. 14490.* doi:10.3386/w14490

Henry-Sanchez, B. L., & Geronimus, A. T. (2013). Racial/ethnic disparities in infant mortality among U.S. Latinos. *Du Bois Review: Social Science Research on Race, 10*(01), 205–231. doi:10.1017/S1742058X13000064

Heron, M. P., Schoeni, R. F., & Morales, L. (2003). *Health status among older immigrants in the United States.* Population Studies Center, University of Michigan.

Huang, Z. J., Stella, M. Y., & Ledsky, R. (2006). Health status and health service access and use among children in US immigrant families. *American Journal of Public Health, 96*(4), 634–640.

Immigration Policy Center. (2010). *Immigrant women in the United States: A portrait of demographic diversity*. Retrieved from http://www.immigrationpolicy.org/just-facts/immigrant-women-united-states-portrait-demographic-diversity

Jasso, G., Massey, D. S., Rosenzweig, M. R., & Smith, J. P. (2004). The US new immigrant survey: Overview and preliminary results based on the new-immigrant cohorts of 1996 and 2003. *Immigration Research and Statistics Service Workshop on Longitudinal Surveys and Cross-Cultural Survey Design: Workshop Proceedings.* London, UK: Crown Publishing.

Kaushal, N., & Kaestner, R. (2007). Welfare reform and health of immigrant women and their children. *Journal of Immigrant and Minority Health, 9*(2), 61–74.

Kim, M., Van Wye, G., Kerker, B., Thorpe, L., & Frieden, T. (2006). The health of immigrants in New York City. *New York City Department of Health and Mental Hygiene*, Retrieved March 1, 2015 from http://www.nyc.gov/html/doh/downloads/pdf/episrv/episrv-immigrant-report.pdf

Leach, M. A., & Bean, F. D. (2008). The structure and dynamics of Mexican migration to new destinations in the United States. In D. S. Massey (Ed.), *New faces in new places: The changing demography of American immigration* (pp. 51–74). New York: Russell Sage Foundation.

Lichter, D. T., Parisi, D., Taquino, M. C., & Grice, S. M. (2010). Residential segregation in new Hispanic destinations: Cities, suburbs, and rural communities compared. *Social Science Research, 39*(2), 215–230.

Massey, D. S. (1999). Why does immigration occur? A theoretical synthesis. In C. Hirschman, P. Kasinitz, & J. DeWind (Eds.), *The handbook of international migration: The American experience* (pp. 34–52). New York: Russell Sage Foundation.

Massey, D. S., Arango, J., Hugo, G., Kouaouci, A., Pellegrino, A., & Taylor, J. E. (1993). Theories of international migration: A review and appraisal. *Population and Development Review, 19*(3), 431–466.

Massey, D. S., & Capoferro, C. (2008). The geographic diversification of American immigration. In D. S. Massey (Ed.), *New faces in new places: The changing demography of American immigration* (pp. 25–50). New York: Russell Sage Foundation.

Massey, D. S., Durand, J., & Malone, N. J. (2002). *Beyond smoke and mirrors*. New York: Russell Sage Foundation.

Mathews, T., & MacDorman, M. F. (2010). Infant mortality statistics from the 2006 period linked birth/infant death data set. *National Vital Statistics Reports: From the Centers for Disease Control and Prevention, National Center for Health Statistics, National Vital Statistics System, 58*(17), 1–31.

Orrenius, P. M., & Zavodny, M. (2012). Economic effects of migration: Receiving states. In M. R. Rosenblum, & D. J. Tichenor (Eds.), *Oxford handbook of the politics of international migration* (pp. 105–152). Oxford: Oxford University Press.

Oza-Frank, R., & Narayan, K. M. V. (2008). Overweight and diabetes prevalence among US immigrants. *American Journal of Public Health, 100*(4), 661–668. doi:10.2105/AJPH.2008.149492

Pandey, S. K., Cantor, J. C., & Lloyd, K. (2014). Immigrant health care access and the affordable care act. *Public Administration Review, 74*(6), 749–759.

Pérez-Escamilla, R. (2011). Acculturation, nutrition, and health disparities in Latinos. *The American Journal of Clinical Nutrition, 93*(5), 1163S–1167S.

Peri, G. (2010). The effect of immigrants on US employment and productivity. *FRBSF Economic Letter, 26*, 1–5.

Peri, G. (2012). Immigration, labor markets, and productivity. *Cato Journal, 32*, 35.

Perlmann, J. (2005). *Italians then, Mexicans now: Immigrant origins and the second-generation progress, 1890–2000*. New York: Russell Sage Foundation.

Pollitt, R., Rose, K., & Kaufman, J. (2005). Evaluating the evidence for models of life course socioeconomic factors and cardiovascular outcomes: A systematic review. *BMC Public Health, 5*(1), 7.

Population Reference Bureau. (2013). Elderly immigrants in the United States. *Today's Research on Aging, 29*, 1–9.

Portes, A., & Rumbaut, R. G. (2014). *Immigrant America: A Portrait*. Oakland: University of California Press.

Portes, A., & Walton, J. (2013). *Labor, Class, and the International System*. Philadelphia: Elsevier.

Portes, A., & Zhou, M. (1993). The new second generation: Segmented assimilation and its variants. *The Annals of the American Academy of Political and Social Science, 530*(1), 74–96. doi:10.1177/0002716293530001006

Read, J. G., Emerson, M. O., & Tarlov, A. (2005). Implications of black immigrant health for US racial disparities in health. *Journal of Immigrant Health, 7*(3), 205–212.

Roshania, R., Narayan, K. M. V., & Oza-Frank, R. (2008). Age at arrival and risk of obesity among US immigrants. *Obesity, 16*(12), 2669–2675. doi:10.1038/oby.2008.425

Rumbaut, R. G. (1997). Assimilation and its discontents: Between rhetoric and reality. *International Migration Review, 31*(4), 923–960.

Rumbaut, Ruben. (2005). Immigration, incorporation and generational cohorts in historical contexts. In K. W. Schaie & G. Elder (Eds.), *Historical influences on lives and aging* (pp. 43–88). New York: Springer Publishing.

Sassen, S. (1990). *The mobility of labor and capital: A study in international investment and labor flow.* Cambridge: Cambridge University Press.

Seto, S., & Bogan, V. L. (2013). Immigrant household investment behavior and country of origin: A study of immigrants to the United States. *International Journal of Finance & Economics, 18*(2), 128–158. doi:10.1002/ijfe.464

Sevak, P., & Schmidt, L. (2014). Immigrants and retirement resources. *Social Security Bulletin, 74*, 27.

Silverstein, M., & Attias-Donfut, C. (2010). Intergenerational relationships of international migrants in developed nations: The United States and France. In C. Phillipson & D. Dannefer (Eds.), *The SAGE handbook of social gerontology* (pp. 177–189). London: Sage Publications Ltd.

Singh, G. K., & Miller, B. A. (2004). Health, life expectancy, and mortality patterns among immigrant populations in the United States. *Canadian Journal of Public Health. Revue Canadienne De Sante Publique, 95*(3), I14.

Singh, G. K., & Siahpush, M. (2001). All-cause and cause-specific mortality of immigrants and native born in the United States. *American Journal of Public Health, 91*(3), 392.

Singh, G. K., & Yu, S. M. (1996). Adverse pregnancy outcomes: Differences between US- and foreign-born women in major US racial and ethnic groups. *American Journal of Public Health, 86*(6), 837–843.

Treas, J. (2008a). Four myths about older adults in America's immigrant families. *Generations, 32*(4), 40–45.

Treas, J. (2008b). Transnational older adults and their families. *Family Relations, 57*(4), 468–478.

United States Census Bureau. (2014). Annual estimates of the resident population for selected age groups by sex for the United States, states, counties, and Puerto Rico commonwealth and municipios: April 1, 2010 to July 1, 2013. Retrieved March 1, 2015, from http://factfinder.census.gov/faces/tableservices/jsf/pages/productview.xhtml?src=bkmk

United States Census Bureau. (2015). American fact finder—selected characteristics of the foreign-born population by region of birth, 2009–2013 American Community Survey 5-Year Estimates. Retrieved April 24, 2015, from http://factfinder.census.gov/faces/tableservices/jsf/pages/productview.xhtml?pid=ACS_13_5YR_S0503&prodType=table

Usita, P., & Shakya, H. (2012). Aging families and immigration. In R. Blieszner, & V. H. Bedford (Eds.), *Handbook of families and aging* (2nd ed., pp. 337–362). Santa Barbara, CA: Praeger.

Wakabayashi, C. (2010). Effects of immigration and age on the health of older people in the United States. *Journal of Applied Gerontology, 29*(6), 697–719.

Wilmoth, J. (2012). A demographic profile of older immigrants in the United States. *Public Policy and Aging Report,* 22(2), 8–11.

Zhou, M. (1997). Growing up American: The challenge confronting immigrant children and children of immigrants. *Annual Review of Sociology*, 23(1), 63–95.

Zhou, M. (2009). Conflict, coping, and reconciliation: Intergenerational relations in Chinese immigrant families. In N. Foner (Ed.), *Across Generations: Immigrant Families in America* (pp. 21–46). New York: New York University Press.

Zong, J., & Batalova, J. (2015). Frequently requested statistics on immigrants and immigration in the United States. Retrieved on April 24, 2015, from http://www.migrationpolicy.org/article/frequently-requested-statistics-immigrants-and-immigration-united-sstates#TOP

CHAPTER TEN

Marital Status and Living Arrangements over the Life Course

Judith Treas and Tanya Sanabria

Over our lives, we look to our close personal ties for companionship, social support, practical assistance, financial help, and many other rewards. At least for some part of adulthood, most of us will find these things in our intimate romantic partnerships, especially in the comparatively permanent relationship of marriage. The pathways into and out of these partnerships define the course of our lives and differentiate our life circumstances in predictable ways. We also look to others with whom we live, whether a partner or not, to meet emotional and pragmatic needs. As we grow up and grow older, our living arrangements change, offering insights into the changes in needs and resources over our lives.

In this chapter, we describe recent historical changes, point to life-course patterns, and describe how well-being is associated with marital status and living arrangements. We begin by examining marital status as a window on the trends and differentials in Americans' lives. Most Americans intend to marry and most will achieve this goal. Heterosexual marriage, however, is no longer the only acceptable arrangement for couples, as seen by the rise in unmarried cohabitation and same-sex marriage. With age at marriage rising, people are spending more of their lives being never-married. By middle age, the ranks of the married are thinned by divorce and in old age by widowhood. Turning to living arrangements, two developments stand out. On the one hand, the share of married-couple households with children has plummeted over the last 40 years. On the other hand, living alone has become remarkably more common for two groups, older women and younger men. In both cases, the trend is to smaller households with fewer people living together. These trends were consequential for the well-being of Americans. Persons not living in households, including younger incarcerated adults and older adults in nursing homes, raise other important issues for the U.S. population.

Marital Status

At one time, the progression of Americans through a series of marital statuses was so predictable that family researchers called it the family life cycle (Duvall, 1962; Glick, 1955). The movement was from singlehood to marriage, where children were born, raised and then sent forth, and eventually to widowhood. While the family life cycle was a useful schema, researchers began to notice how many people deviated from this pattern. Over their lives, some never married. Increasingly, unmarried persons cohabited, living together in intimate domestic arrangements that were once largely restricted to married people. More and more people had children outside of marriage. Of those who did marry, many divorced and some went on to marry again. In recognition of all the variations on the family life cycle, as well as the potentially stigmatizing effects of celebrating one developmental path over the others, family sociologists abandoned discussions of the family life cycle for the multiple pathways of the life course (Elder, Johnson, & Crosnoe, 2003).

Despite the growing emphasis on life-course diversity, marital status never lost its importance as a concept (see Hollingshead, 1975; Umberson et al., 2005). Marriage remained an ideal to which most people aspired, even if not everyone achieved a lasting union. Even as cohabitation became more common, people told pollsters of their intentions to marry someday (Wang & Parker, 2014). Gays and lesbians won over most Americans with their compelling case for marital equality (Pew Research Center, 2013). Marriage, particularly the situation of married couples with their own children, remained the baseline against which other arrangements were gauged. Single parents raising children, for instance, were hard put to match the economic advantages that two married parents were able to provide (Bianchi, 1994). Furthermore, marriage was never just a personal matter. It was a social institution—a nexus of social expectations, practices, and social structures—that brought with it legal and social rights and obligations. Until 2013 when the U.S. Supreme Court ruled a provision of the Defense of Marriage Act (DOMA) unconstitutional, Social Security did not recognize same-sex partners for the survivor pensions to which heterosexuals were entitled (*US v. Windsor*, 2013). Last, marriage was the lightning rod for moral debates ranging from gender equality to sexual freedom to assisted reproductive technology. For instance, in most U.S. states and in contrast to the case with married parents, children born to unmarried parents via alternative insemination are not assured that their mother's partner will be their legal parent (Joslin, 2010).

Noting changes such as the rise in cohabitation and two-earner couples, Cherlin (2004) famously concluded that marriage was becoming deinstitutionalized, shorn of a supporting scaffolding of normative expectations and cultural understandings that had long guided behavior. Lauer and Yodanis (2010) insist that deinstitutionalization would require changes in marriage itself, not just changes in behavior outside marriage. Following this argument, Treas, Lui, and Gubernskaya (2014) analyze changes in attitudes between the late 1980s and the early 2000s in the United States and 20 other industrialized countries. They do find growing acceptance of cohabitation, premarital sex, and single parents—that is, behavior outside marriage. Except for the decline in disapproval of working wives, there was no retreat from traditional beliefs about what marriage is or what married people should do. In fact, there was increased support for sexual fidelity in marriage. After decades of tumultuous debate about changes in family life, surprisingly little had changed in terms of beliefs about the institution of marriage.

The bottom line is that marriage continues to be surprisingly important even as people marry later or perhaps not at all. Marital status—being married, never-married, or previously married—still matters. If different sorts of people take different marital pathways, marital status also continues to be a force that shapes the life styles and life chances of individuals (Fincham & Beach, 2010). People are hardly passive with regard to these most intimate of choices. In their personal lives, Americans have challenged conventions, bringing greater acceptance to new arrangements including unmarried cohabitation and same-sex marriages.

After 30, married is the most common marital status, as Figure 10.1 shows. The ranks of the never-married drop sharply into the 30s when married becomes the dominant marital status. The percentage divorced rises gradually for advancing age groups although divorce is not as high for the oldest Americans as for the baby boomers who came after them. Widowhood is largely found among older adults, particularly women who are more likely to outlive spouses and less likely to remarry.

Marriage. Marriage is no longer the definitive milestone in the passage to adulthood. Americans marry later after they have realized a number of adult aspirations. They usually have finished their schooling, found a full-time job, moved out of their parents' home, cohabited, and sometimes had children. They have time to pack in all these accomplishments

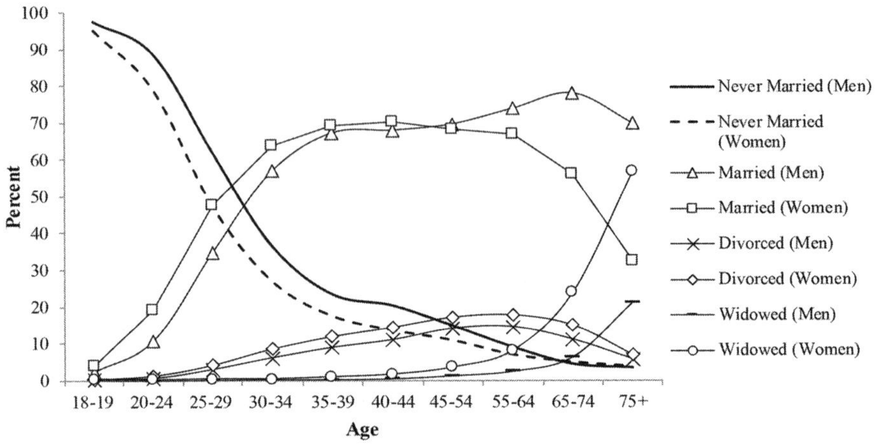

Figure 10.1 Marital status by age and sex. (U.S. Census Bureau, Statistical Abstract of the United States, 2012)

because of the rise in the age at first marriage. Between 1980 and 2010, the median age for women rose from 23.9 to 26.6 years (Cohn, Passel, Wang, & Livingston, 2011). For men, who marry later than women, it rose from 26.1 to 28.7 years, surpassing even the late marriage age of the nineteenth century.

Today, young people experience more adult experiences, such as living apart from parents, before marrying, because they put off marriage longer. They put off marriage longer, because they need the time to make those transitions, such as finishing their schooling, that give them the personal and economic security needed to marry. Blacks and Hispanics are even more likely than whites to insist that a steady job is a very important criterion for a partner (Wang & Parker, 2014). Particularly during the recent recession, some young adults delayed marriage in response to economic uncertainty. Until they meet the economic requirements of marriage, say, by paying off their student loans, cohabitation offers many of marriage's advantages—from companionship to shared household expenses to a regular sexual partner (Smock, Manning, & Porter, 2005).

The significance of finances is seen in the socioeconomic status of those who do marry. In the past, the relatively few highly educated women were passed over for marriage in favor of less-educated women who had a greater need for a husband's support (Qian & Preston, 1993). Today, when dual-earner couples are the norm, highly educated women with strong earning potential are in high demand (Blossfeld, 2009). And, women's remarkable increase in higher education enrollments makes it easier for college-educated singles to meet one another in college and the workplace. Thus, well-educated people marry one another, leaving less privileged individuals to build married life around their mutual disadvantages or, alternately, to not marry at all. Economic inequality between couples has grown as likes marry likes (Schwartz, 2013).

Married persons are drawn from a particularly advantaged population. This points to the difficulty of inferring the benefits that come from marrying. Married people and their children enjoy longer lives, better mental and physical health, higher incomes, and greater life satisfaction than unmarried people and their children (Nock, 2005). While marriage itself may be the cause of these advantages, people who are able to marry have a more favorable situation to begin with. Take married people's superior health. A loving spouse might encourage a lifestyle that promotes the partner's health, but people in poor health may never be able to attract a spouse. Research tends to show benefits to marriage, but this sort of selection into marriage also plays a role in the advantages the married have over others.

Delaying marriage does not mean that marriage is not valued. In 2014, a majority of never-married Americans said that they want to marry; only 13 percent stated definitively that they did not want to marry (Cohn et al., 2011). The reasons given for not being married differ by age (Wang & Parker, 2014). The top reason for 18–24-year-olds is that they are too young or not ready to settle down. In 1960, when the median age at first marriage was 20.3 years for women and 22.8 for men (Cohn et al., 2011), few young adults would have thought they were too young! Focused on establishing a strong economic foundation for marriage, 25-to-34-year-olds today point to not being financially prepared (Wang & Parker, 2014). Among never-married adults, 35 and older, 41 percent say they have not found what they were looking for in a mate yet.

Since the 1960s, the percent that is married has declined among all racial and ethnic groups although the numbers, then and now, are lower for blacks than for whites or Hispanics (Cohn et al., 2011). Only 55 percent of whites were married in 2010, a decline from 74 percent in 1960. Among Hispanics, 48 percent were married, compared with 72 percent in 1960. Among blacks, only 31 percent were married, compared with 61 percent in 1960. These differences may be attributed, in part, to the fact that the Hispanic and black population is younger than whites.

Cohabitation. Cohabitation is not usually tabulated as a marital status. Cohabiters who live together in an intimate relationship are counted as never-married, divorced, separated, widowed—or even married—to someone else. Although some cohabiting unions gain legal recognition as registered partnerships, this arrangement has not really caught on in the United States, at least in comparison with informal cohabitation.

Nonetheless, it is hard to talk about trends in marriage without considering the remarkable rise of cohabitation. At one time, cohabitation was a relatively uncommon experience limited largely to those too poor to marry and to bohemians who rejected societal conventions. Today, cohabitation is so common that it helps explain why people marry at older ages. In 2009–2010, nearly three-fifths of 19-to-24-year-old women in a union were in a cohabiting one instead of a legal marriage (Manning, 2013). Twenty industrialized countries saw a significant decline in disapproval of unmarried cohabitation, with or without intentions to marry, between 1994 and 2002 (Treas, Lui, & Gubernskaya, 2014).

Some explanations for the rise in cohabitation are economic. Women's labor-force participation makes them less dependent on marriage for their livelihood. The changing demand for labor makes it harder for young men to establish a career that can support a family (Oppenheimer, Kalmijn, & Lim, 1997). Other explanations pointed to cultural roots. Sociologists have emphasized the influence of long-term social changes, such as the sexual revolution that diminished the stigma of premarital sex (Bumpass & Lu, 2000; Cherlin, 2004). According to the Theory of the Second Demographic transition, cohabitation is only one of a number of changes in family life, ranging from greater nonmarital childbearing to divorce, that reflect the growing importance of individual freedom over responsibilities to family and community (Lesthaeghe & Meekers, 1986).

As recently as 1987, only one-third of women, aged 19–44, had cohabited at one time or another (Manning, 2013). By 2010, three-fifths had lived in an unmarried cohabitation. Although some still marry directly without cohabiting, each successive generation has been more likely to live together first before marrying. All demographic categories were touched by the rise in cohabitation. Between 1989 and 2010, white women cohabiting went from 32 percent to 62 percent, while Hispanics increased from 30 percent to 59 percent (Manning, 2013). Although black women have traditionally been more likely to cohabit, white women have surpassed them in the share that has ever lived in an unmarried relationship. Cohabitation has increased across educational groups as well, and the educational gap is increasing. In 2009–2010, nearly three-quarters of women without a high school degree had cohabited at some point, in contrast to only half of women with a college degree. Compared to married persons, cohabiters are drawn from those who are at a socioeconomic disadvantage.

Cohabitation is now the typical pathway into marriage. Two-thirds of women who were first married between 2000 and 2009 had cohabited before marriage (Manning, 2013). Although some couples live together with no intention of making their relationship permanent, others treat cohabitation as a courtship stage on the way to the altar. About two-fifths of cohabiters report they were engaged or had definite plans to marry their partner before they began living together (Guzzo, 2009). For those looking to marry, cohabitation is a serious proving ground for marital compatibility or a practical arrangement for building up the resources for marriage. Young adults view cohabitation as a way to test the waters by living with the partner. Others are less deliberate in their planning. They simply drift from cohabitation to marriage after they become locked into a routine, have children, or sign a long-term lease together.

Despite cohabiters who go on to marry, cohabiting unions have features that make them more prone than marriages to breakups. Cohabiters are less committed to their relationship than their married counterparts are. They are less likely to pool all their money together in a shared bank account and less willing to trust that unequal contributions will balance out over the long haul (Brines & Joyner, 1999). Cohabiting partners also have less in common with one another in terms of age, education, and race-ethnicity. Cohabiters do not have the stabilizing education and income advantages of married couples. Their attitudes toward sex and marriage are less traditional (Clarkberg, Stolzenberg, & Waite, 1995). All these factors predispose unmarried couples who live together to go their separate ways.

Today, over one-in-five children are born to cohabiting parents (Lichter, 2012). Besides the children born to them, 63 percent of cohabiting parents report having at least one child born before they started living with their present partner. In the Fragile Families study that followed couples after a birth, 26 percent of cohabiting parents were still cohabiting five years later and another 26 percent had married; 45 percent, however, were no longer romantically involved (Center for Research on Child Well-Being, 2007). Not surprisingly, the quality of the couple's relationship deteriorated with the breakup, leading to weaker father-child relationships. Only 43 percent of fathers who were not romantically involved with the mother had seen their child in the last month compared to 100 percent of the still cohabiting fathers. In short, children growing up with cohabiting, rather than married, biological parents are at a disadvantage because of the parents' initial disadvantages and the danger that the parents' breakup will deprive the child of father's support.

Because cohabitation is still associated with young people who have never-married, it may be surprising to learn that unmarried cohabitation is a popular arrangement for middle-aged and older adults who have been widowed or divorced (Yi Zeng et al., 2012). In later life, unmarried unions are more stable and long lasting, and cohabitation appears to operate as a long-term alternative to marriage instead of as a trial marriage (Brown, Bulanda, & Lee, 2006). While many younger adults may cohabit with the intention to marry their partner, older adults choose cohabitation for reasons relevant to their stage in life. The legal niceties of marriage are less compelling when couples will not be having babies. For older people who want to leave their money to their children when they die, cohabiting offers economies and companionship without legal entanglements. Others may want to keep their Social Security survivor's benefits or the alimony they would lose if they remarried. Family members' objections may influence decisions. Besides cohabitating, however, older adults are also observed to form intimate lasting relationships while maintaining their own homes—a phenomenon referred to as LAT, or living apart together. This has advantages for those who enjoy their privacy or do not want to risk becoming a round-the-clock caregiver to a sick partner.

Same-Sex Unions. Although same-sex cohabitation is a long-standing arrangement, the recognition of same-sex marriages added an important dimension to conversations about the future of marriage. Since the early 1980s, Americans have grown more accepting of same-sex relations (Treas, 2002). Legal recognition has tracked changing attitudes. In 2004, Massachusetts became the first U.S. state to legalize same-sex marriage. Fully 37 states and the District of Columbia had legalized it by February, 2013. By 2013, a majority of all Americans supported same-sex marriage, and fully 72 percent considered it inevitable (Pew Research Center, 2013). Because individual states write their own marriage laws, a uniform policy legalizing same-sex marriage would await the Supreme Court 2015 ruling on constitutional protections.

Marriage equality is not just a sentimental or political issue for same-sex couples. Among the federal rights, protections, and benefits that have been at stake in the definition of marriage have been Social Security for a surviving partner, taxation on the money from a home sale, and the ability to sponsor a partner's immigration to the U.S. (U.S. General Accountability Office, 2004). Marriage could bring other pragmatic benefits to same-sex couples, too. Even controlling for socioeconomic resources, same-sex cohabiters report having health that is not as good as the health of married persons in heterosexual relationships (Liu, Reczek, & Brown, 2013). This raises the possibility that the access to marriage might improve the health of gays and lesbians.

The Census Bureau has worked to count the number of same-sex couples. The estimates have not been very precise, if only because people in the many heterosexual couples sometimes inadvertently report their partner as being of the same sex (DiBennardo & Gates, 2014). Other same-sex couples may be missed because they are reluctant to report their relationship. Revised 2010 figures from the Census Bureau put the number of same-sex couple households at 646,464. Of those, 131,223 involved married same-sex couples, split fairly evenly between 67,506 women and 64,223 men.

More research is needed to place the experience of same-sex couples in life-course context. In previous generations, sodomy laws and social stigma discouraged relationships, such as cohabitations, that might call attention to sexual orientation (Rosenfeld, 1999). Researchers ignored the family relationships of gays and lesbians, who were assumed not to share the everyday family concerns of heterosexuals. As the rise in same-sex marriage testifies, gays, lesbians, and transgendered people increasingly have life-course experiences much like other Americans. For example, more same-sex parents are raising children in same-sex couple households. This is especially true for lesbian mothers, who are apt to bring children from an earlier, heterosexual union to their same-sex relationship. For children raised by same-sex couples, same-sex marriage could translate into greater social acceptance for their families, more stable households, and greater financial well-being.

Divorce. Divorce has important implications for the well-being of individuals and families. After divorce, families can experience substantial declines in economic welfare, particularly for women and their children (Smock, Manning, & Gupta, 1999). The strains and deprivations of divorce lead to poorer health, especially in terms of chronic conditions and disability (Hughes & Waite, 2009). The loss of health insurance, combined with other stresses of the divorce process, increases health risks for women (Lavelle & Smock, 2012). Being uninsured can worsen health conditions and illnesses for women, because the uninsured are less likely to seek routine or emergency medical care (McWilliams, 2009). Men and children are also affected. Although joint custody has become more popular in recent years, children's relationship with the noncustodial parent—usually the father—tends to deteriorate. This pattern leads eventually to less support from grown children to aging fathers (Shapiro & Cooney, 2007). The effects of parental divorce can be felt on children's mental well-being even into adulthood (Cherlin, Chase-Lansdale, & McRae, 1998).

From 1970 to 1975, when new no fault divorce laws ended the legal requirement of wrongdoing, the annual divorce rate for women jumped from 15 to 20 divorces per 1,000 (Kennedy & Ruggles, 2014). Today, tabloid accounts of celebrity divorces fuel the widespread impression that divorce is still on the rise. The picture is complex, but current evidence suggests that divorce rates since 1990 have diverged: They have increased for middle-aged Americans but declined for younger adults, possibly because married people in recent cohorts are selected for positive characteristics that stabilize marriage. Fewer people are marrying, and they are marrying at older ages when they are better prepared for the emotional and financial responsibilities. In the baby boom cohort, nearly one in two marriages ended in divorce, but baby boomers were unusual. They married at young ages when the risk of divorce is highest, and rebellious boomers had little patience for the tradition that couples should stick it out in unhappy relationships.

The early years of marriage are the most divorce-prone, perhaps because spouses acquire the most unsettling information about each other early on (Becker, 1981). The chance of divorce is higher for those with less schooling, particularly for adults who did not complete high school (Stevenson & Wolfers, 2007). Black and native-born Hispanic adults experience more divorce than whites do. In 2012, black and native-born Hispanic women had the highest rates of divorce—25.4 and 26.8 divorces per 1,000 first marriages, respectively, compared to 16.1 per 1,000 among whites (Stykes, Gibbs, & Payne, 2014). Black and Hispanic couples are more likely to have experienced pronounced socioeconomic disadvantages and a premarital birth, thus contributing to higher divorce rates (Bulanda & Brown, 2007).

Older adults are no longer immune to divorce. Even in later life, baby boomers' high rates of divorce continue (Kennedy & Ruggles, 2014). In contrast to the general trend to lower divorce rates, the divorce rate for Americans, 50 and older, doubled between 1990 and 2010 (Brown & Lin, 2012). Today, about a quarter of divorces occur to these middle-aged and older adults. Once divorced, older adults are less likely than others to remarry (Shapiro & Cooney, 2007), so the proportion of older men and women who are divorced will likely rise in the coming years. The late-life divorce boom is not fully understood, but several explanations have been suggested.

Having lived through an era of higher divorce rates, older adults have remarried, and second and higher order marriages are less stable than first marriages are. Having a longer employment history than earlier cohorts, older women are no longer as financially dependent on a husband. Declining mortality means an increase in the number of years of life and, hence, the years at risk of getting a divorce. Other explanations point to the unique strains on marriages in later life. Retirement, health declines, and the empty nest can all lead couples to reevaluate their relationship (Davey & Szinovacz, 2004).

There are social and economic differences in the likelihood of divorce. As we noted above, marrying later gives couples a chance to become financially secure, and the better off have been marrying at higher rates than other Americans. These trends should work against the risk of divorce. For those born since 1980, the leveling off of divorce may reflect this sort of increase in the selectivity of who marries (Ruggles, 1997). The college-educated are much less likely to divorce than those with less education (Stevenson & Wolfers, 2007). In addition, higher earnings and employment protect against divorce (Amato, 2010). Besides individual characteristics, community affluence also matters. Women living in neighborhoods with low levels of poverty, welfare receipt, and unemployment, as well as high levels of education, are less likely to experience separation or divorce (Bramlett & Mosher, 2002).

Remarriage. Remarriage compensates for some of the losses associated with divorce or widowhood, but the remarried do not make up enough lost ground to catch up with the continuously married (Sweeney, 2010). With remarriage, income increases but still falls below that of first marriages. Although marrying again largely closes the gap in depressive symptoms vis-à-vis the continuously married, remarriage cannot completely reverse the deterioration in physical health that occurs with divorce and widowhood (Hughes & Waite, 2009). Remarried adults do report higher psychological well-being than divorced or unmarried adults, particularly for men (Marks & Lambert 1998). However, intense stress associated with the breakup of a marriage or a spouse's death seem to do physiological damage to body systems that remains even after a new partner is found. Whatever the effect of remarriage on partners, children living with a stepparent, instead of two biological parents, do not do as well on academic, behavioral, cognitive, and other measures (McLanahan & Sandefur, 1997).

Four out of every 10 marriages in 2013 involved at least one partner who had been previously married (Livingston, 2014). In two out of ten marriages, both partners had been married before. Women are less likely to remarry than men. Among the previously married, 64 percent of eligible men had remarried but only 52 percent of their female counterparts. In part, this reflects personal preferences. Fully 54 percent of women, but only 30 percent of the men, say that they do not want to get married again. Although the gender difference in remarriage rates narrows at younger ages, it remains especially large for adults, 65 and older, among whom women outnumber men three to two due to sex differences in mortality. Whites are more likely to wed again than are blacks and Hispanics.

Given the relative youth of divorcing persons, many go on to second marriages. A divorced woman is more likely to remarry if she is under the age of 40 and does not have children from a prior marriage (Coleman, Ganong, & Fine, 2000). Some widows and widowers, contemplating better health and longer life expectancies, also marry again. Because widowhood generally occurs in old age, marital prospects are not as good as they are for divorced persons. In fact, the widowed are slower to remarry than their divorced counterparts, half of whom are wed again within four years of divorcing (Kreider & Ellis, 2011).

Trends in remarriage for younger and older adults have moved in different directions. In 2013, only 42 percent of previously married Americans, 25–34, had remarried—down from 75 percent in 1960 (Livingston, 2014). On the other hand, older adults have become more likely to tie the knot again. Among previously married persons, 55 and older, 57 percent had married again compared to 42 percent a half century earlier.

Remarriages are more divorce-prone than first marriages (Livingston, 2014). One explanation is that they have fewer institutional supports, and expectations for second and higher order marriages are weaker. Authority over stepchildren, for instance, may be in doubt, introducing stress into families. Furthermore, the remarried are selected from people with a higher divorce risk. Their prior experience ending a marriage indicates that they are already familiar with the process and perhaps simply more open to the whole idea of divorce. They are also at a socioeconomic disadvantage that predisposes them to divorce.

Widowhood. Of every 1,000 women, aged 15 and older, 7.8 became widowed in 2009 (Elliott & Simmons, 2011). The rate for men was only 3.5 per 1,000. Because of historical declines in mortality, losing a spouse to death almost always occurs later in life. Among widows who lost their husband in the last 12 months, two-thirds were 65 years of age or older. Less than 6 percent were under the age of 45. Because men typically marry women younger than they are and because women live longer, men are less likely to outlive their wives. When they do, they are, on average, older than women when they become widowed.

Given their advanced age, widowed Americans have lower household incomes than their married or divorced counterparts (Elliott & Simmons, 2011). Nearly half of new widows and 35 percent of widowers reported household incomes of less than $25,000 in the last year, and nearly three-quarters were not in the labor force. Having a disability was reported for 39 percent and 36 percent of recently widowed men and women, respectively. If the widowed had an advantage, it was higher rates of homeownership than the adults in other marital circumstances.

Unlikely to remarry, many older adults, especially women, will live out their lives without a partner. The numbers of widows cohabiting are much lower than for divorced persons although the likelihood for the widowed increased fourfold between 1970s and the 1990s (Yi Zeng et al., 2012). For older married people, the death of a spouse is the permanent loss of the major social support in later life. An analysis of the findings from 123 studies on the relationship of widowhood and mortality confirms that widowhood is linked to higher mortality (Shor et al., 2012). All things considered, the risk of dying was 22 percent higher among those who lost a spouse than among their married counterparts. Men experienced more negative effects of widowhood than women. Although the causes are not fully understood, the effect of widowhood on dying has been increasing over time.

Being old, low-income, and disabled, the widowed have higher needs for support than other Americans. Fortunately, children and friends seem to step in as trusted confidants to compensate at least somewhat for the loss of the spouse (Ha, 2008). Mothers, however, are more central to family life than fathers. When widowed, fathers receive less support from children than do mothers (Kalmijn, 2007).

Never Married. Among adults 25 and older in 2013, one in five had never married—up from one in ten in 1960. This rise in singlehood can be traced to the increase in the age of marriage, as well as the growing popularity of unmarried cohabitation. Changing public opinion, hard economic times, and shifting demographic patterns contribute to the rising share of never-married adults. In a 2010 survey, about 39 percent of Americans agreed that marriage as an institution is becoming obsolete (Cohn et al., 2011). Moreover, younger generations were more likely to express this view than those aged 50 and older. Of course, young people also had to put off marriage for college and faced challenges establishing stable careers. Labor-force participation among young men fell significantly—from 93 percent in 1960 to 82 percent in 2012 (Wang & Parker, 2014). Overall wages declined 20 percent since 1980. Increased higher education enrollments may also be keeping young people single. Across most racial and ethnic groups, men were more likely than women to have never married, except among blacks, for whom the percentages are similar.

Most never-married people go on to marry, but some become lifelong singles. In the population, 65 and older, about 4 percent have never married and will most likely stay single (U.S. Census Bureau, 2012). Compared to currently married counterparts, the never-married have greater mobility limitations, poorer self-reported health, and more depression (Hughes & Waite, 2009). Of course, poor health helps to explain why they are unmarried. Older adults, especially women, who have never married are at an economic disadvantage compared to their married counterparts. Nonetheless, those who have not married do not see themselves as disadvantaged. Across seven European countries, the never-married and women are both less likely than the married and men to endorse the view that married people are happier than anyone else (Treas et al., 2014). In fact, this skepticism about the virtues of marriage has grown since the late 1980s.

Living Arrangements

Nearly two-thirds of American households in 2011 consisted of family members living together, as Table 10.1 shows. The remainder—nonfamily

Table 10.1 Percent Distribution of Household Types by Householder Age: U.S. Households, 2011

Characteristic	All Households	Family Households			Nonfamily Households	
		Married Couple	Male Householder	Female Householder	Male Householder	Female Householder
Age of householder						
15–24 years	4.1	0.7	0.3	0.8	1.1	1.2
25–34 years	15.4	6.6	1.0	2.7	3.0	2.1
35–44 years	18.3	9.9	1.2	3.3	2.4	1.5
45–54 years	21.2	11.3	1.1	2.9	3.2	2.7
55–64 years	18.9	10.1	0.6	1.6	2.9	3.6
65+ years	22.0	9.6	0.5	1.8	3.1	7.1
All households	100.0	48.2	4.7	13.1	15.7	18.2

Source: U.S. Census Bureau, American Community Survey, 2011.

households—were made up of individuals living alone or with unrelated persons. Nearly half of U.S. households involved married couples.

As a closer look would show, for every two married-couple households with minor children, there were about three without them. Not only was mom, dad, and offspring not the most popular household form, they were not even the most common type of married-couple household. With only about one-in-five households fitting the married-with-children model, this living arrangement was only half as popular as it had been in 1970.

There are many reasons for this startling decline in households with married couples raising children. Fertility has declined since the days when baby boom youngsters were growing up. Furthermore, the U.S. population has aged. With the baby boomers middle-aged or older, their own children are mostly grown with homes of their own. Given the rising age of marriage, the younger generation has been slower to form married-couple households with children.

Also contributing to the decline in married-with-children households are the changes in the residential experience of children. Today, children spend more of their childhoods growing up in households with a single parent or with two unmarried parents. Mothers, often never-married ones, make up the large majority of single parents. Fathers, who are more often divorced, have increased their share of all single parents with children in the home. In recent years, courts have been more willing to award shared custody to divorcing parents (Cancian, Meyer, Brown, & Cook, 2014). The change in children's living arrangements has led to concerns about the social and economic well-being of American youngsters. Married parents have higher incomes than single parents, particularly single mothers. For example, 39 percent of mother-only families with children under 18 are in low-income households receiving food stamps (Vespa, Lewis, & Kreider, 2013). This compares to only 9 percent of youngsters whose parents are still married. Although single mothers confront challenging circumstances, they are also stigmatized. In 2010, when 12 percent of families consisted of single mothers with children under 18 years, 69 percent of Americans surveyed said that a single woman having children was a bad thing (Horowitz, 2010).

Living Alone. Another big change in living arrangements has to do with the increase in nonfamily households. This increase is driven by growing numbers of one-person households. More Americans live alone. In fact, the percent of households with only one person climbed from 17 percent in 1970 to 27 percent in 2012 (Vespa et al., 2013). Initially, this category of one-person households was dominated by older women. Social Security gave elderly widows enough income to live alone after their husband died instead of moving in with grown children (McGarry & Schoeni, 2000). Being less likely to survive a typically younger wife, older men were less likely to live alone, but this gender gap has narrowed in recent years as men's life expectancy has improved. Among single-person households, women 65 and older are outnumbered by men under the age of 65. In part, higher divorce rates contribute to men living alone before old age (Vespa et al., 2013). Nonelderly women, being more likely to get custody of the children, continue to live in family households after divorce well into middle age (Cancian & Meyer, 1998). Thus, they are less affected by the trend toward solitary living.

Among both whites and Asians, family households built around a married couple amounted to about 80 percent. The comparable figure for blacks was only 44 percent and for Hispanics 62 percent (Vespa et al., 2013). Another racial and ethnic difference has to do with multigenerational households, where three or more generations in a family live together. In about two-thirds of these households, an adult child and grandchild lives in the home owned or rented by an older parent. In the other cases, it is the grown child who provides the housing for both the older and the younger generation—a pattern common among Asian families. Although only 3 percent of non-Hispanic white households were multigenerational, 6 percent of Asian and 8 percent of black or Hispanic households had three or more generations. Because the households of immigrant families are more likely to be multigenerational, it is easy to assume that residential choices simply reflect cultural preferences and family-oriented values. Multigenerational households, however, are overrepresented among the population living in poverty, suggesting that shared housing is a way of coping with greater economic need (Taylor et al., 2010). Of course, multigenerational households also offer noneconomic advantages such as companionship, help with household chores, and assistance with childcare (Treas & Mazumdar, 2004).

The economic tribulations of the recent recession had an effect, forcing many young adults to reclaim the childhood bedrooms that they had abandoned earlier when they left home (Fry, 2013). The 25-to-34-year-old group saw the biggest increase in multigenerational living. Even before the recession, however, young Americans with no more than a high school education were less likely to have left the nest for good than their counterparts who had graduated from college. Young women are less likely to live in the parental home than young men are. This trend used to be attributed to women marrying at younger ages than men. Today, it is attributed, in part, to women's higher rates of college attendance.

Household Size. Consistent with the growth in individuals living alone and the decline in married parents with children, the number of people living in the average household has fallen over time. The mean size of households dropped from 3.1 persons in 1970 to 2.6 in 2012 (Vespa et al., 2013). By 2012, households with five or more members made up only 10 percent of all households; 40 years earlier, their share of households had been twice as large. Over the same period, households consisting of just one or two people climbed from 21 percent to 46 percent.

Of course, household size changes predictably over the life course. With time, children move out and spouses pass away. Households empty out with the aging of the householder, that is, the person in whose name the residence is owned or rented. With increasing time in the United States, immigrant households become less crowded (Myers & Lee, 1996). Not only do children grow up, but income rises so families no longer have to double up or squeeze into small dwellings to make ends meet. An exception to this rule of diminished crowding, however, has occurred for Mexican immigrants. Their incomes do not rise as much, and departing household members have often been replaced by new immigrants.

Larger households signal greater economic needs to be met, but larger size also brings advantages. Having more members raises the odds that someone in an immigrant household, probably a younger person, will be able to speak English well—thus, protecting against what is called linguistic isolation. If adults live together, there are apt to be more people who can contribute money to support the household. Of course, not all households are share-and-share-alike arrangements with rich exchanges and resource transfers that benefit less well-off members.

Especially in nonfamily households where members do not have feelings of responsibility and emotional ties based kinship, coresidence may be a strictly economic expedient among unrelated persons who are not involved in one another's lives. Roommates may share the rent but little else. Because unrelated persons are not likely to feel very strong obligations to subsidize one another's lifestyle and living standard, their shared living arrangements are more lasting when they contribute equally (Glick & Hook, 2011). Parents and grown children have stronger commitments to one another. Those who live together adopt more permanent relationships when their incomes are unequal and when one generation relies financially on the other for support.

Not in Households. Not everyone lives in households. Some Americans live in institutions where their custody or care is formally supervised. Two types of institutions have received a great deal of attention lately, namely, prisons and facilities for older adults.

Since the 1970s War on Drugs, the U.S. incarceration rate has shot up and ranks as the highest in the world (Wakefield & Uggen, 2010). About 2.3 million adults are incarcerated. The prison population is disproportionately young, male, black, and poorly educated. Because of the stigma of imprisonment and limited job skills, ex-offenders have poor employment prospects when they are released. They are often barred from public assistance. If rejected by landlords and family members, they can wind up living on the streets. About half who leave prison are reincarcerated within three years.

Incarceration not only punishes felons, but also hurts their families. Grandparents, for example, may find themselves raising grandchildren, because the middle generation is in prison. Mass incarceration has been implicated in the rise in low-income, female-headed households, especially in the African American community where the shortage of marriageable men makes it hard for women to find acceptable partners. The separation of incarceration leads couples to break-up. Most prisoners have children. The effects of a parent's imprisonment on youngsters are complex. Removing an abusive parent from the home may be a positive development for children, but prison may also mean the loss of the principal breadwinner. Often, parental incarceration ripples through the family impacting, for example, grandparent-grandchild relations (Turney, 2014a) as well as children's learning and conduct (Turney, 2014b).

Considering a different sort of specialized institution, some older adults live apart from private households and communities. Among the U.S.

population, 65 and older in 2012, 3.6 percent or 1.3 million resided in nursing homes and other institutions (Administration on Aging, n.d.-b). The institutionalized population rises to 11 percent of Americans, 85 and older. These age differences reflect the greater disability and the greater needs among the oldest old for ongoing medical care, daily assistance, and supervision. Although nursing home use is notoriously difficult to project, it is estimated that 35 percent of 65-year-olds living in 2005 will spend at least a year in a nursing home at some point in their lives (Houser, 2007). If only because of the high costs associated with institutionalized care, there is growing interest in keeping older adults in households in the community.

Older adults live in nursing homes, because they need skilled nursing care, require intensive help with ordinary activities such as bathing and eating, or have severe cognitive impairments such as Alzheimer's Disease (Administration on Aging, n.d.-a). In fact, half of nursing home residents have dementia, and half are confined to a bed or wheelchair (Houser, 2007). Because they live to older ages, have higher rates of disability, and are more likely to be widowed, women are more likely than men to live in nursing homes (Houser, 2007). Marital status is a critical factor in the institutionalization of older adults. When admitted, half of the residents of nursing homes are widowed as compared to only 20 percent who are married or partnered. This point underscores the key role of family members in helping older adults to continue to live in their homes even if they become frail or disabled.

Conclusion

The conventional categories used to describe marital status and living arrangements often seem inadequate to capture contemporary experience. Being never-married or in a married-couple family household fails to characterize the rich variety of family and interpersonal relationships over the life course. Exhaustive and mutually exclusive, these categories are well-suited to demographic accounting exercises. They leave much unsaid when it comes to the nature and quality of relationships between, say, husband and wife or unrelated people who share a household together. It is, nonetheless, surprising how much marital status and living arrangements reveal about the changing circumstances of lives. Historical shifts, life-course patterns, and associated advantages and disadvantages are all evident in the trends and differences in marital status and living arrangements.

Categorical frameworks illustrate historical changes. For example, the introduction of Social Security increased the economic security of widows, and this development registered in the long time series of data tracking the rise in older women who are householders living independently from kin. The historical decline in married-couple households has kept pace with other important developments, including the contemporary tendency of Americans to cohabit and to defer first marriages to later ages.

Similarly, marital status and living arrangements not only make clear the regularities in the life course as we grow up and grow older, but also demonstrate the diverse pathways in intimate lives. Getting married is no longer the definitive marker of adulthood that it once was. Most people do marry, but shifts in the timing of first marriages and the looser coupling of marriage and childbearing both define contemporary patterns in the temporal organization of lives. The recognition of these life-course changes invites a much broader examination of the ways that individual lives are dictated by cultural expectations, economic opportunities, legal constraints, and other factors.

Our marital status and domestic arrangements would matter much less if they were not associated with advantage and disadvantage. Despite the considerable variation within marital categories, just knowing marital status can convey useful information about one's age, socioeconomic circumstances, and risks to physical and emotional well-being. Married persons prove to be advantaged on most counts. The challenge for researchers has been to tease out how much of this advantage is due to the privileged status of those most likely to marry and how much is due to the beneficial dynamics of marriage itself. Partnering and household arrangements continue to permit us to monitor historical developments, the organization of the life course, and the sources of personal well-being.

References

Administration on Aging. (n.d.-a). A profile of older Americans: 2012. Washington, DC: U.S. Department of Health and Human Services.

Administration on Aging. (n.d.-b). A profile of older Americans: 2020. Washington, DC: U.S. Department of Health and Human Services.

Amato, P.R. (2010). Research on divorce: Continuing trends and new developments. *Journal of Marriage and Family, 72*, 650–666.

Becker, G. (1981). *A treatise on the family*. Cambridge, MA: Harvard University Press.

Bianchi, S. M. (1994). The changing demographic and socioeconomic characteristics of single parent families. *Marriage & Family Review, 20*, 71–97.

Blossfeld, H. P. (2009). Educational assortative marriage in comparative perspective. *Annual Review of Sociology, 35*, 513–530.

Bramlett, M. D., & Mosher, W. D. (2002). Cohabitation, marriage, divorce, and remarriage in the United States. *National Center for Health Statistics. Vital and Health Statistics, 23*(22), 1–32.

Brines, J., & Joyner, K. (1999). The ties that bind: Principles of cohesion in cohabitation and marriage. *American Sociological Review, 64*, 333–355.

Brown, S. L., & Lin, I.-F. (2012). The gray divorce revolution: Rising divorce among middle-aged and older adults: 1990–2010. *Journals of Gerontology, Series B: Psychological Sciences and Social Sciences, 67*, 731–741.

Brown, S. L., Bulanda, J. R., & Lee, G. R. (2005). The significance of nonmarital cohabitation: Marital status and mental health benefits among middle-aged and older adults. *The Journals of Gerontology Series, B: Psychological Sciences and Social Sciences,60*, S21–S29.

Bulanda, J. R., & Brown, S. L. (2007). Race–ethnic differences in marital quality and divorce. *Social Science Research, 36*, 945–967.

Bumpass, L., & Lu, H. H. (2000). Trends in cohabitation and implications for children s family contexts in the United States. *Population Studies, 54*, 29–41.

Cancian, M., & Meyer, D. R. (1998). Who gets custody? *Demography, 35*(2), 147–157.

Cancian, M., Meyer, D. R., Brown, P. R., & Cook S. T. (2014). Who gets custody now? Dramatic changes in children's living arrangements after divorce. *Demography, 51*, 1381–1396.

Center for Research on Child Well-Being. (2007). Parents' relationship status five years after a non-marital birth. *Fragile Families Research Brief* (Vol. 39, pp. 1–4). Princeton, NJ: Center for Research on Child Well-Being.

Cherlin, A. J. (2004). The deinstitutionalization of American marriage. *Journal of Marriage and Family,66*, 848–861.

Cherlin, A. J., Chase-Lansdale, P. L., & McRae, C. (1998). Effects of parental divorce on mental health throughout the life course. *American Sociological Review, 63*, 239–249.

Clarkberg, M., Stolzenberg, R. M., & Waite, L. J. (1995). Attitudes, values, and entrance into cohabitational versus marital unions. *Social Forces, 74*, 609–633.

Cohn, D-V., Passel, J. S., Wang, W., & Livingston, G. (2011). Barely half of U.S. adults are married—A record low. *Social and Demographic Trends*, Retrieved from http://www.pewsocialtrends.org/2011/12/14/barely-half-of-u-s-adults-are-married-a-record-low/

Coleman, M., Ganong, L., & Fine, M. (2000). Reinvestigating remarriage: Another decade of progress. *Journal of Marriage and Family, 62*, 1288–1307.

Davey, A., & Szinovacz, M. E. (2004). Dimensions of marital quality and retirement. *Journal of Family Issues, 25*, 431–464.

DiBennardo, R., & Gates, G. L. (2014). U.S. Census same-sex couple data: Adjustments to reduce measurement error and empirical implications. *Population Research Policy and Review, 33*, 603–614.

Duvall, E. M. (1962). *Family development* (2nd ed.). Philadelphia, PA: Lippincott.

Elder, G. H., Jr., Johnson, M. K., & Crosnoe, R. (2003). The emergence and development of life course theory. In J. Mortimer & M. Shanahan (Eds.), *Handbook of the life course* (pp. 3–19). New York: Springer.

Elliott, D. B., & Simmons, T. (2011) Marital events of Americans: 2009. *Vol. ACS13. American Community Survey Reports*. Washington, DC: U.S. Census Bureau.

Fincham, F.D., & Beach, S.R. (2010). Marriage in the new millennium: A decade in review. *Journal of Marriage and Family, 72*(3), 630–649.

Fry, R. (2013). Long-term changes in young adult living arrangements. *Social and Demographic Trends*, Retrieved from http://www.pewsocialtrends.org/2013/08/01/long-term-changes-in-young-adult-living-arrangements/

Glick, J.E., & Hook, J.V. (2011). Does a house divided stand? Kinship and the continuity of shared living arrangements. *Journal of Marriage & Family, 73*, 1149–1164.

Glick, P.C. (1955). The life cycle of the family. *Marriage and Family Living, 17*, 3–9.

Guzzo, K.B. (2009). Marital intentions and the stability of first cohabitations. *Journal of Family Issues, 30*, 179–205.

Ha, J.-H. (2008). Changes in support from confidants, children, and friends following widowhood. *Journal of Marriage & Family, 70*, 306–318.

Hollingshead, A.B. (1975). Four factor index of social status. Unpublished working paper, Department of Sociology, Yale University.

Horowitz, J.M. (2010). Section 4: Children. In P. Taylor (Ed.), *The Decline of Marriage and the Rise of New Families*, Retrieved from http://www.pewsocialtrends.org/2010/11/18/the-decline-of-marriage-and-rise-of-new-families/.

Houser, A. (2007). Fact sheet: Nursing homes. Washington, DC: AARP Public Policy Institute.

Hughes, M.E., & Waite, L.J. (2009). Marital biography and health at did-life. *Journal of Health and Social Behavior, 50*, 344–358.

Joslin, C.G. (2010). Protecting children (?): Marriage, gender, and assisted reproductive technology. *Southern California Law Review,* 83, 1177–1229.

Kalmijn, M. (2007). Gender differences in the effects of divorce, widowhood and remarriage on intergenerational support: Does marriage protect fathers? *Social Forces, 85*, 1079–1104.

Kennedy, S., & Ruggles, S. (2014). Breaking up is hard to count: The rise of divorce in the United States, 1980–2010. *Demography, 51*, 587–598.

Lavelle, B., & Smock, P.J. (2012). Divorce and women's risk of health insurance loss. *Journal of Health and Social Behavior, 53*, 413–431.

Lauer, S., & Yodanis, C. (2010). The deinstitutionalization of marriage revisited: A new institutional approach to marriage. *Journal of Family Theory & Review,* 2, 58–72.

Lesthaeghe, R., & Meekers, D. (1986). Value change and the dimensions of familism in the European Community. *European Journal of Population,* 2, 225–268.

Liu, H., Reczek, C., & Brown, D. (2013). Same-sex cohabitors and health:The role of race-ethnicity, gender, and socioeconomic status. *Journal of Health and Social Behavior, 54*, 25–45.

Livingston, G. (2014). Four-in-ten couples are saying "I Do," again. *Social and Demographic Trends,* Retrieved from http://www.pewsocialtrends.org/2014/11/14/four-in-ten-couples-are-saying-i-do-again/

Manning, W.D. (2013). Trends in cohabitation: Over twenty years of change, 1987–2010. (FP-13–12). National Center for Family & Marriage Research. Retrieved from http://ncfmr.bgsu.edu/pdf/family_profiles/file130944.pdf

Marks, N. F., & Lambert, J. D. (1998). Marital status continuity and change among young and midlife adults longitudinal effects on psychological well-being. *Journal of Family Issues, 19*, 652–686.

McGarry, K., & Schoeni, R. F. (2000). Social security, economic growth, and the rise in elderly widows' independence in the twentieth century. *Demography, 37*(2), 221–236.

McLanahan, S., & Sandefur, G. (1997). *Growing up with a single parent: What hurts, what helps.* Cambridge, MA: Harvard University Press.

McWilliams, J. M. (2009). Health consequences of uninsurance among adults in the United States: Recent evidence and implications. *Milbank Quarterly, 87*, 443–494.

Myers, D., & Lee, S. W. (1996). Immigration cohorts and residential overcrowding in Southern California. *Demography, 33*, 51–65.

Nock, S. L. (2005). Marriage as a public issue. *The Future of Children, 15*, 13–32.

Oppenheimer, V. K., Kalmijn, M., & Lim, N. (1997). Economic aspects of marriage and cohabitation: Men's career development and marriage timing during a period of rising inequality. *Demography, 34*, 311–330.

Pew Research Center. (2013). Changing attitudes on same sex marriage, gay friends and family. *US Politics and Policy*, Retrieved from http://www.people-press.org/2013/06/06/changing-attitudes-on-same-sex-marriage-gay-friends-and-family/

Qian, Z., & Preston, S. H. (1993). Changes in American marriage, 1972 to 1987: Availability and forces of attraction by age and education. *American Sociological Review, 58*, 482–495.

Ruggles, S. (1997). The rise of divorce and separation in the United States, 1880–1990. *Demography, 34*, 455–466.

Rosenfeld, D. (1999). Identity work among lesbian and gay elderly. *Journal of Aging Studies, 13*, 121–144.

Shapiro, A., & Cooney, T. (2007). Divorce and intergenerational relationships across the life course. In T. J. Owens & J. J. Suitor (Eds.), *Advances in life course research* (Vol. 12, pp. 191–219). Oxford: Elsevier.

Schwartz, C. R. (2013), Trends and variation in assortative mating: Causes and consequences. *Annual Review of Sociology, 39*, 451–470.

Shor, E., Roelfs, D. J., Curreli, M., Clemow, L., Burg, M. M., & Schwartz, J. E. (2012). Widowhood and mortality: A meta-analysis and meta-regression. *Demography, 49*, 575–606.

Smock, P. J., Manning, W. D., & Gupta, S. (1999). The effect of marriage and divorce on women's economic well-being. *American Sociological Review, 64*, 794–812.

Smock, P. J., Manning, W. D., & Porter, M. (2005). "Everything's there except money": How money shapes decisions to marry among cohabitors. *Journal of Marriage and Family, 67*, 680–696.

Stevenson, B., & Wolfers, J. (2007). Marriage and divorce: Changes in their driving forces. *Journal of Economic Perspectives, 21*, 27–52.

Stykes, B., Gibbs, L., & Payne K. K. (2014). First Divorce Rate, 2012. (FP-14–09). National Center for Family & Marriage Research. Retrieved from http://www.bgsu.edu/content/dam/BGSU/college-ofarts-and-sciences/NCFMR/documents/FP/FP-14–09-divorcerate-2012.pdf

Sweeney, M.M. (2010). Remarriage and stepfamilies: Strategic sites for research in the 21st century. *Journal of Marriage & Family, 72*, 667–684.

Taylor, P., Passel, J., Fry, R., Morin, R., Wang, W., Velasco, G., & Dockterman, D. (2010). The return of the multi-generational family household. *Pew Research Center. A Social & Demographic Trends Report,* Retrieved from http://pewsocialtrends.org/files/2010/10/752-multi-generational-families.pdf

Treas, J. (2002). How cohorts, education and ideology shaped a new sexual revolution on American attitudes toward nonmarital sex, 1972–1998. *Sociological Perspectives, 45*, 267–283.

Treas, J., Lui, J., & Gubernskaya, Z. (2014). Attitudes on marriage and new relationships: Cross-national evidence on the deinstitutionalization of marriage. *Demographic Research, 30*, 1495–1526.

Treas, J., & Mazumdar, S. (2004). Caregiving and kinkeeping: Contributions of older people to America's immigrant families. *Journal of Comparative Family Studies, 35*, 105–122.

Turney, K. (2014a). The intergenerational consequences of mass incarceration: Implications for children's co-residence and contact with grandparents. *Social Forces, 93*, 299–327.

Turney, K. (2014b). Stress proliferation across generations? Examining the relationship between parental incarceration and childhood health. *Journal of Health and Social Behavior, 55*, 302–319.

Umberson, D., Williams, K., Powers, D.A., Chen, M.D., & Campbell, A.M. (2005). As good as it gets? A life course perspective on marital quality. *Social Forces, 84*(1), 493–511.

US v. Windsor. (2013), 133 S. Ct. 2675, 570 U.S. 12, 186 L. Ed. 2d 808.

U.S. Census Bureau. (2012). Marital status of the population by sex and age: 2010 [Table 57]. In *2012 Statistical Abstract, Section 1: Population,* Retrieved from http://www.census.gov/prod/2011pubs/12statab/pop.pdf

U.S. General Accountability Office. (2004). Defense of Marriage Act: An update to prior report. Washington, DC.

Vespa, J., Lewis, J.M., & Kreider, R.M. (2013) America's families and living arrangements: 2012. *Current Population Reports* (Vol. P20–P570). Washington, DC: U.S. Census Bureau.

Wakefield, S., & Uggen, C. (2010). Incarceration and stratification. *Annual Review of Sociology, 36*, 387–406.

Wang, W., & Parker, K. (2014). *Record share of Americans have never married as values, economics, and gender patterns change.* Washington, DC: Pew Research Center. Retrieved from http://www.pewsocialtrends.org/2014/09/24/record-share-of-americans-have-never-married/

Yi Zeng, S., Morgan, P., Wang, Z., Gu, D., & Yang, C. (2012). A multistate life table analysis of union regimes in the United States: Trends and racial differentials, 1970–2002. *Population Research and Policy Review, 31*, 207–234.

CHAPTER ELEVEN

Grandparenthood: A Developmental Perspective

Bert Hayslip Jr. and Heidemarie Blumenthal

That becoming a grandparent is a common experience for many adults is underscored by the fact that as life expectancy has increased, the chances of becoming a grandparent have also increased (Hayslip & Page, 2012). Seventy-five percent of those born in 2000 can expect to have at least one grandparent still living when they reach age 30. Nearly 60 percent of older adults have at least one grandchild, and 80 percent of middle-aged and older adults are grandparents (AARP, 2002).

The focus of this chapter is to examine the *developmental* aspects of grandparenting. In this context, it is important to note that grandparenthood has many existential advantages: it can buffer an older person's fears about isolation, loneliness, dying, or not feeling valued as a person. This is supported by the work of Friedman, Hechter, and Kreager (2008), who found grandparents who invested themselves more fully into the grandparent role to be less uncertain about the end of life.

The Nature of Grandparenting and Grandparent-Grandchild Relationships

As middle-aged and older adults, grandparents are in a unique position to positively influence their grandchildren. They can transmit values to a younger grandchild (Pratt et al., 2008), and in serving as a support for that child and his/her family in times of crisis, grandparents can also positively influence their grandchildren; such grandparents experience greater well-being (Won, 2010). Likewise, middle-aged and older grandparents who are more highly educated tend to positively impact their grandchildren's academic abilities (Ferguson & Ready, 2011) and their emotional/ego development (Scholl, 1997). Additionally, both greater emotional and financial involvement by grandparents longitudinally predict their grandchildren's prosocial behavior and school involvement (Yorgason et al., 2011). Indeed, in some cases, the *symbolic* nature of a grandparent's role—what grandparenting means or represents in a given family system—may be an influence on a grandchild's educational or career goals (see Mansson, 2013).

Another example of the positive influence middle-aged or older grandparents can have on their grandchildren is in terms of how they are seen by such persons. In this respect, adolescent and young adult grandchildren's perceptions of their closeness to a grandparent varies with grandchild-grandparent frequency of contact, grandparent age, health and level of education (see Hokoyama & MaloneBeach, 2013), as well as the grandparent's particular personality attributes (Hokoyama & MaloneBeach, 2013). Yet, emotional closeness to an older grandparent predicts the goals that grandchildren set for themselves as well as the likelihood of such goal attainment (Wise, 2010). Indeed, meaningful frequent contact with a grandparent can mitigate the effect of a parent's divorce, mental illness, or death on a grandchild (Henderson et al., 2009).

The Dyadic Nature of Grandparenthood

A central theme of this chapter is that developmentally, grandparents and grandchildren are best thought of in *dyadic* terms; their influence on one another is *dynamic* and *bidirectional*, wherein the *developmental trajectories* of both grandparents and their grandchildren coexist and, indeed, are superimposed upon one another (Combrinck-Graham, 1985). That is, in addition to being influenced by one's grandparent(s), it is likely that at least some grandchildren might also help socialize their grandparents to matters of contemporary culture, such as using modern technology, violence in the schools, or assistance in learning about aspects of culture particular to the child's world, such as music, new scientific discoveries, fashion, drug use, or sexuality.

In the context of a life span approach to developmental trajectory emphasizing its multiple antecedents (see Baltes, 1997; Baltes, Reese, & Nesselroade, 1988), we argue that reaching an understanding of grandparent-grandchildren dyads *must* be accomplished in a *developmental context*. This assumption about grandparent-grandchild dyads is critical to understanding such relationships in *normative age-related* terms, where roles and relationships evolve over time; this is consistent with normal changes in physical and social-emotional functioning experienced by both the grandparent and the grandchild. In addition, acknowledging *cohort-related* influences on each generation's influence upon the other is essential to understanding grandparent-grandchild relationships, as each is uniquely shaped by the historical context in which they have grown up. Additionally, recognizing departures from what would be considered normative, such as *nonnormative* variations on typical grandparent-grandchild interactions, is also essential to fully understand and capture the complexity of such dyadic relationships.

In light of the above age-graded, history-graded, and nonnormative influences, it follows that the experience of grandparenting, and consequently the nature of the influence grandparents have on their grandchildren as well as the grandchild's impact upon a grandparent, is largely *unique* to each grandparent-grandchild dyad, wherein the emotional complexities particular to each dyad have been noted by Fingerman (1998).

This uniqueness is explained by numerous factors, wherein (Hayslip & Page, 2012), grandparent-grandchild relationships are impacted by (1) the *meaning* that grandparenting has for the individual, wherein there are advantages to middle-aged and older persons whose identities centralize the role of grandparent; (2) the particular behavioral *style* derived from this meaning that persons enact; (3) the cultural context in which the grandparent-grandchild relationship exists; (4) *how* that grandparent is perceived by the grandchild, whether negatively or positively, subject to the gender of the grandchild and the health of the grandparent; or (5) the *nature and extent of grandparent-grandchild contact*, as mediated by one's children or son/daughter-in-laws and geographic distance, and (6) each person's particular place along a *developmental continuum of youth to later life*, where changing life circumstances may alter the nature of this relationship, as when family dynamics are altered by events such as death or illness, or when grandchildren become independent (Bangerter & Waldron, 2014).

In this respect, the seeds of a continued close relationship with a grandparent in adulthood are often sown in childhood (Geurts, Van Tilburg, & Poortman, 2012). Yet, Villar et al. (2010) found that grandparents perceived greater positive changes in their relationships with their grandchildren as the latter grew older.

Grandparenthood and Development

At the minimum, a developmental life-course perspective suggests that grandparent-grandchild relationships are likely to be different when grandchildren are young and grandparents are in good health versus when grandchildren are adults and grandparents are older or frail (Boon, Shaw, & McKinnon, 2008; Coali & Hertwig, 2011). For instance, when grandchildren are young, grandparents may focus on play and childcare, while during adolescence, grandparents' roles often revolve around listening, supporting, and serving as family historians (Hayslip & Page, 2012). While their contact with grandparents lessens as grandchildren get older and become more independent, older grandparents often provide emotional support or offer advice to adult grandchildren (Connidis, 2010). Indeed, reciprocal and ongoing grandparent-grandchild relationships in childhood are a precursor of close relationships in adulthood (Guerts, van Tiburg, & Poortman, 2012; Sigurdardottir & Julursdottir, 2013). Yet, grandparents who are ill, impaired, retired, or widowed may be viewed differently by grandchildren who expect their grandparents to be physically active, have the resources to travel, or expect to have both grandparents still living. In adulthood, grandchildren expect grandparents to buffer parental relationships and be a role model and a financial advisor (see Boon, Shaw, & Mackinnon).

From a developmental point of view, key to grandparenting is a *life course change* perspective (MacMillan & Copher, 2005), which stresses the changing intergenerational family system, centralizing the embeddedness of the grandparent in this system, which itself changes as grandparents' and grandchildren's lives change over time (Combrinck-Graham, 1985; Hayslip & White, 2008). Insight into the normative nature of such changes can be facilitated by framing them in terms of *developmental theory*, for example Erikson's (1968) psychosocial approach stressing such constructs as trust/mistrust, identity/role confusion, intimacy/isolation, generativity/stagnation, or integrity/despair, or upon *key points of developmental change* in the grandchild's life, such as early and middle childhood, adolescence, early/emerging adulthood. Additionally, developmental change points in the lives of grandparents are often pivotal to grandparent-grandchild relationships, as when grandparents experience health-related or cognitive decline, or when they are dying (see Bangerter & Waldron, 2014).

It is worth noting that the majority of work examining the grandparent-grandchild relationship has included data drawn solely from the grandparent (Attar-Schwarts, Tan, & Buchanan, 2009) or grandchild retrospective report (e.g., Soliz, 2008). Importantly, preliminary work indicates that child perspectives may differ from that reported by their caregivers (e.g., Lussier et al., 2002; Triadó et al., 2005), and retrospective reports may be prone to affective and memory bias (Nisbett & Ross, 1980). Accordingly, in discussing grandparenting and development, we will focus on work utilizing grandchild reports on their *current* relationship with close and/or living grandparents.

Childhood and Early Adolescence

While the majority of the literature examining the content and nature of grandparent-grandchild relations has focused on families with young children, very little work has been conducted addressing the child's or adolescent's perspective (e.g., Dunifon, 2013). In one exception, Creasey and Kaliher (1994) collected data from 169 third, fifth, and seventh graders. Overall, these youth described the relationships with their grandparents as a source of great satisfaction. Although high levels of intimacy or self-disclosure were not typically reported, most youth did characterize their relationships as low in conflict and high in affection, respect, instrumental aid, and stability. Further, offspring age (as indexed by grade), frequency of contact, and grandparent health all played a role in the quality of the relationships reported. For example, third graders reported greater intimacy, instrumental support, and sense of approval as compared to older participants; seventh graders indicated lower levels of companionship and stability as compared to younger participants. Of note, significant age differences were *not* found in terms of frequency of contact, affection, conflict, or support of the grandparent by the child; this suggests continuity over time in such relationships. Frequency of contact evidenced the most consistent influence, relating positively to affection, intimacy, respect/approval, grandparent-directed support, as well as overall satisfaction. Finally, grandparent health also was related to increased child-reported support behaviors and was negatively related to companionship and instrumental support. Together, these findings indicate that grandchildren view their grandparents as playing several key roles in their lives and highlight the importance of grandparent contact and availability in maintaining these relationships in addition to (if not beyond) maturation-related changes across childhood and early adolescence (see Hurme, Westerback, & Quadello, 2010; Sims & Rofail, 2013).

Other work indicates that grandparents may take on a special role in aiding healthy adjustment among young grandchildren in risk-related situations (e.g., Bridges et al., 2007; Sheridan, Haight, & Cleeland, 2011). For instance, Sheridan, Haight, and Cleeland (2011) examined the role of grandparents in a sample of youth aged 6–14 years whose parents used methamphetamine. Overall, most children reported that their grandparents provided important social-emotional support, and many indicated that they enjoyed positive leisure activities together. Approximately 10–15 percent of children indicated that grandparents were a key source of psychological support (e.g., comfort, advice) as well as material goods (e.g., school supplies, books, musical instruments). However, just under 10 percent also expressed quite negative relationships, indicating that their grandparents were harsh and/or also were using drugs. Of note, grandparents were the *only* source of support significantly related to child behavioral problems in this study, wherein children who reported social-emotional support from their grandparents evidenced lower overall externalizing problems, social problems, and aggression problems; no other adult figure in this study (e.g., parents, service professionals, school officials, siblings) evidenced a significant impact on these outcomes.

Children's perspectives on the grandchild-grandparent relationship require further study. Although preliminary data indicate that children view their relationship and respective roles with grandparents in congruence with the grandparent report, related work also suggests that differences do exist (e.g., Triadó et al., 2005), wherein this discrepancy has been termed the *generational stake* (Harwood, 2001)—that grandparents assign more importance to their roles in their grandchildren's lives than the grandchildren themselves report, hence the greater stake in the relationship as reported by the older generation. In addition to efforts incorporating child self-report, creative research designs such as dyadic interaction observation and interview (e.g., Kenner et al., 2007) will be required in efforts designed to further understand the dynamic relationship between children and their grandparents across a variety of contexts.

Adolescence

Adolescence is characterized by rapid biopsychosocial maturation (especially those associated with puberty, for example secondary sexual characteristics; Petersen et al., 1998). Gains in cognition (Schwartz, Maynard, & Uzelac, 2008), emotion (Zimmermann & Iwanski, 2014), and risk-related behaviors (Albert, Chein, & Steinberg, 2013) also normatively occur during this period. Of note, adolescence also is characterized by important shifts in interpersonal relationships, including sources of support and conflict (Albert, Chein, & Steinberg, 2013; Paikoff & Brooks-Gunn, 1991). Observed distancing and conflict between adolescent offspring and parents also may extend to relationships with grandparents. Indeed, Dellmann-Jenkins, Papalia, and Lopez (1987) found that adolescents' self-disclosure to grandparents reliably decreased across the high school years. Triadó et al. (2005) found that neither adolescents nor grandparents ($n = 154$) characterized the relationship as one of intimacy, mutual understanding, or mutual trust. Further, grandchildren (but not grandparents) also reported that trust in the relationship decreased over time. As seen in the work conducted with children described above, frequency of contact was an important predictor in how the dyad viewed their relationship, and both parties characterized the grandparent as one who can provide history and context for the family. Complementing this work, Van Ranst, Verschueren, and Marcoen (1995) examined a sample of over 500 adolescents, also finding consistent differences in the grandchild-grandparent relationship as a function of age. Specifically, participant age was used to establish three categories: early adolescence (average age = 12.5 years), middle adolescence (average age = 15.7 years), and late adolescence (average age = 18.9 years). Across the sample, participants described their relationships with their grandparents as primarily characterized by emotional support, reassurance of worth, stability, and the role of the grandparent as a mentor/role model. However, participants in early adolescence rated each of these characteristics, as well as financial support and caregiving, significantly higher than those in middle and late adolescence, suggesting that grandparents' actual or perceived influence does indeed lessen across adolescence. Despite these shifts, all participants rated their grandparents as supportive and perceived the relationship to be close overall.

Taking a systems perspective, Attar-Schwartz, Tan, and Buchanan (2009) examined the additive and interactive influence of several offspring, parent, and grandparent variables in the grandchild-grandparent relationship among almost 1,500 adolescents aged 11–16 years. Consistent with the work described above, age was negatively related to emotional closeness and importance of the grandparent; however, once relevant grandparent (e.g., grandparent age; frequency of contact) and parent (e.g., closeness with grandparent; encouragement of the relationship) variables were taken into account, this relation was no longer significant. Indeed, *grandparent* characteristics contributed the largest amount of variance to the models; specifically, grandparent age was negatively related, and frequency of contact and grandparent involvement were positively related to child-reported emotional closeness and importance of the relationship. It also is important to note that across the entire sample, the majority of participants described the relationship as emotionally close, important, and one of respect for the grandparent. Finally, existing work supports the contention that grandparents also may play an important role in buffering the effects of negative life events (e.g., Flouri et al., 2010). For instance, Botcheva and Feldman (2004) found that grandparent support moderated the relation between harsh parenting and adolescent depression; specifically, harsh parenting predicted adolescent depression among those reporting nonsupportive grandparents, but not among those indicating grandparental support. Qualitative analyses highlighted the role of grandparents in providing both instrumental and emotional support.

Collectively, these data indicate that changes in family dynamics during adolescence also may effect relationships with grandparents; however, the nature and impact of these changes are far from simple. From a research perspective, future efforts including several key past and current variables, for example, grandchild psychopathology, parent-grandparent relationships, additional contextual factors, clearly are required to better understand the role of grandparents during this complex, significant period of development.

Emerging Adulthood

Although previously regarded solely as an artifact of convenience sampling (e.g., Roberto & Skoglund, 1996), a burgeoning literature highlights the importance of examining psychosocial functioning among college students from a developmental perspective (e.g., Arnett, 2000; Arnett & Tanner, 2006). The years encompassing the late teens and twenties have been referred to as a period of *psychosocial moratorium* (Erikson, 1968), the *novice phase* (Levinson, 1978), and most recently as one of *emerging adulthood* (Arnett, 2000). Indeed, in his seminal work on emerging adulthood, Arnett (2000) presents compelling theoretical and empirical work underscoring the distinctive psychological, behavioral, and sociodemographic characteristics of this period for many individuals in industrialized societies.

Several key characteristics of this developmental phase may have direct bearing on the dynamic relationship between emerging adult grandchildren and their grandparents. For instance, college students may be living outside of the family home for the first time, many in a different city, state, or country from their childhood friends and family (Arnett & Tanner, 2006). Several studies indicate that emerging adult grandchildren desire to maintain regular contact with their grandparents (Kornhaber & Woodward, 1981), and many are quite successful at doing so despite physical distance via electronic assistance (Hodgson, 1992; Taylor, Robila, & Lee, 2005). That noted, research also indicates that physical distance may have a direct effect on several aspects of the grandchild-grandparent relationship (e.g., Brussoni & Boon, 1998). In an examination of 171 undergraduate students in western Canada, physical distance not only was strongly correlated with frequency of contact, but also evidenced modest, though statistically significant correlations with current relationship strength, perceived benefits from, and overall importance of, participants' relationships with their closest grandparent (Brussoni & Boon, 1998). Further, Mills et al. (1998) found that frequency of contact with a grandparent was positively correlated with sensitivity to potential elder abuse in a vignette study including over 100 college students.

Emerging adulthood also is characterized by the opportunity for continued identity development (Arnett, 2000, 2007a; Arnett & Tanner, 2006). Although the emphasis on self-focus (Arnett, 2007b) and potential increase in physical distance might suggest a limited role for grandparents, college students still see their grandparents as key contributors in the course of self-exploration (e.g., Roberto & Skoglund, 1996; Taylor, Robila, & Lee, 2005). For example, Brussoni and Boon (1998) found that despite the negative impact of physical distance on several features of the grandchild-grandparent relationship, distance was *not* related to the role that college students perceived their grandparents to play in the shaping of their values. In a sample of 70 United States college students from 27 different countries, Taylor, Robila, and Lee (2005) found that international students reported that they viewed their grandparents as mentors, historians, and role models, and that for many students the influence of these relationships was maintained despite currently living in a different country. There are of course certain aspects of identity that students report are minimally influenced by grandparents; almost 90 percent of students reported that grandparents did not play a strong role in their sexual identity or political beliefs (Brussoni & Boon, 1998). However, given that a high proportion of college students indicate that their grandparents are a valuable source of advice and family history (e.g., Sanders & Trygstad, 1989) and are influential in shaping their family ideals, moral beliefs (Brussoni & Boon, 1998), and ethical standards (Perry & Nixon, 2005), it stands to reason that one of the key developmental tasks of this period, that of identity exploration and formation, continues to benefit from close relationships with living grandparents.

Finally, alongside the increased autonomy of emerging adulthood comes a sense of instability (e.g., Arnett, 2000). On average, emerging adults will change jobs, living arraignments, and romantic partners more frequently during this period than any other point in their lives (Arnett & Tanner, 2006). The stability and support provided by close relationships with grandparents may help offset the peak in loneliness experienced by many emerging adults (Rokach, 2000). Indeed, college students report that close grandparents continue to serve as important attachment figures, providing a secure base and sense of emotional connection (e.g., Taylor, Robila, & Lee, 2005). For example, Creasey and Koblewski (1991) examined a sample of 142 college students, finding that students characterized their relationships with their grandparents as including a very low level of conflict, high warmth/affection, and a strong sense of stability/consistency. Further, research indicates that many emerging adults report that their grandparents treat them with respect (Creasey & Koblewski, 1991), evidence trust in their independent decisions, and generally treat them like an adult (Sanders & Trygstad, 1989). Given that individual responsibility and independent decision making typically are key features of the transition from adolescence to adulthood, as reported by emerging adults (Arnett, 1997, 1998), close relationships with grandparents may play a special role in helping emerging adults not only navigate their current developmental needs, but further support the successful transition into adulthood proper.

One key area requiring attention includes the forgotten half (Arnett, 2000) of this period. The emerging adulthood period described above is not entirely a maturationally based one, and thus is not experienced by all in their late teens-twenties. Indeed, even in industrialized countries only about half of those in this age-group experience this environmentally created period. Unfortunately, little work has sought to include, let alone compare, data across these distinct developmental experiences, and none has been conducted in terms of grandchild-grandparent relationships. From a research perspective, in addition to more sophisticated assessments of the relationships described above via dyadic interaction, multi-informant, multimodal assessments, work addressing the forgotten half, those persons not experiencing emerging adulthood, will be required in an effort to better understand maturational versus contextual influences in the young adult grandchild-grandparent relationship.

Historical-/Cohort-Related Aspects of Grandparenthood

Despite the fact that grandparents may be able to anticipate some aspects of their role while their grandchild is still in utero (Somary & Stricker, 1998), grandparents frame their expectations for their grandchild in light of their own *cultural traditions* (see Cole, 1999). That grandparents and their grandchildren will have grown up in distinctly different historical contexts underscores the relevance of seeing grandparenthood in cultural-historical terms. This cohort-related shift in the nature of grandparenting has been nicely expressed by Uhlenberg (2004, 2009) and Uhlenberg and Kirby (1998), who document a variety of sociodemographic influences (e.g., the number of grandchildren one has as well as their timing, one's longevity) on grandparenting that not only affect the nature of the role, but also influence grandparents' interactions with their grandchildren, supporting the contention that the grandparent role has indeed changed over historical time.

Hurme, Westerback, and Quadrelle (2010) found that as the physical proximity between grandparents and grandchildren increases, there were fewer face-to-face contacts and phone calls, but more letters and cards. Even given the accessibility of text messaging, this form of contact from grandchildren lessened with greater physical proximity. To the extent that there is lessened contact between grandparents and grandchildren, the potential for *identity gaps* via identifying with one's own cohort increases the likelihood for poorer communication and lessened relationship quality (Kam & Hecht, 2009). In such cases, grandparents may need to be especially proactive in maintaining meaningful contacts with their grandchildren. At the same time, some families are able to maintain close intergenerational bonds despite changes in persons' lives and family circumstances, such as divorce or remarriage (Kemp, 2007).

Such experiential gaps between persons of different generations challenge each to find ways to meaningfully communicate with one another and also reinforce grandparents as persons whose life histories may reflect tradition, who can serve as transmitters of family history, and who can serve as role models to their grandchildren (Kahana et al., In Press). They may represent a living ancestor who teaches grandchildren ethnic traditions, experience, culture, and history (Reitzes & Mutran, 2004a), or advocate for/participate in school-related activities on behalf of their grandchildren (Watson, 2010). At the same time, grandchildren may bring to their interactions with grandparents representations of a culture where gender roles have changed, where technology is ever presently influential, and where mores and norms for child-rearing/parenting, sex roles, sexual behavior, drug use, and even violence reflect more historically recent cultural expectations. Key to such meaningful intergenerational communication are the lessening of age segregation, the sharing of personal concerns between generations, changing views about older adults as unproductive, an emphasis on adolescents as agents in the reconnection between generations, and an emphasis on maintaining emotional closeness and the family's identity in the face of change and in the face of adult role transitions among grandchildren (Soliz & Harwood, 2006; Mills, Wakeman, & Rea, 2001; Strom & Strom, 2015).

In this respect, the nature and extent of grandparents' contact with their grandchildren and, consequently, the nature of their relationship to a grandchild is primarily *mediated* by the quality of the grandparent's relationship to the grandchild's parent (see Connidis, 2010). This mediational role impacts the quality of the grandparent-adult child relationship, where the adult child serves as a *gatekeeper*. Consequently, how the adult child functions as a gatekeeper influences whether disagreements with adult children regarding the nature and extent of contact with grandchildren exist, and if they exist, how they are handled. Relatedly, intergenerational and intercultural differences in expectations about a grandparent's involvement or about issues relating to child care and discipline and/or values in raising a child can result in family conflicts, particularly when such expectations are unclear or not mutually agreed upon prior to the birth of a grandchild (Maiden & Zuckerman, 2008). Indeed, it is out of the interaction of grandparents and their children (as well as their interactions with adult children) that these distinct perspectives are shared and in some cases modified. That is, consistent with a dialectical perspective on developmental change, persons both change and are changed via their interactions with others (Riegel, 1976).

Nonnormative/Idiosyncratic Aspects of Grandparenthood

To the extent that grandparenting is a normative age-graded experience, it is instructive to observe that most people become a grandparent in their late 40s or early 50s. On the other hand, for others it is nonnormative; they do not become grandparents until their 60s or 70s. Likewise, grandparents who must cope with the death or disability of a grandchild, those who must raise a grandchild due to the death, divorce, or drug use of an adult child, or those whose physical or cognitive skills have been compromised via illness or dementia and who are cared for by their grandchildren all experience the grandparent role in a uniquely nonnormative manner. In this respect, Stelle et al. (2010) found that grandparents' gender, sexual orientation, and extent of physical or mental decline accounted for the great diversity they observed in grandparent-grandchild relationships. Indeed, the essential nonnormativeness of grandparenting is underscored by its *countertransitional* nature; it is a role persons assume that is based upon the actions of *others* (Hagestad, 1985).

In emphasizing departures from grandparenthood as an age-graded normative role, it should be made clear that many persons enjoy their roles as grandparents and maintain happy and fulfilling relationships with their grandchildren and the parents of these children. Indeed, grandparents who can clearly and actively express their affection toward a grandchild positively influence that child's social-interpersonal development (Mansson, 2013). Complementarily, whether grandparents feel they are important in the lives of their grandchildren and consequently influence them in many ways influences and is influenced by how grandparents define their roles (as central or peripheral). This role definition lays the groundwork for their self-efficacy as grandparents, how (and if) they will aid in their grandchild's development as well as how they will influence the family as a whole.

As discussed by Hayslip et al. (2015), grandparents at risk for unsatisfying experiences in this role and/or mental health/communicative difficulties with their children and grandchildren may have experienced unanticipated role changes for which they are unprepared such as a serious illness or a divorce, having to cope with the divorce of their adult children, the death of a grandchild, or having to assume full-time care of a grandchild. Still others must cope with the birth of a grandchild with a disability, teenage pregnancy, challenges in relationships with daughters- or sons-in-law who discourage their involvement, and unfulfilled expectations about the nature and degree of their involvement in a grandchild's life. Still others may have difficulty defining their roles as grandparent in the context of their roles as workers, retirees, or as caregivers for an ill spouse or older parent (see Hayslip et al., 2015). Indeed, even well-meaning and well-adjusted grandparents face numerous adjustments in dealing with the divorce/separation of an adult child (Christiansen & Smith, 2002; Doyle, O'Dywer, & Timonen, 2010), the serious illness of a grandchild (Wakefield e al., 2014), in discovering that a grandchild has been exposed to domestic violence (Semberg, 2013), or in dealing with the fact that a grandchild is GLBQ (Scherrer, 2012).

Culture and Grandparenting

While our focus here is to examine the developmental aspects of grandparenting, it is of note to observe that culture impacts grandparenting as well. Studying the cultural context in which grandparenting occurs can enhance our understanding of what is likely a normative life transition for most middle-aged and older adults. Culture is a fundamental factor in shaping the grandparent-grandchild relationship, and the grandparent-grandchild relationship is an integral part of intergenerational cultural transmission—the passing on of ideas for successful adaptation. The daily family interactions, practices and structure, which are heavily influenced and patterned by culture, shape the way developing children come to know and understand the world.

Culture pervades all aspects of life; it organizes perceptions, cognitions, and behaviors (Cole, 1999). Culture influences the way that grandparents experience aging and grandparenting, as well as the ways that grandchildren influence their grandparents and their own development. For these reasons, there must be an appreciation for the relevant cultural context in order to fully understand the meaning and function of interactions in the grandparent-grandchild relationship over time.

Strom et al. (2008) discussed how changes in China over the past 20 years (e.g., the end of martial law and media censorship) have dramatically changed Taiwanese culture and daily life (e.g., increases in women working and income, youth more immersed in Western culture) and thereby affected grandparent-grandchild relationships. Strom et al. (2008) explored how sociocultural changes put a strain on traditional cultural values (e.g., moving away from intergenerational cohabitation and hierarchical structure), intergenerational relationships, and how they influenced each generation's perceptions of grandmothers' role and functioning.

Sharing culture has been described as one of the primary functions of grandparenting (Wiscott & Kopera-Frye, 2000). In a study of ethnically diverse students, grandchildren in general felt that it was typical to engage in cultural activities with grandparents including sharing stories and family photos, and learning about family traditions (Wiscott & Kopera-Frye, 2000). They also reported a moderate influence of their grandparents, particularly on issues of religion, family, morality, and personal identity (Wiscott & Kopera-Frye, 2000). While ethnicity was related to sharing everyday and cultural activities, as well as positive affect toward grandparents and culture, grandparent-grandchild relationship quality did not differ by ethnicity (Wiscott & Kopera-Frye, 2000).

Pratt, Norris, Hebblethwaite, and Arnold (2008) found that adolescents that rated themselves as having more close relationships with their maternal grandparents were more likely to tell stories about experiences of the grandparents' value teaching, and these stories were more likely to be interactive, specific, and caring. Telling stories with these characteristics was related to higher generativity scores for the adolescents, indicating higher concern about contributing to future generations. These results suggest that closeness to grandparents relates to more elaborate and positive perceptions of their value teaching, which would intuitively seem to be important for intergenerational cultural transmission.

Given that American culture is typically considered more individualistic and both African American and Hispanic cultures are typically more collectivistic, it is relevant to note that one cultural value that is central to African American and to Hispanic cultures is *familism*, which is characterized by "the desire to maintain strong family ties [nuclear and extended], the expectation that the family will be the primary source of instrumental and emotional support, the feeling of loyalty to the family, and the commitment to the family over individual needs and desires" (Halgunseth, Ispa, & Rudy, 2006, p. 1285). Familism influences Hispanic family structure in emphasizing intergenerational relationships, frequent shared activities and high levels of interaction and coresidency with older family members (Silverstein & Chen, 1999). Among Mexican American grandparents, the amount of shared activity time with grandchildren relates to increased satisfaction, feelings of success in family role performance, less difficulty with grandparent obligations, and importantly greater teaching involvement with grandchildren among Mexican American grandparents (Strom, Buki, & Strom, 1997). In a study comparing Euro-American grandchildren and Mexican American grandchildren, ratings of grandparent-grandchild affection were generally moderate to high; but ratings were relatively higher for Mexican American grandchildren than Euro-American grandchildren (Giarusso et al., 2001; Wiscott & Kopera-Frye, 2000). Euro-American grandparents report more affection for and similarity with their grandchildren than the grandchildren report, while gaps are much closer among Mexican American dyads (Giarusso et al., 2001).

For grandparents, grandchild age and value of family responsibility, grandparent education, and grandparent acculturation predict grandparent affection for their grandchild (Silverstein & Chen, 1999). Among Mexican Americans, greater acculturation and grandchild's perception of similarity predict a larger gap between the affection reported by grandparent and grandchild toward each other (Giarusso et al., 2001). Thus, for both Mexican American grandparents and grandchildren, collectivistic values and lack of acculturation predict more affectionate and interactive relationships. In turn, affectionate relationships with adult grandchildren predict greater life satisfaction for older Mexican American grandparents (Markides & Krause, 1985).

Race and ethnicity, as reflections of culture, also affect grandparenting styles, where grandparents serve as mentors for younger parents, as transmitters of cultural values and heritage, as persons who are agents of socialization for and influence over their grandchildren, or as persons who can simply enjoy their grandchildren but not be responsible for raising them. Whether one's cultural or ethnic background uniquely define one's role as a grandparent depends upon whether this role is a valued one (see Hayslip, 2009; Hayslip & Page, 2012; Hayslip et al., 2015). For example, there are differences in grandparenting styles between African Americans and Whites, wherein African American grandparents have almost twice the degree of involvement with their grandchildren than whites. Compared to whites, African American grandmothers' parenting involvement is substantial, especially in the areas of control, support, and punishment (Cherlin & Ferstenberg, 1986; Pearson et al., 1990). Indeed, Mexican Americans belonging to larger, more multigenerational families, report higher satisfaction relating to their grandchildren, and have a greater degree of intergenerational contact (Schmidt & Padilla, 1983).

Race and ethnicity are also powerful influences on how the grandparent is viewed by one's grandchildren. For example, African Americans see the grandparent role as a more active one in the family than do Whites, reflecting racial and cultural differences in perceptions of the extended family network (Kornhaber, 1996). Among African American and white grandfathers, it seems to be that (1) the grandfather role is more affectionate than functional, (2) the grandfather role is more central among older African

Americans, and (3) other than geographic proximity, other factors are of little importance in the grandfather-grandchild relationship. This gender-specific role definition appears to be related to (a) the African American family's flexibility in expanding and contracting sources to meet the specialized needs of various extended family members, and (b) the flexibility of African American male family roles (see Kornhaber, 1996).

The Uniqueness of Grandparent-Grandchild Relationships

Beyond developmental, cohort-related, and cultural perspectives on grandparenthood, to an extent, each grandparent-grandchild is unique. In this respect, in times of family stress, maternal grandmothers are the most likely to be involved (Condon et al., 2013). Additionally, grandparents can aid in establishing and maintaining patterns of communication with a deafblind child (Shaw, 2005), in helping to care for an autistic child (Kahana et al., In Press), assist parents who have a child who is disabled (Findler, 2014; Lee, 2010), or in opening up communication on matters relating to sexuality (Cornelius, LeGrand, & Jemmot, 2009). On the other hand, *remote or distant* grandparents (Cherlin & Furstenberg, 1986) may cause additional stress to parents by bringing up long-standing family conflicts or insisting on being involved in decision making (Silverstein & Parrott, 1997). Grandparents can indeed foster maladaptive behavior in their grandchildren (Bailey et al., 2009) and can also contribute to marital discord or model pathological behaviors which grandchildren may internalize, reflecting the latter's response to underlying family conflict (Hayslip et al., 2015). Even investing oneself *too* heavily into a grandchild's life, such as spending more nights with a grandchild, can have counterintuitive and negative effects on a grandparent's self-esteem (Won, 2010). Thus, as there is much variability in grandparenting, the responsibility for child discipline, financial assistance, patterns of visitation, giving advice to the parents, sharing religious faith, and supporting the parents in decision-making are salient dimensions of the grandparent role for *some* persons but not others. Such variability contributes to differences in grandparent-grandchild dyads' contact, emotional closeness, and influence upon one another.

Just as grandparents may provide many types of support to a single, divorced, widowed, or never-married child, grandchildren may be called upon to care for an impaired or dying grandparent, wherein filial obligation and the need to prepare for the future helped make caring for a grandparent meaningful (Fruhauf, Jarrott, & Allen, 2002). Moreover, grandchildren caring for a grandparent experience a wide variety of emotions and developed a variety of coping strategies to deal with the demands of caregiving

(Fruhauf & Orel, 2008). Not surprisingly, grandchildren's perceptions of their grandparents' health and the degree to which such impairments affect their own lives each impact the quality of the relationship with the grandparent (Boon, Shaw, & Mackinnon, 2008). For grandparents who need help in managing their everyday affairs, emotional solidarity and frequency of telephone contact predict a grandchild's ability and motivation to provide functional assistance (Even-Zohar, 2011) and providing such assistance is often crucial to the mental health of grandparents. Ihara, Horio, and Tompkins (2012) have underscored the complexity of this caregiving in noting the salience of not only the grandchild's ability to provide care for a grandparent, but also his/her motivation for doing so, as influenced by the strength of the intergenerational bond, caregiver stress and financial hardship, the degree to which the grandchild has time to provide care, and the physical distance from the grandparent. Key however, is that feelings of closeness and affection must *first* exist if grandchildren are to provide help and assistance to a frail grandparent (Even-Zohar, 2011).

Grandparents with dementia present many socioemotional difficulties for grandchildren (Celdran, Tirado, & Villar, 2011), though while demented grandparents and their grandchildren attribute less attitudinal and behavioral importance to the grandparent role, they assigned no less symbolic and emotional salience to the grandparent role versus nondemented grandparents and their grandchildren (Werner & Lowenstein, 2001). Grandchildren caring for a grandparent with dementia may learn new ways of coping, develop patience, and gain insight about the meaning of life in caring for them (Celdran, Tirado, & Villar, 2011; Fruhauf & Orel, 2008). Grandchildren caring for dying grandparents also face unique challenges: dealing with physical and emotional fatigue, coping with the stresses of caregiving, guilt over having survived a grandparent, and the loss of their "grandchild" identity (Boquet et al., 2011). Boquet et al. found that grandchildren caring for a dying grandparent not only experience guilt, stress, and fatigue in doing so, but they also reported losing the role of "grandchild." Smith (2012) not only found that the dynamics of the grandparent-grandchild relationship were influential in affecting the experience of caregiving, but also that such dynamics were altered by the experience of caregiving, consistent with understanding such relationships in a dyadic, fluid manner.

Complementarily, how grandparents respond to a grandchild's disability or illness affects parents' adjustment to such issues (see Kahana et al., In Press; Miller, Buys, & Woodbridge, 2012), wherein previously established relationships and the perception that family members help one another in times of need become quite important (Mirfin-Vietch, Bray, & Watson, 1997).

In the context of nonnormative influences on grandparent-grandchild relationships and grandparenthood more generally, we briefly discuss three examples of such: the death of a grandchild, the divorce of an adult child, and having to raise a grandchild.

Losing a grandchild through death is nonnormative, though its impact on grandparents is substantial. Grandparents' emotional needs when a grandchild dies are twofold; they grieve for their adult child as well as for themselves (Reed, 2000). A grandchild's death can undermine relationships with surviving grandchildren or with an adult child in that the grief that grandparents often experience is *disenfranchised* (Doka, 2002). Disenfranchised grief typically undermines the opportunities grandparents have to share their feelings with others and to get emotional support from them. Complicating matters is the fact that family customs and rituals may not meet a grandparent's needs. While grandparents are often put in the delicate position of supporting their adult child as well as meeting their own needs for support from others, grandparents respond to loss in a similar manner compared to the grandchild's own parents (see Hayslip & White, 2008).

Another salient nonnormative aspect of grandparenthood is when contact is lost with a grandchild because of an adult child's divorce. While there are exceptions (see Holladay et al., 1998), both maternal grandmothers' and paternal grandparents' contact with their grandchildren are diminished when a parent divorces (Ahrons, 2007), and such losses can predispose grandparents to depression (Drew & Silverstein, 2007). Importantly, the impact of divorce on the grandparent depends upon whether the grandparent is an *agent* in the life of a grandchild (in providing support and serving as a role model for a grandchild), or whether the grandparent is seen as a *victim* (where grandparents view grandparenting as compensating for the lack of other sources of life satisfaction; Drew & Smith, 1999).

Taking on the responsibility of raising one's grandchild is a unique aspect of grandparenthood. While the numbers of grandparents raising grandchildren has increased over the last few decades (Hayslip & Kaminiski, 2005), the number of caregiving grandparents has risen again in recent years as a result of the recession of 2008–2009 (Pew Foundation, 2010). Normatively, custodial grandparents tend to be younger, the mother's parents, in worse health, more socially isolated, poorer, less highly educated, and raising boys, all relative to noncustodial grandparents (Generations United, 2009). In some cases, grandparent caregiving exists in a *skipped generation* household, where the adult parent is absent. In contrast, *coparenting* households are defined by the coresidence of the grandparent and adult child. Even in these situations, the grandparent may still have primary caregiving responsibility. Not surprisingly, grandparents in skipped generation households tend to fare worse physically and emotionally, due to their diminished resources and greater comparative isolation from others compared to coparenting grandfamily households (Generations United, 2009). The incidence of skipped generation versus coparenting grandfamily households varies with ethnicity (see Hayslip et al., 2015; Park & Greenberg, 2007), with skipped generation families being more common among Caucasians and coparenting families being more common among African Americans and especially among Hispanics.

Grandparent caregiving may be linked to the divorce, drug use, incarceration, job loss, teenage pregnancy, or death of the adult child, as well as to the abandonment or abuse of the grandchild. These circumstances often stigmatize and isolate grandparents from needed social and emotional support, making it difficult for them to be treated equitably by social service providers and fellow grandparents who are not raising a grandchild (Hayslip & Glover, 2008; Hayslip, Glover, & Pollard, In Press). Indeed, grandparent caregivers often experience health difficulties as a consequence of having neglected their health to the exclusion of their grandchildren's (Baker & Silverstein, 2008). They also sometimes experience difficulties in parenting a grandchild (Hayslip & Kaminski, 2005). Indeed, the impact of grandmothers' distress on grandchildren's adjustment is mediated by dysfunctional parenting (Smith et al., 2008). This distress may be exacerbated by the grandparent's negative attitudes toward child-rearing as well be reflected in the tendency of some grandparents to rely on their grandchildren for emotional support (Kaminski et al., 2008) and their failure to set boundaries on their involvement with grandchildren (Breheny, Stephens, & Spilsbury, 2013). Not surprisingly, disappointment in that adult child as a poor parent are experienced by many grandparent caregivers (Hayslip et al., 2009), and grandparent caregivers grieve over the many losses they have experienced in taking on this responsibility (Backhouse & Graham, 2013), wherein their plans for the future, the quality of their relationship to the grandchild, and even their satisfaction with their marriages are all often undermined. If the relationship with the adult child is ambivalent, conflictual, or poorly structured, the demands on the grandparent caregiver are more debilitating (Hayslip et al., 2009).

Discussion and Future Directions for Research

Examining grandparenthood from a dyadic developmental perspective allows us to understand it in light of its multiple influences, which are interactive (see Baltes, Reese, & Nesselroade, 1988), reflecting the complexity of grandparent-grandchild relationships. Viewed in this manner, we can well understand grandparent-grandchild dyads in light of the age-graded and history-graded contexts in which they exist as well as what is unique and particular to each grandparent-grandchild dyad. Clearly, the developmental issues we have discussed here bearing on grandparenting interact with those related to cohort effects, historical change, and culture.

A major research issue yet to be dealt with is the nature of the interaction between these factors. For example, do the developmental patterns we have presented here vary by cohort membership and/or historical change? To what extent does culture alter these developmental patterns of grandparent-grandchild relationships? What is the relative balance between those aspects of grandparenting which are age-graded and normative and those which are nonnormative in nature?

At a finer grain level of understanding, more attention needs to be paid to how grandparents and grandchildren negotiate and renegotiate their relationships *over time* in light of developmental periods such as emerging adulthood of grandchildren, health-related impairments experienced by grandparents, or the death, divorce, or remarriage of adult children. In each scenario, how do grandparents and grandchildren fare? What is the impact of losing a spouse or divorce on the experience of grandparenthood? Additionally, despite recent attention to this issue (see Hayslip & Kaminski, 2005; Park & Greenberg, 2007) more needs to be learned about grandparents as caregivers, be they raising a grandchild, or caring for an ill spouse or an impaired older parent. What are the long-term effects on such persons who have provided care oftentimes many for years? Complementarily, what are the long-term effects on grandchildren who have either been raised by a grandparent or who have otherwise enjoyed a loving relationship a traditional non-caregiver grandparent?

These and other questions specific to distinct life periods (see above) regarding the developmentally normative and nonnormative aspects of grandparenthood remain to be answered. As more persons live into their 80s and beyond, the experience of grandparents and great-grandparents as significant influences on the lives of their grandchildren will become more salient and perhaps even rival the direct influence that parents have on their children. At the minimum, our understanding of grandparenthood is enhanced via a recognition of the importance of the developmental context in which grandparents and grandchildren are embedded. In a dyadic, developmental sense, grandparents can both influence and are potentially influenced by their grandchildren, to the benefit of both.

References

Ahrons, C. R. (2007). Family ties after divorce: Long-term implications for children. *Family Process, 46*, 53–65.

American Association of Retired Persons (AARP). (2002). *The grandparent study*. Washington, DC.

Albert, D., Chein, J., & Steinberg, L. (2013). The teenage brain peer influences on adolescent decision making. *Current Directions in Psychological Science, 22*, 114–120.

Arnett, J.J. (1997). Young people's conceptions of the transition to adulthood, *Youth & Society, 29*, 3–23.

Arnett, J.J. (1998). Learning to stand alone: The contemporary American transition to adulthood in cultural and historical context. *Human Development, 41*, 295–315.

Arnett, J.J. (2000). Emerging adulthood: A theory of development from the late teens through the twenties. *American Psychologist, 55*, 469.

Arnett, J.J. (2007a). Emerging adulthood: What is it, and what is it good for? *Child Development Perspectives, 1*, 68–73.

Arnett, J.J. (2007b). Suffering, selfish, slackers? Myths and reality about emerging adults. *Journal of Youth and Adolescence, 36*, 23–29.

Arnett, J.J., & Tanner, J.L. (Eds.). (2006). *Emerging adults in America: Coming of age in the 21st century*. Washington, DC: American Psychological Association.

Attar-Schwartz, S., Tan, J.P., & Buchanan, A. (2009). Adolescents' perspectives on relationships with grandparents: The contribution of adolescent, grandparent, and parent–grandparent relationship variables. *Children and Youth Services Review, 31*, 1057–1066.

Backhouse, J., & Graham, A. (2012). Grandparents raising grandchildren: Negotiating the complexities of role identity conflict. *Child and Family Social Work, 17*, 305–315.

Backhouse, J., & Graham, A. (2013). Grandparents raising grandchildren: Acknowledging the experience of grief. *Australian Social Work, 66*, 440–454.

Bailey, J., Hill, K., Oesterle, S., & Hawkins, D. (2009). Parenting practices and problem behavior across three generations: Monitoring, harsh discipline, and drug use in the intergenerational transmission of externalizing behavior. *Developmental Psychology, 45*, 1214–1226.

Baker, L., & Silverstein, M. (2008). Preventative health behaviors among grandmothers raising grandchildren. *Journals of Gerontology: Psychological and Social Sciences, 63B*, S304–S311.

Baltes, P.B. (1997). On the incomplete architecture on human ontogeny: Selection, optimization, and compensation of developmental theory. *American Psychologist, 52*, 366–379.

Baltes, P., Reese, H., & Nesselorade, J. (1988). *Life span developmental psychology: Introduction to research methods.* Hillsdale, NJ: Erlbaum.

Bangerter, L., & Waldron, V. (2014). Turning points in long distance grandparent–grandchild relationships. *Journal of Aging Studies, 29*, 88–97.

Boon, S., Shaw, M., & MacKinnon, S. (2008). Grandparent health and young adults' judgments of grandparent–grandchild relationships. *Journal of Intergenerational Relationships, 6*, 155–173.

Boquet, J., Oliver, D., Wittenberg-Styles, E., Doorenbos, A., & Demiris, G. (2011). Taking care of a dying grandparent: Case studies of grandchildren in the hospice caregiver role. *American Journal of Hospice and Palliative Medicine, 28*, 564–568.

Botcheva, L. B., & Feldman, S. S. (2004). Grandparents as family stabilizers during economic hardship in Bulgaria. *International Journal of Psychology, 39*, 157–168.

Breheny, M., Stephens, C., & Spilsbury, L. (2013). Involvement without interference: How grandparents negotiate intergenerations expectations in relationship with grandchildren. *Journal of Family Studies, 19*, 174–184.

Bridges, L. J., Roe, A. E., Dunn, J., & O'Connor, T. G. (2007). Children's perspectives on their relationships with grandparents following parental separation: A longitudinal study. *Social Development, 16*, 539–554.

Brussoni, M. J., & Boon, S. D. (1998). Grandparental impact in young adults' relationships with their closest grandparents: The role of relationship strength and emotional closeness. *The International Journal of Aging and Human Development, 46*, 267–286.

Celdran, M., Tirado, C., & Villar, F. (2011). Learning from the disease: Lessons drawn from adolescents having a grandparent suffering from dementia. *International Journal of Aging and Human Development, 68*, 243–259.

Cherlin, A., & Furstenberg, F. (1986). *The new American grandparent.* New York: Basic Books.

Christiansen, F., & Smith, T. (2002). What is happening to satisfaction and quality of relationships between step/grandparents and step/grandchildren? *Journal of Divorce and Remarriage, 37*,117–133.

Coali, D., & Hertwig, R. (2011). Grandparental investment: A relic of the past or reinvestment in the future? *Current Directions in Psychological Science, 20*, 93–98.

Cole, M. (1999). Culture in development. In M. Bernstein & M. Lamb (Eds.), *Developmental psychology: An advanced textbook* (pp. 73–124). Mahwah, NJ: Erlbaum.

Combrinck-Graham, L. (1985). A developmental model for family systems. *Family Process, 24*,139–150.

Condon, J., Corkindale, C., Luszcz, M., & Gamble, E. (2013). The Australian first-time grandparents study: Time spent with a grandchild and its predictors. *Australasian Journal on Ageing, 32*, 21–27.

Connidis, I. A. (2010). *Family ties and aging.* Thousand Oaks, CA: Pine Forge Press.

Cornelius, J., Le Grand, S., & Jemmot, L. (2009). African American grandfamilies' attitudes and feelings about sexual communication: Focus group results. *Journal of the Association of Nurses in AIDS Care, 20*, 133–140.

Creasey, G. L., & Kaliher, G. (1994). Age differences in grandchildren's perceptions of relations with grandparents. *Journal of Adolescence, 17*, 411–426.

Creasey, G. L., & Koblewski, P. J. (1991). Adolescent grandchildren's relationships with maternal and paternal grandmothers and grandfathers. *Journal of Adolescence, 14*, 373–387.

Dellmann-Jenkins, M., Papalia, D., & Lopez, M. (1987). Teenagers' reported interaction with grandparents: Exploring the extent of alienation. *Lifestyles, 8*, 35–46.

Doka, K. J. (Ed.). (2002). *Disenfranchised grief: New directions, challenges, and strategies for practice.* Champaign, IL: Research Press.

Doyle, M., O'Dywer, C., & Timonen, V. (2010). "How can you just cut off a whole side of the family and say move on?" The reshaping of paternal grandparent–grandchild relationships following divorce or separation in the middle generation. *Family Relations, 59*, 587–598.

Drew, L., & Silverstein, M. (2007). Grandparents' psychological well-being after loss of contact with their grandchildren. *Journal of Family Psychology, 21*, 372–379.

Drew, L., & Smith, P. (1999). The impact of parental separation/divorce on grandparent–grandchild relationships. *International Journal of Aging and Human Development, 48*, 191–216.

Dunifon, R. (2013). The influence of grandparents on the lives of children and adolescents. *Child Development Perspectives, 7*, 55–60.

Erikson, E. H. (1968). *Identity: Youth and crisis.* New York: Norton.

Even-Zohar, A. (2011). Intergenerational solidarity between adult grandchildren and their grandparents with different levels of functional ability. *Journal of Intergenerational Relationships, 9*, 128–145.

Ferguson, J., & Ready, D. (2011). Expanding notions of social reproduction: Grandparents' educational attainment and grandchildren's cognitive skills. *Early Childhood Research Quarterly, 26*, 216–226.

Findler, L. (2014). The experience of stress and personal growth among grandparents of children with and without intellectual disability. *Intellectual and Developmental Disabilities, 52*, 32–48.

Fingerman, K. (1998). The good, the bad, and the worrisome: Emotional complexities in grandparents' experiences with individual grandchildren. *The Family Life Coordinator, 47*, 403–414.

Flouri, E., Buchanan, A., Tan, J. P., Griggs, J., & Attar-Schwartz, S. (2010). Adverse life events, area socio-economic disadvantage, and adolescent psychopathology: The role of closeness to grandparents in moderating the effect of contextual stress. *Stress, 13*, 402–412.

Friedman, D., Hechter, M., & Kreager, D. (2008). A theory of the value of grandchildren. *Rationality and Society, 20*, 31–63.

Fruhauf, C., Jarrott, S., & Allen, K. (2002). Grandchildren's perceptions of caring for grandparents. *Journal of Family Issues, 27*, 887–911.

Fruhauf, C., & Orel, N. (2008). Developmental issues of grandchildren who provide care to grandparents. *International Journal of Aging and Human Development, 67*, 209–230.

Generations United. (2009). *Grandfacts: Data, interpretation, and implications for caregivers.* Washington, DC: Author.

Giarusso, R., Feng, D., Silverstein, M., & Bengtson, V. L. (2001). Grandparent–adult grandchild affection and consensus. *Journal of Family Issues, 22*, 456–477.

Geurts, T., Van Tilburg, T., & Poortman, A. (2012). The grandparent–grandchild relationship in childhood and adulthood: A matter of continuation? *Personal Relationships, 19*, 267–278.

Hagestad, G. O. (1985). Continuity and connectedness. In V. L. Bengtson & J. F. Robertson (Eds.), *Grandparenthood* (pp. 31–48). Beverly Hills, CA: Sage.

Halgunseth, L. C., Ispa, J. M., & Rudy, D. (2006). Parental control in Latino families: An integrated review of the literature. *Child Development, 77*, 1282–1297.

Harwood, J. (2001). Comparing grandchildren's and grandparent's stake in their relationship. *International Journal of Aging and Human Development, 53*, 195–210.

Hayslip, B. (2009). Ethnic and cross cultural perspectives on custodial grandparenting. In J. Sokolovsky (Ed.), *The cultural context of aging: Worldwide perspectives* (3rd ed., pp. 346–356). Westport, CT: Greenwood Publishing.

Hayslip, B., Glover, R., Harris, B., Miltenberger, P., Baird, A., & Kaminski, P. (2009). Perceptions of custodial grandparents among young adults. *Journal of Intergenerational Relationships, 7*, 209–224.

Hayslip, B., & Kaminski, P. (2005). Grandparents raising their grandchildren: A review of the literature and suggestions for practice. *The Gerontologist, 45*, 262–269.

Hayslip, B., Maiden, R., Page, K., & Dolbin-MacNab, M. (2015). Grandparenting. In P. Lichtenberg, B. Mast, B. Carpenter, & J. Wetherell (Eds.), *APA handbook of clinical geropsychology* (pp. 497–511). Washington, DC: American Psychological Association.

Hayslip, B., & Page, K. (2012). Grandparenthood: Grandchild and great-grandchild relationships. In R. Blieszner & V. Bedford (Eds.), *Handbook of families and aging* (pp. 183–212). Santa Barbara, CA: Praeger.

Hayslip, B., & White, D. (2008). Grandparents as grievers. In M. S. Stroebe, R. O. Hansson, W. Stroebe, & H. Schut (Eds.), *Handbook of bereavement research* (3rd ed., pp. 441–460). Washington, DC: American Psychological Association.

Hayslip, B., Glover, R., & Pollard, S. (In Press). Traditional grandparent peers' perceptions of custodial grandparents: Extent of life disruption and needs for social support, social, and mental health services. In M. H. Meyer (Ed.), *Grandparenting in the US.* Amityville, NY: Baywood.

Henderson, C., Hayslip, B., Sanders, L., & Louden, L. (2009). Grandmother–grandchild relationship quality predicts psychological adjustment among youth from divorced families. *Journal of Family Issues, 30*, 1245–1264.

Hodgson, L. G. (1992). Adult grandchildren and their grandparents: The enduring bond. *International Journal of Aging and Human Development, 34*, 209–225.

Hokoyama, M., & MaloneBeach, E. (2013). Predictors of grandparent–grandchild closeness: An ecological perspective. *Journal of Intergenerational Relationships, 11*, 32–49.

Holladay, S., Lackovich, R., Lee, M., Coleman, M., Harding, D., & Dento, D. (1998). (Re)constructing relationships with grandparents: A turning point analysis of granddaughters' relational development with maternal grandmothers. *International Journal of Aging and Human Development, 46*, 287–303.

Hurme, H., Westerback, S., & Quadello, T. (2010). Traditional and new forms of contact between grandparents and grandchildren. *Journal of Intergenerational Relationships, 8*, 264–280.

Ihara, E., Horio, B., & Tompkins, C. (2012). Grandchildren caring for grandparents: Modeling the complexity of family caregiving. *Journal of Social Service Research, 38*, 629–636.

Kahana, E. et al. (In Press). Childhood autism and proactive family coping: Intergenerational perspectives. *Journal of Intergenerational Relationships.*

Kam, J., & Hecht, M. (2009). Investigating the role of identity gaps among communicative and relational outcomes within the grandparent–grandchild relationship: The young-adult grandchildren's perspective. *Western Journal of Communication, 73*, 456–480.

Kaminski, P., Hayslip, B., Wilson, J., & Casto, L. (2008). Parenting attitudes and adjustment among custodial grandparents. *Journal of Intergenerational Relationships, 6*, 263–284.

Kemp, C. (2007). Grandparent–grandchild ties: Reflections on continuity and change across three generations. *Journal of Family Issues, 28*, 855–881.

Kenner, C., Ruby, M., Jessel, J., Gregory, E., & Arju, T. (2007). Intergenerational learning between children and grandparents in East London. *Journal of Early Childhood Research, 5*, 219–243.

Kornhaber, A. (1996). *Contemporary grandparenting*. Thousand Oaks, CA: Sage.

Kornhaber, A., & Woodward, K. L. (1981). *Grandparents, grandchildren: The vital connection*. Piscataway, NJ: Transaction Publishers.

Lee, M. (2010). Grandparents' involvement and support in families with children with disabilities. *Educational Gerontology, 36*, 467–499.

Levinson, D. J. (1978). *The seasons of a man's life*. New York: Ballantine.

Lussier, G., Deater-Deckard, K., Dunn, J., & Davies, L. (2002). Support across two generations: Children's closeness to grandparents following parental divorce and remarriage. *Journal of Family Psychology, 16*, 363–376.

MacMillan, R., & Copher, R. (2005). Families in the life course: Interdependencies of roles, role configurations, and pathways. *Journal of Marriage and the Family, 67*, 858–879.

Maiden, R. J., & Zuckerman, C. (2008). Counseling grandparents parenting their children's children: Case studies. In B. Hayslip Jr. & P. Kaminski (Eds.), *Parenting the custodial grandchild: Implications for clinical practice* (pp. 197–214). New York: Springer.

Mansson, D. (2013). Affectionate communication and relational characteristics in the grandparent–grandchild relationship. *Communication Reports, 26*, 47–60.

Markides, K. S., & Krause, N. (1985). Intergenerational solidarity and psychological well-being among older Mexican–Americans: A three-generations study. *Journal of Gerontology, 40*(3), 390–392.

Miller, L., Buys, L., & Woodbridge, S. (2012). Impact of disability on families: Grandparents' perspectives. *Journal of Intellectual Disability Research, 56*, 102–110.

Mills, R. B., Vermette, V., & Malley-Morrison, K. (1998). Judgments about elder abuse and college students' relationship with grandparents. *Gerontology & Geriatrics Education, 19*, 17–30.

Mills, T., Wakeman, M., & Rea, C. (2001). Adult grandchildren's perceptions of emotional closeness and consensus with their maternal and paternal grandparents. *Journal of Family Issues, 22*, 427–455.

Mirfin-Vietch, B., Bray, A., & Watson, M. (1997). "We're just that sort of family": Intergenerational relationships in families including children with disabilities. *Family Relations, 46*, 305–311.

Nisbett, R., & Ross, L. (1980). *Human inference: Strategies and shortcomings of social judgment*. Englewood Cliffs, NJ: Prentice Hall.

Paikoff, R. L., & Brooks-Gunn, J. (1991). Do parent–child relationships change during puberty? *Psychological Bulletin, 110*, 47–66.

Park, H., & Greenberg, J. (2007). Parenting grandchildren. In J. Blackburn & C. Dumus (Eds.), *Handbook of gerontology: Evidence-based approaches to theory, practice, and policy* (pp. 397–425). New York: Wiley.

Pearson, J., Hunter, A., Ensminger, M., & Kellam, S. (1990). Black grandmothers in intergenerational households: Diversity in family structure and parenting involvement in the Woodlawn community. *Child Development, 61*, 434–442.

Perry, G. M., & Nixon, C. J. (2005). The influence of role models on negotiation ethics of college students. *Journal of Business Ethics, 62*, 25–40.

Petersen, A. C., Crockett, L., Richards, M., & Boxer, A. (1998). A self-report measure of pubertal status: Reliability, validity, and initial norms. *Journal of Youth and Adolescence, 17*, 117–133.

Pew Foundation. (2010). *Since the start of the great recession, more children raised by grandparents.* http://pewreseacrh.org/pubs/1724

Pratt, N., Norris, J. E., Hebblethwaite, S., & Arnold, M. (2008). Intergenerational transmission of values: Family generativity and adolescents' narratives of parent and grandparent value teaching. *Journal of Personality, 76*, 171–198.

Reed, M. L. (2000). *Grandparents cry twice: Help for bereaved grandparents.* Amityville, NY: Baywood Publishing Company.

Reitzes, D. C., & Mutran, E. J. (2004). Grandparent identity, intergenerational family identity, and well-being. *The Journal of Gerontology: Social Sciences, 59B*, S213–S219.

Riegel, K. (1976). The dialectics of human development. *American Psychologist, 31*, 689–700.

Roberto, K. A., & Skoglund, R. R. (1996). Interactions with grandparents and great-grandparents: A comparison of activities, influences, and relationships. *The International Journal of Aging and Human Development, 43*, 107–117.

Rokach, A. (2000). Loneliness and the life cycle. *Psychological Reports, 86*(2), 629–642.

Sanders, G. F., & Trygstad, D. W. (1989). Stepgrandparents and grandparents: The view from young adults. *Family Relations, 38*, 71–75.

Scherrer, K. (2012). The intergenerational family relationships of grandparents of GLBQ grandchildren. *Dissertation Abstracts International: Humanities and Social Sciences, 72*(12-A), 4762 (abstract).

Schmidt, A., & Padilla, A. M. (1983). Grandparent–grandchild interaction in a Mexican–American group. *Hispanic Journal of Behavioral Sciences, 5*, 181–198.

Scholl, P. (1997). Relationships among adolescents' ego development, their academic achievement, and the amount of contact and social distance from grandparents. *Dissertation Abstracts International, 57*(8-B), 5391 (abstract).

Schwartz, P. D., Maynard, A. M., & Uzelac, S. M. (2008). Adolescent egocentrism: A contemporary view. *Adolescence, 43*, 441–448.

Semberg, L. (2013). Be there for my grandchild–grandparents' responses to their grandchildren's exposure to domestic violence. *Child and Family Social Work, 18*, 23–30.

Shaw, S. (2005). Grandparent involvement and communication development of children who are deaf blind. *Educational Gerontology, 31*, 51–71.

Sheridan, K., Haight, W.L., & Cleeland, L. (2011). The role of grandparents in preventing aggressive and other externalizing behavior problems in children from rural, methamphetamine-involved families. *Children and Youth Services Review, 33*, 1583–1591.

Sigurdardottir, S., & Julursdottir, S. (2013). Reciprocity in relationships and support between grandparents and grandchildren: An Icelandic example. *Journal of Intergenerational Relationships, 11*, 118–133.

Silverstein, M., & Chen, X. (1999). The impact of acculturation in Mexican American families on the quality of adult grandchild–grandparent relationships. *Journal of Marriage and the Family, 61*, 188–198.

Silverstein, M., & Parrott, T.M. (1997). Attitudes toward public support of the elderly does early involvement with grandparents moderate generational tensions? *Research on Aging, 19*, 108–132.

Sims, M., & Rofail, M. (2013). The experience of grandparents who have limited or no contact with their grandchildren. *Journal of Aging Studies, 27*, 377–386.

Smith, G.C., Palmieri, P., Hancock, G., & Richardson, R. (2008). Custodial grandmothers' psychological distress, dysfunctional parenting, and grandchildren's adjustment. *International Journal of Aging and Human Development, 67*, 327–358.

Smith, T. (2012). Adult grandchildren providing care to frail elderly grandparents. *Dissertation Abstracts International: Section A: Humanities and Social Sciences, 72*(11-A), 4320 (abstract).

Soliz, J. (2008). Intergenerational support and the role of grandparents in post-divorce families: Retrospective accounts of young adult grandchildren. *Qualitative Research Reports in Communication, 9*, 72–80.

Soliz, J., & Harwood, J. (2006). Shared family identity, age salience, and intergroup contact: Investigation of the grandparent–grandchild relationship. *Communication Monographs, 73*, 87–107.

Somary, K., & Stricker, G. (1998). Becoming a grandparent: A longitudinal study of expectations and early experiences as a function of age and lineage. *The Gerontologist, 38*, 53–61.

Stelle, C., Fruhauf, C., Orel, N., & Landry-Meyer, L. (2010). Grandparenting in the 21st century: Issues of diversity in grandparent–grandchild relationships. *Journal of Gerontological Social Work, 53*, 682–701.

Strom, R.D., Buki, L.P., & Strom, S.K. (1997). Intergenerational perceptions of English speaking and Spanish speaking Mexican-American grandparents. *International Journal of Aging and Human Development, 45*, 1–21.

Strom, R.D., Lee, T., Strom, P.S., Nakagawa, K., & Beckert, T.E. (2008). Taiwanese grandmothers: Strengths and learning needs as perceived by grandmothers, mothers, and granddaughters. *Educational Gerontology, 34*, 812–830.

Strom, P.S., & Strom, R.D. (2015). Assessment of intergenerational communication and relationships. *Educational Gerontology, 41*, 41–52.

Taylor, A.C., Robila, M., & Lee, H.S. (2005). Distance, contact, and intergenerational relationships: Grandparents and adult grandchildren from an international perspective. *Journal of Adult Development, 12*, 33–41.

Triadó, C., Villar, F., Solé, C., Osuna, M.J., & Pinazo, S. (2005). The meaning of grandparenthood: Do adolescent grandchildren perceive the relationship and role in the same way as their grandparents do? *Journal of Intergenerational Relationships, 3*, 101–121.

Uhlenberg, P. (2004). Historical forces shaping grandparent–grandchild relationships: Demography and beyond. *Annual Review of Gerontology and Geriatrics, 26*, 77–97.

Uhlenberg, P. (2009). Children in an aging society. *Journal of Gerontology: Social Sciences, 64B*, S489–S496.

Uhlenberg, P., & Kirby, J. (1998). Grandparent over time: Historical and demographic trends. In M. Szionovacz (Ed.), *Handbook on grandparenthood* (pp. 23–39). Westport, CT: Greenwood Press.

Van Ranst, N., Verschueren, K., & Marcoen, A. (1995). The meaning of grandparents as viewed by adolescent grandchildren: An empirical study in Belgium. *The International Journal of Aging and Human Development, 41*, 311–324.

Villar, F., Triado, C., Piazo-Hernandis, S., Cedlran, M., & Sole, C. (2010). Grandparents and their adolescent grandchildren: Generational stake or generational complaint? A study with dyads in Spain. *Journal of Intergenerational Relationships, 8*, 281–297.

Wakefield, C., Drew, D., Ellis, S., Doolan, E., McLoone, J., & Cohn, R. (2014). "What they're not telling you": A new scale to measure grandparents' information needs when their grandchild has cancer. *Patient Care and Counseling, 94*, 351–355.

Watson, M. (2010). The facilitators and inhibitors for grandparents raising grandchildren in relation to parental involvement in school on behalf of their grandchildren. *Dissertation Abstracts International: Humanities and Social Sciences, 70*(7-A), 2839 (abstract).

Werner, P., & Lowenstein, A. (2001). Grandparenthood and dementia. *Clinical Gerontologist, 23*, 115–129.

Wiscott, R., & Kopera-Frye, K. (2000). Sharing of culture: Adult grandchildren's perceptions of intergenerational relations. *International Journal of Aging and Human Development, 51*, 199–215.

Wise, R. (2010). Intergenerational relationship characteristics and grandchildren's perceptions of grandparent goal influence. *Journal of Intergenerational Relationships, 8*, 54–68.

Won, S. (2010). The closeness between grandparents and grandchildren and its impact on grandparents' well-being. *Dissertation Abstracts International Section A: Humanities and Social Sciences, 71*(2-A), 717 (abstract).

Yorgason, J., Padilla-Walker, L., & Jackson, J. (2013). Nonresidential grandparents emotional and financial involvement in relation to early adolescent grandchild outcomes. *Journal of Research on Adolescence, 21*, 552–558.

Zimmermann, P., & Iwanski, A. (2014). Emotion regulation from early adolescence to emerging adulthood and middle adulthood age differences, gender differences, and emotion-specific developmental variations. *International Journal of Behavioral Development, 38*, 182–194.

CHAPTER TWELVE

The Transformation of Aging Politics and Policy in the United States

Robert B. Hudson

Aging-related issues have found an increasingly prominent place on the nation's political agenda in recent years. After several decades of growing slowly and accompanied by little controversy, aging policies have more recently expanded dramatically and have yielded a more highly charged politics than had earlier been the case. This chapter speaks to three factors, dating from the New Deal period to the present, that lie at the heart of this transformation: (1) changes in the political standing of the older population over time and understanding of what are its collective policy needs; (2) an imposing political presence of older Americans in Washington, a presence created in part by programs enacted on their behalf; and (3) constraints in the economic and political environment impinging on elders' emergent policy domain. Taken together, these developments have served to expand the scope of conflict around aging policy whereby the heightened political and policy presence of the old is now encountering a series of countervailing economic and political pressures.

Early Years and Growth of Aging Policy and Politics

At least in historical perspective, the first 50 years of aging policy and politics were relatively benign. The older population was small in size and uniquely vulnerable, the larger social and economic environment was largely favorable, and there was little political resistance to promoting programs to address older persons' needs.

Vulnerable Elders

Dating back to the early 1900s, most elders led a precarious existence, one marked by lack of income, marginal health status, and a presumed inability to work. The great fear of late life was outliving one's income and, in the absence of individual wealth or family supports, people in old age were left to mercies of private charity or public alms. Such data as exist point to this host of perilous circumstances. Writing in the first issue of the *Social Security Bulletin*, Shearon (1938) reported some two-thirds of the older population to be dependent on others, but found—perhaps more striking—that one-half of those she was able to categorize as self-dependent were reliant on family or friends for additional income. Addressing the same period, Upp (1982) estimated that three-quarters of elders' income had come from their adult children.

Illness and disability were a second great concern of older people, both because they made work difficult or impossible and because there were few health and social supports to address those needs. Failed public health insurance initiatives during the Roosevelt and Truman years and restrictive private insurance provisions had left half of the older population with no form of health insurance at the time of Medicare's enactment in 1965. In the case of chronic illness and disability, elders were reliant principally on the care of family, friends, and private charities, with those of modest means occasionally gaining access to early "mom and pop" nursing homes (Vladeck, 1980). As late as 1961, a husband, testifying before the Senate Special Committee on Aging, asked what would happen if either he or his wife became ill, lamented that "I will have to seek come charity institution . . . and pronounce to the whole world that I am a pauper, a beggar" (Sundquist, 1968, p. 288).

Finally, there was a presumption that older people either could not work (due to illness) or should not work (in order than younger people might have jobs). That older people did work was frequently seen as unfairly burdensome to them, inefficient for employers, and unjust for unemployed younger workers (Graebner, 1980). As such, for many years Social Security was seen as much as labor market policy (encouraging retirement) as it was understood to be social welfare policy (assuring adequate income in old age). Until 2000, there was an earnings test under Social Security which served as a work disincentive by essentially taxing benefits above a modest income disregard. The formulas in defined-benefit pension plans, which grew dramatically in the immediate postwar years, also contained major disincentives to continued work. Only recently has eliminating the earnings test and the movement toward 401(k)-type retirement savings plans recognized and promoted continued work among older adults.

The Politics of Vulnerability

The political importance of these early understandings of elders as systematically at risk was its having lent significant legitimacy to their needs, that is, it granted elders the critical status that they *should* be supported through some public policy mechanism (Sherman & Kolker, 1987). Social insurance pioneer Isaac Rubinow (1934) spoke of the unquestioned needs of older people as "the final emergency"; Franklin Roosevelt opined that poverty in old age was not a result of a lack of thrift but was a "mere by-product of modern industrial life" (cited in Rimlinger, 1971, p. 212); and Gordon (1998) writes that, compared to single mothers in the early twentieth century, elders were a "group to be quintessentially deserving" of public support. These conditions lay at the heart of what Binstock (1983) identified as the long-standing "compassionate stereotype" of older adults. If one is understood as not being able or expected to work, pensions or savings vehicles should be put in place; if older people are understandably more ill than young people; and if the private market will not serve them, provision should be made for publicly sponsored health insurance.

A policy typology put forth by Schneider and Ingram (1993) neatly captures this reality. Interested in how different "target populations" fare in the public policy world, the authors suggest that populations be ranged along two dimensions: social construction (positive or negative) and political power (high or low). Four population types result from this configuration: Dependents (positive construction, low power), Advantaged (positive construction, high power), Contenders (negative construction, high power), and Deviants (negative construction, low power).

This typology has great utility in tracing the origins and evolution of aging politics and policy. As suggested by the preceding material, positive construction (or legitimacy) was an early hallmark of elders' social standing: they appeared deserving and in need of a variety of supports. At the same time—being relatively few in number and possessing few material resources—elders constituted a weak, bordering on nonexistent, political constituency. This combination of positive construction and low political power rendered them as Dependents as seen through the Schneider and Ingram construct.

Elders' needs generated both sympathy and political support from advocates for social reform and from policy makers sympathetic to those needs. Three critical legislative episodes speak to the political utility of their marginal social standing. The original Social Security Act featured seniors in both Title I (Old-Age Assistance) and Title II (Old-Age Insurance). A federal-state public assistance program, OAA was the sweetener to introduce the more controversial social insurance titles directed to both elders and to the unemployed (Title V). Driving these developments were the desperate conditions produced by the Depression, the leadership of Franklin Roosevelt, and the workings of a small group of policy reformers constituting the Committee on Economic Security. While economic circumstances set the stage for major policy initiatives, it was key elite actors invoking the plight of seniors that brought agency to those circumstances and led to Social Security's enactment (Witte, 1962).

The second policy episode centered on Medicare represents an equally clear example of elders' standing and agendas which it serves. Attempts by Presidents Roosevelt and Truman to enact national health insurance having failed in the 1930s and 1950s, policy advocates turned toward older Americans as a politically sympathetic target population in devising Medicare proposals in the early 1960s. Elders' health-care needs and their limited resources were beyond question; as put by Medicare architect Wilbur Cohen, "massing statistical data to prove that the aged were sicker, poorer, and less insured than other adult groups was like using a steamroller to crush an ant of opposition" (quoted in Marmor, 1970, p. 17). In conjunction with intense lobbying by organized labor and its retirees, Medicare became law in 1965 (Sundquist, 1968). In no other country have older people served as either the sole or primary beneficiaries of national health insurance initiatives.

A third instance of the political utility of elders' vulnerability is found in the enactment of Supplemental Security Income in 1973. In 1970, President Richard Nixon proposed a fundamental restructuring of the Aid to Families with the Dependent Children program, calling for creation of a national minimum cash benefit and ending a so-called services approach to welfare dependency among young families (Moynihan, 1973). The proposal made considerable legislative headway until it was finally defeated in the Senate Finance Committee, conservatives appalled by the income guarantee and liberals finding the actual amount woefully low. Because the underlying idea of an income guarantee was dear to reform-minded officials, they set about to see if it would find acceptance directed to a different population. They concluded that such might be the case with regard to the so-called adult public assistance categories, those directed to the old, the blind, and the disabled, the Old-Age Assistance program being by far the largest of the three. In a remarkable turn of legislative fortune, the proposal was redirected to those groups and enacted shortly thereafter. Health, Education, and Welfare Secretary Wilbur Cohen, seated in the House chamber at the time of passage, exclaimed, "do you realize what they're doing? It's not even controversial, it's not even controversial!" (quoted in Burke and Burke, 1974, p. 198). Again, the policy legitimacy of the aged held center stage, and the nation's first public income guarantee, as a supplement to low Social Security benefits, was enacted as SSI.

The remainder of the remarkable 1965–1974 policy decade saw additional policy activity on behalf of older Americans: enactment of Medicaid, the Older Americans Act, the Age Discrimination in Employment Act, and the Employee Retirement Income Security Act. As well, an Institute on Aging was created within the National Institutes of Health, and, importantly, Social Security benefits were increased by 58 percent between 1967 and 1973 (U.S. Office of Management and Budget, 2013). To be sure, elders were not alone in enjoying policy gains during these years, but they were disproportionately favored. This is seen perhaps most dramatically in a comparison in expenditure differences between aging programs the much heralded War on Poverty of the late 1960s. Expenditures for the latter never exceeded $2 billion per year whereas outlays for Social Security alone totaled $30 billion in 1970.

Policy Benefits and Political Activism

By the mid-1970s, these policy gains began generating positive both personal and political outcomes. The poverty rate among older Americans fell from 35 percent in 1959, to 25 percent in 1969, and to 15 percent in 1979 (U.S. Bureau of the Census, 2012). By the early 1980s, Social Security benefits constituted two-thirds of all income for one-half of older Americans. Median income among seniors increased from $19,900 in 1970 to $33,800 in 2001 (U.S. Bureau of the Census, 2002). Private pension coverage doubled between 1945 and 1980 (Employee Benefit Research Institute, 1998). Medicare and Veterans benefits resulted in over 95 percent of elders having health insurance coverage. These and other developments helped to both create retirement as a fully institutionalized life stage (Ekerdt, 1989) and, more broadly, to allow Treas and Bengtson (1982) to represent them as nothing less than "the democratization of aging."

These gains translated into the political as well as the social and economic spheres. A new Senate Select Committee on Aging trumpeted during the mid-1970s that seniors had gone from one-in-eleven to one-in-ten and then to one-in-nine, speaking to their new prominence (Brotman, 1977). Yet more to the point, elders were being transformed from a demographic cluster to a political constituency, evolving from "a category created by policy analysts" (Heclo, 1988) to one held together by a common characteristic, being distinct policy beneficiaries (Campbell, 2003).

After the rise and fall of the Townsend Movement of the 1930s and the postwar lull in organized activity, political involvement of the old ratcheted up beginning in the 1970s. To this point the policy gains made by elders had resulted largely from their indisputable needs and advocates' desire to both assist them and promote progressive social policy. Now, a new period dawned in which needs were translated into interests and newly aware elders attracted the attention of business, service, and research organizations eager to associate with their new prominence. In rough cut, the need-to-demand part of the equation manifested itself principally in the birth of elder participation in politics; the organized interest element was seen in the formation of new advocacy groups targeting aging issues.

This extent of this transformation of elders' involvement in politics is remarkable on several counts. First, older people's rate of voting has not only increased over the ensuing years but has done so to the point that older Americans now vote at a higher rate than any other age group. This is in stark contrast to the pre-1970s scenario wherein seniors voted less than any group other than those aged under 24. Older people's high levels of voting have become even more pronounced in off-year elections, and presumably even more so in primaries where candidates for elective office are chosen. Beginning in 1986, elders voted at a higher level in off-year elections than other age groups, doing so at a rate twice that of the youngest voters and considerably more than the middle-aged (Campbell, 2003).

Elders' increasing involvement in politics extended beyond the formal act of voting. From a time when Schmidhauser (1970) suggested that older people ranked lowest in sense of political efficacy and among the lowest in "sense of citizen duty," elders have dramatically elevated their political game: they have quadrupled their rate of campaign contributing since 1952 (catching up to 35–64-year-olds in the 1980s), increased their level of campaigning (now equaling the 35–64-year-old group), and are increasingly in contact with Congressional representatives from the mid-1970s to the mid-1990s (whereas all nonsenior groups were in less frequent contact) (Campbell, 2003).

Elders' success in developing and attracting organized political support is perhaps even more stunning than their heightened levels of individual involvement. The birth and growth of contemporary aging interest groups began with the founding of the National Retired Teachers Association (NRTA) by an insurance executive creating a new market for his policies; NRTA later expanded into the American Association of Retired Persons, the name since abbreviated to AARP (Binstock, 2005). This group's reach now extends to over 40 million members with an operating budget in hundreds of millions of dollars, much of it centered on service provision and reduced-rate travel and kindred packages for members. A second mass-membership group—today named the Alliance for Retired Americans—began as Senior Citizens for Kennedy in

1960 and later became the National Council of Senior Citizens, where as an offshoot of organized labor it played a major role in the promotion of Medicare legislation in the early 1960s.

A host of additional groups sprang up in the wake of the late 1960s/early 1970s, watershed years of aging policy. Some are self-standing, others are sections within larger professional organizations such as law, nursing, or medicine. Yet others are more directly involved in the implementation of federal and state aging policy, notably the National Association of State Agencies on Aging and Disability and the National Association of Area Agencies on Aging (N4A). The number of such groups has continued to grow, and they came together in 1980 to form the Leadership Council of Aging Organizations, a confederation consisting of new fewer than 64 organizational members. Under the LCAO umbrella, these groups promote and defend aging policy provisions, both on behalf of elders themselves but especially around service contracts, research grants, and professional advancement opportunities (Lowi, 1969; Binstock, 1972; Walker, 1983).

Political and Policy Advantage: Elders

By the 1980s, this combination of policy benefits and political activity had introduced a new stage to aging politics. Abject need had generated policies that in the prosperous post–World War II years had begun to grow substantially. These policy benefits, in turn, had led to a dawning of political awareness among older people. What resulted was a symbiotic relationship between the policies and the politics that—in the Schneider and Ingram formulation—transformed elders from being a Dependent to an advantaged target population. While still maintaining their legitimate or deserving political standing, they had now emerged as a formidable political constituency.

In unraveling this connection, conventional wisdom would suggest that political activity came first, being requisite to public policy formation. Given the voting and lobbying presence of older Americans and their advocates, the necessary ingredients were surely in place. Yet, the picture is more complicated, and there is today strong evidence that the causal connection was largely in the other direction, that is, that the policies themselves helped generate elder political involvement. This dynamic has become a major focus of policy studies in recent years, referred to variously as "path dependency" (Pierson, 1993) or "bringing the state back in" (Skocpol, 1985). Looking at the policy process through this lens, policy at Time 1 is an independent factor shaping subsequent political activity at Time 2. In Campbell's (2012) words: "The central insight was that public policies are not merely products of politics but also shape the political arena and the possibilities for further policymaking" (p. 334). This relationship has been documented in the cases of the GI Bill of the 1940s and 1950s (Mettler, 2005), Disability Insurance in the 1950s and 1960s (Soss, 2000), and welfare reform in the 1990s (Soss and Schram, 2007).

However, there may be no arena other than aging policy where this dynamic is seen more clearly. Examining the interplay in the particular case of aging policy during and in the wake of the 1960s–1970s growth of aging policies, Walker (1983) determined that more than one-half of the 46 aging-related interest groups emerging during this period were formed after 1965, the year in which Medicare, Medicaid, and the Older Americans Act were enacted. Walker concludes that:

> In all of these cases, the formation of new groups was one of the *consequences* of major new legislation, not one of the *causes* of its passage. A pressure model of the policymaking process in which an essentially passive legislature responds to positions from groups of citizens who have spontaneously organized because common social or economic concerns must yield to a model in which influences for change come as much from inside the government as from beyond its institutional boundaries. (p. 403; emphasis in original)

The most direct piece of evidence in support of the policy's independent role in aging politics was the creation of the two trade associations whose state and local affiliates were brought into existence by federal legislation. The Older Americans Act mandated creation of State Units on Aging across the country in 1965, and Amendments passed in 1973 required creation of substate planning bodies, designated as Area Agencies on Aging. Within a year of each of these enactments, both the National Association of State Units on Aging (NASUA) and the N4A had established offices in Washington through which they continued to bring the social service needs of older persons to the attention of Congress and federal agencies (Hudson and Strate, 1985).

The most compelling application of this model to aging policy centers on the role of Social Security in helping to create a sense of political identity among older people. In her book, *How Policies Make Citizens: Senior Political Activism and the American Welfare State*, Campbell (2003) establishes a clear connection between the dramatic expansion of Old-Age and Survivors benefits under Social Security and the heightened participation by older Americans in the political process. She juxtaposes Social Security liberalization—involving both eligibility for benefits and benefit increases—against measures of participation—voting, contributing, campaign work, contacting—and finds increases in each of these types of activity in the wake of Social Security expansion and, more recently, in the wake of perceived threats to existing benefits. While broadening concern from a few score groups to millions of individuals, Campbell's conclusions are very reminiscent of Walker's:

> Absent Social Security, senior citizens are a disparate group of people whose common characteristic, age, has little political meaning. Once governmental benefits are conferred, however, the group has political relevance and is ripe for mobilization by policy entrepreneurs, interest groups, and political parties. (p. 36)

As a result of this interplay of critical aging-centric forces—demographic (growing population), social (heightened self-identification), economic (increasing prosperity), and political (imposing presence)—older Americans had clearly achieved Schneider and Ingram's Advantaged status by the turn of the century. They had largely maintained their legitimacy based on a deeply held, though somewhat suspect, belief in their universal vulnerability, and they had attained major standing in domestic politics, at one point seen as "America's most powerful lobby" (Van Atta, 1998). It is hard to overstate the magnitude of this transformation over little more than half a century, and it is nearly as important to highlight the role of public policy in bringing it about.

Emergence of a Transformed Aging Policy Environment

Elders, attaining an Advantaged status, were a function of a supportive environment and the improvements in life circumstances fostered by that environment. Emerging in the late-1970s, however, was a different set of forces which introduced new and unprecedented pressures into the aging policy domain. In the years since, this newly constrained environment has greatly expanded the scope of conflict around age-related policy and, as a consequence, has fundamentally transformed its dynamics.

A Downshifting Economy

The United States enjoyed a period of virtually uninterrupted economic expansion in the quarter-century following World War II. The Depression had suppressed economic growth, and the war had diverted resources from the domestic economy. Moreover, these two climactic events had led to a dramatic decline in birth rates over a 15-year period. In the postwar years, a combination of pent-up consumer demand, arrival of the baby boom, and the United States' domination of the international economy yielded enormous economic gains. During the century's fourth quarter, however, major changes occurred in each of these realms, with economic growth slowing, birth rates declining, and international economic competition exploding.

The significant slowdown in economic growth impacted both the larger economy and government revenues. Between 1950 and 1973, growth in the gross domestic product (GDP) averaged 4.25 percent annually; between 1974 and 2013, that average had fallen to 2.65 percent annually, a decline of more than one-third (U.S. Bureau of Economic Analysis, 2012). Persistent and increasing federal budget deficits also represented a great divide between the two periods. In constant 2005 dollars, the average annual deficit (including periodic surpluses in the calculation) from 1950 to 1973 was $37 billion, or 0.71 percent of GDP; for the period 1974–2013, annual deficits (also in constant dollars) averaged $320 billion, equal to 3.37 percent of GDP (U.S. Office of Management and Budget, 2013), with the deficit at 9.8 percent of GDP at the height of the recession in 2009 (U.S. Congressional Budget Office, 2013). The accumulated federal debt level also accelerated during this period, today totaling $17 trillion.

The combination of slowed economic growth and federal budget deficits has had clear relevance to aging policy. Social Security and Medicare constitute the second and third largest federal budget items after national defense. Not all of these dollars are directed to older Americans—Disability and Survivors Insurance constitute roughly one-third of Social Security outlays, and Medicare beneficiaries include individuals with disability and end-stage renal disease. Nonetheless, in much political parlance it is assumed that older people are virtually the sole recipients of these expenditures, and federal expenditures on behalf of seniors from all federal government sources are very large. The Congressional Budget Office calculated the amount to be $615 billion in 2000 (U.S. Congressional Budget Office, 2002), and a more recent calculation by Isaacs (2009) placed the figure at $767 billion. In broader perspective, CBO found expenditures for individuals aged 65 and over to constitute 35 percent of federal spending and projected it to be 43 percent by 2010; Isaacs estimates that such spending may constitute no less than 47 percent of spending by 2050. This contrasts with spending on behalf of older Americans during the earlier period to have equaled 22 percent of the budget in 1971, or $46 billion (U.S. Congressional Budget Office, 2002).

Political Realignments

The political context in which old-age policy found itself also underwent fundamental changes beginning in the late 1970s. Rising levels of inflation and unemployment, the travails of the Nixon/Ford (Reeves, 1975) and Carter presidencies (Johnson, 1980), and a rising conservative movement assailing the Great Society programs of the 1960s brought new players into the political arena. Conservative think tanks (Cato Institute, Heritage Foundation), new journals (*The Public Interest*, *Commentary*, *National Review*), and nationally syndicated columnists (William F. Buckley, George Will, Robert Samuelson, Charles Krauthammer) all joined the fray.

The election of Ronald Reagan in 1980 solidified the rise of conservatism. Its encompassing attack on federal social policy was captured by three of the President's stock phrases promoting his alternative agenda: privatization ("getting the government off your back"), decentralization ("bringing government closer to the people"), and individualization ("promoting traditional family values") (Palmer & Sawhill, 1984). Hacker (2006) captured the totality of this agenda, labeling it "the great risk shift." From a time when government offered protection against selected risks of modern life—old age, disability, illness—and large companies provided guaranteed pensions and health-care coverage—defined-benefit plans and employee and retiree health insurance—the emergent conservative agenda stressed the roles of families, communities, and the private sector. More generally, the entire domestic political agenda moved to the right post-Reagan, as captured by Thrush (2011), contending during the 2011 federal debt ceiling debate that "the center has shifted to the right" and that in today's politics "there is no such thing as a liberal victory."

Aging Policy and the New Environment

Prior to this period, aging policy had enjoyed—by the prevailing standards of American social policy—a charmed existence. From a time when "you couldn't do enough for the elderly," older Americans entered a more contested arena captured in the title of Derthick's (1979) seminal article "How Easy Votes for Social Security Came to an End." Similar analyses abounded, as in Estes (1979) critiquing "the aging enterprise," Hudson (1978) cautioning advocates around "the graying of the federal budget," and Samuelson (1978) bemoaning the challenge of "shouldering the growing burden" of aging-related expenditures. Indeed, expenditures did continue to grow despite new clouds on the aging horizon, whether automatically (Weaver, 1988), unsustainably (Concord Coalition, 2003), or understandably (Ball, 2000). Social Security benefits rose 67 percent between 1967 and 1973, and spending under the nascent Medicare program jumped from $33 billion in 1971 to $105 billion in 1980.

Pressures began to rise against these and other aging expenditures. Early in his administration, Reagan proposed major Social Security cuts which, while rescinded in the face of fierce resistance, were unprecedented in their intent (Palmer & Sawhill, 1984). Seven years later, the Administration proposed a liberalization of Medicare benefits through the Medicare

Catastrophic Coverage Act, but with the catch that—unlike all previous social insurance benefits for seniors—these would have to be paid for by seniors themselves (Himelfarb, 1995). Vocal opposition led to the law being repealed, but the intragenerational funding mechanism spoke to an entirely new aging politics playing field. Some years later, President Clinton fought a successful two-year battle against Congressional Republicans trying to enact major cuts in Medicare and Medicaid, but once again elder interests were defending turf they already occupied rather than expanding benefits in a manner seen in the earlier years (Smith, 2002).

The contested politics around aging continued after the turn of the century. The results were mixed, but in no way were the politics benign. Republicans and Democrats came to a grudging agreement to add a prescription drug benefit to Medicare, with Republicans putting in place an entirely private insurance delivery system and Democrats claiming credit for a benefit that they had long advocated (Pear, 2003). In 2005, the Bush Administration sought to partially privatize Social Security as well, but was defeated by opposition from elders, their organizations, and a wide array of progressive policy interests (Weisberg, 2005).

There have been fewer policy fireworks than these in the Obama years, but two somewhat tangential episodes, both centered on Medicare, speak to the tensions that continue to surround aging policy. Passage of the Affordable Care Act (aka "Obamacare") in 2009 dominated the domestic policy agenda at the end of the decade. While the ACA's benefits and requirements are directed exclusively at working-age and younger Americans, negative reaction to the legislation resonated loudly among older Americans and politicians seeking their support. Republicans, who had pressed for Medicare cuts in the 1990s, suddenly rushed to the program's defense, arguing that major cuts were being made to Medicare to fund the ACA (Nagourney, 2009). The ACA's defenders contended that the cost savings would come from providers, not beneficiaries, but many older voters were convinced that the ACA was an attack on their program. Indeed, support for the ACA was lower among older voters than any other age group, and analysts associated gains made by Republicans in the 2010 off-year election to elders' concerns (Binstock, 2012).

In 2012, Representative Paul Ryan of Wisconsin, arguing that competition would hold down rising Medicare costs, proposed converting Medicare into a voucher program whereby elders would get a fixed-amount "premium support" to take into the private insurance market. Opponents argued that this was a clear example of risk-shifting and that elders (and providers) would be penalized by what was certain to be failure of the voucher amounts to keep up with utilization and cost growth (Morgan, 2014).

The dual conclusion to be drawn from this series of legislative episodes is that new political, economic, and budgetary pressures are now growing on aging programs but that elders and their advocates have emerged as a potent political force willing and usually able to withstand these growing pressures, It is in that sense that aging politics has moved into a third of Schneider and Ingram's (1993) categories, that of Contenders: a population whose legitimacy has come into question but whose power has been maintained or increased. In the specific case of older Americans, the lessened legitimacy has resulted in new questions about their collective needs and the seeming political consequence that seniors seem to be perfectly able to take care of themselves. In sum, through the Schneider and Ingram formulation, over the course of some 75 years elders' political life has segued from being that of Dependents, to becoming Advantaged, and most recently as having to do battle as Contenders.

The Challenges of Issue Framing

The positive political news for today's elders is that they are politically powerful; the more cautionary message is that they had better be powerful given the forces and trends that are confronting them. No longer being helped along by others or helping themselves in a supportive environment, elders now must muster their energies to maintain benefits and prepare for future challenges.

Much of their success will revolve around the seemingly abstract notion of issue framing. When groups can largely control their policy agendas, as seniors long could, issue framing was a nonissue. But when political actors with different and/or opposing agendas are in place, whose issues are placed on the political agenda and how they are framed becomes all important. In recent years, older Americans have faced three such framing challenges that have tested their political mettle.

The first frame to reconfigure understandings of aging policy centered on the notion of intergenerational equity. Beginning in the late-1980s, various commentators argued that public benefits being weighted so heavily in favor of older people was putting an unfair burden on younger people and threatening their very future. Article and book titles such as "The Tyranny of America's Old" (Smith, 1992) and "Meet the Greedy Grandparents" (Chapman, 2003) suggested the rise of some of kind of generational warfare as old and young would be pitted against each other. *Washington Post* columnist Robert Samuelson has captured this framing repeatedly with articles over the decades such as "The withering freedom to govern" (1978), "Why are we in this debt fix? It's the elderly, stupid," (2011) and "We need to stop coddling the elderly" (2013). Most notorious was Alan Simpson's (Co-Chair of the Simpson–Bowles Deficit Reduction Commission of 2010), declaring "people on Social Security milk it to the last degree. . . . We've reached a point now where it's like a milk cow with 310 million tits. Call when you get honest work" (Simpson, 2010).

Two substantive arguments are made in defense of this alleged intergenerational injustice. First, the federal government spends a great deal more money on behalf of elders than it does of children, estimated to be seven times as much (Isaacs, 2009). Second, elders are faring much better than has ever been the case. Poverty among the old has been reduced fourfold between 1959 and 2012, and average incomes increased by 50 percent between 1974 and 2010. Moreover, during this time period, the poverty rate for elders fell, remarkably, below that of children, and middle-aged and younger families had much smaller percentage gains in average income and net wealth than did seniors over that time frame (Interagency Forum on Aging-Related Statistics, 2012; Fry, 2011).

Elder advocates have mounted strong rebuttals to these assertions, arguing most fundamentally that there is overwhelming sociological evidence that generations are tightly bound together and that their relationships are more about reciprocity than opposition (Williamson & Watts-Roy, 1999). In addition, on the empirical side, there is a wealth of evidence that conclusions being drawn from these averaged data are highly misleading. Disparities in wealth and well-being among the old are enormous, with non-Hispanic whites being twice as well-off as Hispanics and blacks, and with the differences between older men and women being nearly as large. Social Security may be an expensive program, but half of elders receive more than three-quarters of their income from the program, and the average annual old-age benefit is roughly $15,000, hardly a king's ransom.

More broadly, advocates argue that the entire generational argument is a Trojan horse, used by conservatives to mask their real concern, which is to cut federal social spending. The harshest critics contend that there is no genuine concern for children in this framing, arguing that if age-related spending were substantially reduced, the savings might well result in tax cuts and increased defense spending rather than being directed toward children (Marmor & Hacker, 1997). Nonetheless, the intergenerational frame has put aging policy in a defensive mode in a range of policy venues.

The second frame directed at aging policy and expenditures is centered on benefit and delivery privatization. Private alternatives speak directly to individual ownership rather than publicly pooled trust funds (as an alternative to Social Security), the promotion of market competition (as an alternative to traditional Medicare), and the sanctity of family values and responsibility (the principal home of long-term care services and supports in addition to the means-tested Medicaid program). Whatever the theoretical benefits of private provision, privatizing old-age benefits would represent an enormous assault on overall federal social programs. It is in this vein, that observers occasionally invoke the words of notorious bank robber Willy Sutton who, when asked why he robbed banks, said "because that's where the money is." With the partial exception of the Part D prescription drug program, the privatization tack has not seriously eroded the federal government's central role in aging policy, but ongoing privatization initiatives—including those associated with the Affordable Care Act and its Medicaid provisions—press directly against elders' policy interests. The abrupt repeal of the so-called CLASS Act to create a federal long-term care insurance program illustrated how difficult it will be to see enactment of new public sector initiatives in aging (*Public Policy & Aging Report*, 2010).

The most recent recasting of aging policy has centered on the alleged "entitlement crisis" that the nation has been facing. Once an arcane budgetary term, the entitlement moniker came to suggest people getting something for nothing or at least something for not enough. And because formal entitlements are indeed free from annual appropriation cycles, they could be argued to be growing uncontrollably. Couple this with the state of the Social Security Trust Funds—money presumably set aside for future retirees but which has long been used for general government purposes in exchange for which the U.S. Treasury now owes the Social Security system billions of dollars—and critics argue that the arrangement has reduced the system to little more than a Ponzi Scheme. Defenders retort that of course Treasury will pay back the borrowed funds as it would to any lender, for example, the Chinese government. Moreover, they argue that a modest tweaking of the existing system will resolve any potential shortfalls on the ongoing flow of payroll tax revenues. But the larger argument here is that yet another framing puts aging benefits in political crosshairs, which was seldom the case previously. In short, aging policy has been extended beyond aging by its challengers. Doing so has imperiled aging advocates from setting their own agenda and promoting what they see to be ongoing needs among older Americans.

Political Dynamics and Population Characteristics

This analysis has focused exclusively on the political dynamics surrounding the impressive expansion of aging policy over the course of several decades. In a colloquial phrasing, there is a widespread assumption that these "rising policy tides have lifted most (older) boats." But, not coincidentally, these framings not only place aging advocates into a defensive posture, but they also bring with them the collateral damage of ignoring the harsh realities facing large numbers of older people. Put differently, the battle over these indisputably large aging programs—totaling well over $1 trillion dollars and being largely universal—loses sight of the modest level of benefits that individual elders actually receive from them. Yes, the $760 billion elders receive from Social Security is a great deal of money, but the $1,300 per month received by any one of them is very difficult to live on.

Data speaking to the remaining and ongoing vulnerabilities faced by many elders are voluminous, a very partial enumeration of which finds:

- 48 percent of seniors are economically vulnerable by virtue of having incomes less than two times the Census Bureau's Supplemental Poverty measure for adults (Gould & Cooper, 2013).
- 31 percent of black women living alone are in poverty compared to 11 percent of white men (Gonyea, 2014).
- 45 percent of working-age households have no dedicated retirement savings (Kingson & Checksfield, 2015).
- 39 percent of non-Hispanic black and 27 percent of Hispanic older households have employer-sponsored pensions or IRA/Keogh retirement accounts in contrast to 72 percent of non-Hispanic whites who have such plans (Mudraziija & Angel, 2014).
- 73 percent of women over 85 are widows compared to 35 percent of men (Federal Inter-Agency Forum on Aging-Related Statistics, 2013).
- 54 percent of people 85 and older living in the community reported having functional limitations inhibiting daily activities (U.S. Congressional Budget Office, 2013).
- 7 of the top 10 causes of death are chronic illnesses, a risk addressed only marginally through the means-tested Medicaid program (Carstensen et al., 2015).
- 10 percent of elders are the victims of physical, mental, financial mistreatment or neglect (Kaplan and Pillemer, 2015).

These are grim indicators of structured inequality among the old, where the predictors of vulnerability are distressingly clear. Yet, on the other end of these distributions are elders who are prosperous, healthy, safe, and secure. The richest 10 percent of individuals aged 65 have incomes averaging $87,000 whereas the income for the poorest 10 percent have ones averaging $7,500 (U.S. Bureau of the Census, 2012), and the longevity of the richest 10 percent (born in 1940) is 35 years compared to 25 years for the poorest 10 percent (Bosworth & Burke, 2014). To say that there are shades of gray marking disparities in elders' well-being does not do justice to the differences; the more apt metaphor would be black and white striations.

These dueling political realities bring us back to the Schneider and Ingram (1993) formulation, which has guided much of the discussion here. In the earliest stage, most elders were in fact dependent; in the second stage most, but certainly not all, elders were advantaged. In the current contender stage, the existing policy template seems to be firmly in place, with critics and advocates engaged in much of a policy standoff.

Should the pressures remain and the plight of many baby boomers headed to retirement become the crisis that some are predicting (Ellis, Munnell, & Eschtruth, 2014), we can speculate that a fourth stage may emerge, one which splits the shifting singularity that has captured elders as a target population over time. This fracturing would result in a large subset of elders being recast—politically, at least—as dependents, understood to be in demonstrable need of support from all quarters, with more prosperous elders able to defend existing benefits in a manner consistent with being seen and behaving as contenders.

The policy consequences of such a bifurcation might take one of two forms, and the struggle between them would be intense. Conservative forces would see the logical policy extension of elders understood as Dependent to be devising or expanding means-tested programs, ones that by definition were directed to the neediest individuals. Such public assistance programs would resemble or, in fact, be extensions of existing programs, such as SSI or Medicaid. But, as public assistance programs, they would be funded out of general revenues and would involve formal income and/or functional means-testing. The liberal alternative would follow along the lines of what Skocpol (1995) has labeled "targeting within universalism" through which broad-based social insurance programs, notably Social Security, would have the benefit formula increasingly tilted toward low-income and/or impaired individuals, but all would remain in the same pool. Either system could generate benefits that were more or less generous or more or less progressive, but the underlying philosophies would be very different. The extension of assistance programs represents public charity, whereas the modification of social insurance programs represents contractual reciprocity, albeit in a form that mixes elements of adequacy with insurance's core element of equity.

However future policy debates may play out, the present analysis suggests that the days in which elders were considered politically as singular and legitimate beneficiaries of public benefits may have ended. This singular understanding has long served elders very well, but for it to continue would require that higher-income elders and organizations representing them be open to more progressive allocations benefitting lower-income compatriots. Income and wealth inequalities mark contemporary and emerging aging populations every bit as much as younger ones, and policy will need to recognize this one way or the other.

References

Ball, R. (2000). *Insuring the essentials*. New York: Century Foundation.

Binstock, R. B. (1972). Interest group liberalism and the politics of aging. *Gerontologist, 12*(3), 265–280.

Binstock, R. B. (1983). The aged as scapegoat. *Gerontologist, 23*(2), 136–143.

Binstock, R. B. (2005). Contemporary politics of old age policies. In R. B. Hudson (Ed.), *New politics of old age policy* (pp. 265–293). Baltimore, MD: Johns Hopkins University Press.

Binstock, R. B. (2012). Older voters and the 2010 US election: Implications for 2012 and beyond? *Gerontologist, 52*(3), 408–417.

Bosworth, B., & Burke, K. (2014). *Differential mortality and retirement benefits in the health and retirement study*. Washington, DC: Brookings Institution.

Brotman, H. (1977). The graying of every 10th American or every 9th American. *Developments in aging* (pp. xv–xxiii). Washington, DC: U.S. Senate Committee on Aging.

Burke, V., & Burke, V. (1974). *Nixon's good deed: Welfare reform*. New York: Columbia University Press.

Campbell, A. L. (2003). *How policies make citizens: Senior political activism and the American welfare state*. Princeton, NJ: Princeton University Press.

Campbell, A. L. (2012). Policy makes mass politics. *Annual review of Political Science*, (15), 333–351.

Carstensen, L., Rosenberger, M., Smith, K., & Modrek, S. (2015). Organizing health in aging societies. *Public Policy & Aging Report, 25*(2): 38–42.

Chapman, S. (2003). Meet the greedy grandparents. *Slate*. http://slate.msn.com/id/2092302/%20

Concord Coalition. (2003, March 19). Seniors still come first in the budget. *Facing Facts Alert, 9*(2).

Derthick, M. (1979). How easy votes on Social Security came to an end. *Public Interest, 54*, 94–105.

Ekerdt, D. J. (Ed.) (1989). Retirement comes of age. *Generations, 13*(2), 5–6.

Ellis, C. D., Munnell, A. H., & Eschtruth, A. D. (2014). *Falling short: The coming retirement crisis and what to do about it*. New York: Oxford University Press.

Employee Benefit Research Institute. (1998). *History of pensions*. www.ebri.org/publications/facts/index.cfm?fa=0398afact

Estes, C. (1979). *The aging enterprise*. San Francisco, CA: Jossey-Bass.

Federal Inter-Agency Forum on Aging-Related Statistics. (2013). *Older Americans: Indicators of well-being*. http://www.agingstats.gov/agingstatsdotnet/Main_Site/Data/2012_Documents/Docs/EntireChartbook.pdf

Fry, R. (2011). The rising gap in economic well-being: The old prosper relative to the young. *Pew Research: Social and demographic trends*. New York: Pew Foundation.

Gonyea, J. G. (2014). The policy challenges of a larger and more diverse oldest-old population. In R. B. Hudson (Ed.), *The new politics of old age policy* (3rd ed., pp. 155–181). Baltimore, MD: Johns Hopkins University Press.

Gordon. L. (1998). *Pitied but not entitled: Single mothers and the history of welfare*. New York: Free Press.

Gould, E., & Cooper, D. (2013). *Financial security of elderly Americans at risk*. Washington, DC: Economic Policy Institute. http://www.epi.org/publication/economic-security-elderly-americans-risk/

Graebner, W. (1980). *A history of retirement: The meaning and function of an American institution*. New Haven, CT: Yale University Press.

Hacker, J. (2006). *The great risk-shift*. New York: Oxford University Press.

Heclo, H. (1988). Generational politics. In J. L. Palmer, T. Smeeding, & B. B. Torrey (Eds.), *The vulnerable* (pp. 381–412). Washington, DC: Urban Institute.

Himelfarb, R. (1995). *Catastrophic politics: The rise and fall of the Medicare Catastrophic Coverage Act of 1988*. State College, Pennsylvania State University Press.

Hudson, R. B. (1978). The graying of the federal budget and its consequences for old-age policy. *Gerontologist, 18*(5), 28–40.

Hudson, R. B., & Strate, J. (1985). Aging and political systems. In R. H. Binstock & E. Shanas (Eds.), *Handbook of aging and the social sciences* (pp. 554–588). New York: Van Nostreand Reinhold.

Isaacs, S. (2009). *Spend on children and the elderly*. http://www.brookings.edu/~/media/research/files/reports/2009/11/05-spending-children-isaacs/1105_children_elderly_isaacs.pdf

Johnson, H. (1980). *In the absence of power*. New York: Viking.

Kaplan, D., & Pillemer, K. (2015). Fulfilling the promise of the Elder Justice Act: Priority goals for the White House Conference on Aging. *Public Policy & Aging Report, 25*(2), 63-66.

Kingson, E. R., & Checksfield, M. (2015. Advancing a retirement income security agenda for all ages. *Public Policy & Aging Report, 25*(2), 47-51.

Lowi, T. J. (1969). *The end of liberalism*. Chicago, IL: W.W. Norton.

Marmor, T. R. (1970). *The politics of Medicare*. Chicago, IL: Aldine.

Marmor, T. R., & Hacker, J. (1997). Ends don't justify the means-test. *Los Angeles Times*. http://articles.latimes.com/1997/jul/14/local/me-12570

Mettler, S. (2005). *Soldiers to citizens: The GI Bill and the making of the greatest generation*. New York: Oxford University Press.

Morgan, K. J. (2014). Medicare: Clients, cost controls, and Congress. In R. B. Hudson (Ed.), *The new politics of old age policy* (3rd ed., pp. 201–220). Baltimore, MD: Johns Hopkins University Press.

Moynihan, D. P. (1973). *The politics of a guaranteed income*. New York: Vintage.

Mudraziija, S., & Angel, J. (2014). Diversity and the economic security of older Americans. In R. B. Hudson (Ed.), *The new politics of old age policy* (3rd ed., pp. 38–154). Baltimore, MD: Johns Hopkins University Press.

Nagourney, A. (2009, September 13). Politics and the age gap. *New York Times*, p.1.

Palmer, J. L., & Sawhill, I. (1984). *The Reagan record*. New York: Ballinger.

Pear. R. (2003, November 18). Medicare plan covering drugs backed by AARP. *New York Times*, A1.

Pierson, P. (1993). When effect becomes cause: Policy feedback and political change. *World Politics, 45*(4), 595–618.

Pressman, J., & Wildavsky, A. (1973). *Implementation: How great expectations in Washington are dashed in Oakland*. Berkeley: University of California Press.

Public Policy & Aging Report (2010). Bringing CLASS to long-term care, *20*(2), 3–42.

Reeves, R. (1975). *A Ford, not a Lincoln*. New York: Harcourt.

Rimlinger, G. (1971). *Welfare policy and industrialization in Europe, America, and Russia*. New York: Wiley.

Rubinow, I. (1934). *The quest for security*. New York: Holt.

Samuelson, R.J. (1978, March 5). The withering freedom to govern. *Washington Post*.

Samuelson, R.J. (2011, July 28). Why are we in this debt fix? It's the elderly, stupid! *Washington Post*. http://www.washingtonpost.com/opinions/why-are-we-in-this-debt-fix-its-the-elderly- stupid/2011/07/28/gIQA08LtfI_story.html

Samuelson, R.J. (2013, November 3). We need to stop coddling the elderly. *Washington Post*. http://www.washingtonpost.com/opinions/robert-j-samuelson-we-need-to-stop-coddling-the-elderly/2013/11/03/4063ebc0–430f-11e3-a624-41d661b0bb78_story.html

Schmidhauser, J.R. (1970). The elderly and politics. In A.M. Hoffman (Ed.), *The daily needs and interests of older people* (pp. 72–89). Springfield, IL: Charles C Thomas.

Schneider, A., & Ingram, H. (1993). Social construction of target populations. *American Political Science Review, 87*, 333–347.

Shearon, M. (1938). The economic status of the aged. *Social Security Bulletin, 1*, 5–16.

Sherman, A.K., & Kolker, A. (1987). *The social bases of politics*. Belmont, CA: Wadsworth.

Simpson, A. (2010). http://money.cnn.com/2010/08/25/news/economy/alan_simpson_fiscal_commission/

Skocpol, T. (1985). Bringing the state back in. In P. Evans, D. Rueschemeyer, & T. Skocpol (Eds.), *American society and politics* (pp. 3–37). New York: Cambridge University Press.

Skocpol, T. (1995). Targeting within universalism: Politically viable strategies to fight poverty in the United States. In T. Skocpol (Ed.), *Social policy in the United States* (pp. 250–274). Princeton, NJ: Princeton University Press.

Smith, D.G. (2002). *Entitlement politics: Medicare and Medicaid 1995–2001*. New York: Aldine.

Smith. L. (1992). The tyranny of America's old. *Fortune, 125*(1), 68–72.

Soss, J. (2000). *Unwanted claims: The politics of participation in the U.S. welfare system*. Ann Arbor: University of Michigan Press.

Soss, J., & Schram, S.F. (2007). A public transformed? Welfare reform as policy feedback. *American Political Science Review, 101*(1), 111–127.

Sundquist, J.L. (1968). *Politics and policy: The Eisenhower, Kennedy, and Johnson years*. Washington, DC: Brookings Institution.

Thrush, G. (2011). The summer of liberal discontent. *Politico*. http://dyn.politico.com/printstory.cfm?uuid=9D50ABF4–22CE-4945-B01B-9CAF16F5C9B8

Treas, J., & Bengtson, V. L. (1982). The demography of mid- and late-life transitions. *Annals of the American Academy of Political and Social Science, 446*, 11–21.

Upp, M. (1982). A look at the economic status of the aged then and now. *Social Security Bulletin, 45*, 16–20.

U.S. Bureau of the Census. (2002). *Current population survey, annual social and economic supplement.* Washington, DC.

U.S. Bureau of the Census. (2012). *Current population survey, annual social and economic supplement*, Table PINC 01.

U.S. Bureau of Economic Analysis. (2012). *U.S. GDP by year since 1929 compared to major events*. Washington, DC: U.S. Department of Commerce.

U.S. Congressional Budget Office. (2002). *Federal spending for the elderly and children.* http://www.cbo.gov/sites/default/files/cbofiles/ftpdocs/23xx/doc2300/fsec.pdf

U.S. Congressional Budget Office. (2013). *The budget and economic outlook, fiscal years 2013 to 2023 and supplementary data.*

U.S. Office of Management and Budget. (2013). *Summary of Receipts, Outlays, Surpluses and Deficits Table 1.1.* http://www.whitehouse.gov/omb/budget/Historicals

Van Atta, D. (1998). *Trust betrayed: Inside the AARP*. New York: Regnery Press.

Vladeck, B. (1980). *Unloving care: The nursing home tragedy*. New York: Basic Books.

Walker, J. (1983). The origins and maintenance of interest groups in America. *American Political Science Review, 77*(2), 390–406.

Weisberg, J. (2005, March 31). Bush's first defeat: The president has lost on social security. *Slate*. www.slate.com/id/2115141

Weaver, R. K. (1988). *Automatic government: The politics of indexation*. Washington, DC: Brookings Institution.

Williamson, J. B., & Watts-Roy, D. (1999). Framing the generational equity debate. In J. B. Williamson, D. Watts-Roy, & E. R. Kingson (Eds.), *The generational equity debate* (pp. 3–37). New York: Columbia University Press.

Witte, E. (1962). *Development of the Social Security Act*. Madison: University of Wisconsin Press.

Index

About the Editors and Contributors

Editors

Madonna Harrington Meyer, PhD, is chair of sociology, Laura J. and L. Douglas Meredith Professor of Teaching Excellence, and faculty associate of the Aging Studies Institute, at Syracuse University. She is co-editor, with Ynesse Abdul-Malak, of the forthcoming *Grandparenting in the United States*. She is author of *Grandmothers at Work: Juggling Families and Jobs*, winner of the 2014 GSA Kalish Book Award. She is co-author with Pamela Herd of *Market Friendly or Family Friendly? The State and Gender Inequality in Old Age*, winner of the 2008 GSA Kalish Book Award. She is also editor of *Care Work: Gender, Labor, and the Welfare State*.

Elizabeth A. Daniele, MS, is a PhD student and fellow in sociology at Syracuse University. She is a co-editor of *Student Involvement and Academic Outcomes: Implications for Diverse Student Populations* (2015). She also co-authored a chapter about diversity in American graduate education in *International Perspectives in Higher Education Admission Policy: A Reader* (2015). She has a BA from Smith College and an MS in higher education administration from the University of Rochester.

Contributors

Ynesse Abdul-Malak, MA, MPH, is a doctoral candidate in sociology at Syracuse University. Her work focuses on understanding how social structures impact the aging processes of individuals over the life course with a special emphasis on U.S. Caribbean immigrants. She is the coeditor of *Grandparenting in the U.S.* (in press). She is currently coauthoring a book manuscript, *Grandparenting Children with Disabilities*.

Vern L. Bengtson, PhD, is research professor in the Edward R. Royal Institute on Aging at the University of Southern California. A Past President of the Gerontological Society of America, he has published 17 books and over 250 articles in the sociology of aging and family sociology. He is author of *Families and Faith: How Religion Is (and Isn't) Passed Down Across Generations* (2013), winner of the 2015 GSA Kalish Book Award, and editor (with Richard Settersten) of the *Handbook of Theories of Aging* (2016).

Heidemarie Blumenthal, PhD, is an assistant professor in the Department of Psychology at the University of North Texas. She is the director of the Teen St. A.R. Laboratory at the University of North Texas; as a developmental psychopathologist, her work reflects an intersection between traditional developmental and clinical domains.

Evan Chartier, BA, is a Colgate University graduate where he majored in sociology, anthropology, and women's studies. Evan is also a student affairs professional, social justice educator, and is currently pursuing a master's degree in global studies and international relations.

Marguerite DeLiema, PhD, is a postdoctoral research fellow at the Stanford Center on Longevity. She received her doctorate in gerontology from the University of Southern California in 2015 and has authored numerous publications on elder abuse and neglect. Her current work at Stanford University centers on measuring the cost and prevalence of financial fraud in the United States, with a particular focus on protecting vulnerable adults from exploitation. She works with fraud investigatory agencies and financial institutions to develop fraud prevention strategies.

Sarah Desai, MA, is a PhD student in sociology at the University at Buffalo, SUNY. She coauthored a chapter, "Planning for Old Age," in the *Handbook of the Sociology of Aging* (2011). She has a BS from Houghton College and an MA in sociology from the University at Buffalo.

Nicole Etherington is a PhD candidate in the Department of Sociology at the University of Western Ontario. Her dissertation research focuses on gender and well-being over the life course, with particular interests in intersectionality, childhood poverty, and the cumulative effects of disadvantage in women's lives. Her recent work on the intersections of race and gender in shaping women's psychosocial resources and subsequent health outcomes is available in *Women & Health*. Nicole's commitment to gender- and feminist-based research has been recognized with an Ontario Women's Health Scholars Award.

Bert Hayslip Jr., PhD, is Regents Professor Emeritus at the University of North Texas. He is a fellow of the American Psychological Association, the Gerontological Society of America, and The Association for Gerontology in Higher Education. An associate editor of *Experimental Aging Research* and of *Developmental Psychology,* his coauthored books include *Emerging Perspectives on Resilience in Adulthood and Later Life* (2012), *Resilient Grandparent Caregivers: A Strengths-Based Perspective* (2012), *Adult Development and Aging* (2011), and *Parenting the Custodial Grandchild* (2008). He is co-PI on an NINR-funded project exploring interventions to improve the functioning of grandparent caregivers.

Robert B. Hudson, PhD, is professor of social policy at Boston University School of Social Work, where he directs the Lowy-GEM Program in Gerontological Studies. He has served as editor-in-chief of *Public Policy & Aging Report*, the quarterly publication of the National Academy on an Aging Society since 1996. The third edition of his volume *The New Politics of Old Age Policy* was published in 2014. He received his doctorate in political science from the University of North Carolina at Chapel Hill.

Meika Loe, PhD, is professor of sociology and women's studies and director of the Women's Studies Program at Colgate University in New York, where she teaches courses on aging, gender, culture, and medicine. She is the author of *Aging Our Way: Lessons for Living from 85 and Beyond* (2011) and *The Rise of Viagra: How the Little Blue Pill Changed Sex in America* (2004). She is coeditor (with Kelly Joyce) of *Technogenarians: Studying Health and Illness through an Aging, Science, and Technology Lens* (2010).

Andrew S. London, PhD, is professor of sociology and affiliated with the Aging Studies Institute, Center for Policy Research, and Institute for Veterans and Military Families at Syracuse University. His research focuses on the health, care, and well-being of stigmatized and vulnerable populations. His research on veterans is published in *Archives of Sexual Behavior*; *Disability and Health Journal*; *Journal of Aging and Health*; *Journal of Family Issues*; *Journal of Gerontology, Social Sciences*; *Journal of Marriage and Family*; *Population Research and Policy Review*; *Research on Aging*; and *Sociology & Social Welfare*. With Janet M. Wilmoth, he edited *Life-Course Perspectives on Military Service* (2013).

Jan E. Mutchler, PhD, is professor of gerontology and director of the Center for Social and Demographic Research on Aging at the University of Massachusetts Boston. Recent publications include "The Elder Economic

Security Standard Index: A New Indicator for Evaluating Economic Security in Later Life" (*Social Indicators Research*, 2015) and "The Role of Aging and Disability Resource Centers in Serving Adults Aging with Intellectual Disabilities and Their Families: Findings from Seven States" (*Journal of Aging and Social Policy*, forthcoming). She is the research lead on the Age-Friendly Boston Initiative, a collaboration with the City of Boston and AARP Massachusetts.

Tanya Sanabria is a PhD student in sociology at University of California, Irvine. She is currently a NLSY Postsecondary Research Network fellow. Her research interests focus on the consequences of failure in education, including impacts on marriage and family, through a life-course perspective. She has authored a related entry in *The Sage Encyclopedia of Economics and Society* (2015) and coauthored an entry about Asian for-profit after school programs (termed "hagwons") in *Asian American Society: An Encyclopedia* (2014). She received her BA from California State Polytechnic University, Pomona.

Ariel Sherry, BA, is a graduate from Colgate University where she majored in psychology and religion. She is an entrepreneur focusing on innovation in eldercare. She is currently working on a venture she founded called Age Together.

Michael Silverstein, MD, MPH, is clinical professor at the University of Washington School of Public Health. He previously was Washington State Health Officer, director of Policy for the U.S. Occupational Safety and Health Administration, director of Washington State OSHA and assistant director for Occupational Health and Safety with the United Automobile Workers Union. He is board certified in occupational medicine and practiced occupational medicine with degrees from Harvard, Stanford, and the University of Michigan. He also chaired the National Advisory Committee on Occupational Safety and Health and served on several Institute of Medicine panels.

Ceara R. Somerville, MS, is a PhD student in Gerontology at the University of Massachusetts Boston. She is a McCormack Scholar in the McCormack Graduate School of Policy and Global Studies at UMass Boston and has spent time as both president and treasurer of the Gamma Upsilon chapter of Sigma Phi Omega—the national academic and professional honor society in gerontology. She completed her undergraduate studies at Salem State University in 2013, where she received her BS in mathematics with minors in physics, English, and education studies. She recently completed her MS in gerontology at UMass Boston.

Debra Street, PhD, is professor and chair of sociology at the State University of New York at Buffalo. She is editor, with Áine Ní Léime, Sarah Vickerstaff, Clary Krekula, and Wendy Loretto of the forthcoming book *Gender and Extended Working Lives: Cross National Perspectives* and with Jay Ginn and Sarah Arber, edited *Women, Work and Pensions: International Issues and Prospects* (2001). Street is the recipient of the Janice L. Moritz Distinguished Lecture Award (UB Gender Institute) and the SUNY Chancellor's Award for Excellence in Teaching.

Judith Treas, PhD, is professor of sociology and director of the Center for Demographic and Social Analysis at the University of California, Irvine. Her latest book, coedited with Jacqueline Scott and Martin Richards, is the *Wiley-Blackwell Companion to the Sociology of Families* (2015). The ASA Section on Aging and the Life Course honored her with its Matilda White Riley Distinguished Scholar Award. It also recognized her 2015 *American Sociological Review* paper with Anja-Kristin Abendroth and Matt Huffman ("The Parity Penalty in Life Course Perspective: Motherhood and Occupational Status in 13 European Countries") with the Outstanding Publication Award.

Rebecca Wang, MA, is a doctoral candidate in sociology at Syracuse University, where she is also a graduate research associate at the Aging Studies Institute and Center for Policy Research. Rebecca holds a BA in sociology from the University of California, Irvine, and an MA in sociology from San Jose State University. Rebecca has coauthored publications in *Public Policy and Aging Report* with Merril Silverstein, PhD, and *Wiley-Blackwell Encyclopedia of Sociology*, 2nd Edition (forthcoming) with Janet M. Wilmoth, PhD.

Andrea E. Willson, PhD, is an associate professor and director of the Centre for Population, Aging and Health at the University of Western Ontario. Her research interests include studies of social inequality over the life course, particularly social disparities in health. Her ongoing research includes an investigation of health inequality over the life course and its transmission across generations. Her recent work has appeared in *Advances in Life Course Research* and *International Sociology*.

Janet M. Wilmoth, PhD, is professor of sociology and director of the Aging Studies Institute at Syracuse University. Professor Wilmoth has authored of over 50 articles and book chapters and coedited *Gerontology: Perspectives and Issues* (2nd and 3rd Editions) and *Life Course Perspectives on Military Service*. Her research examines older adult migration, living arrangements, and health status, and explores how military service shapes various life-course outcomes related to marriage and family, economic well-being, and disability.

Jeanette M. Zoeckler, MPH, is a PhD student of social science in the Maxwell School of Citizenship and Public Affairs at Syracuse University. She was lead author of a report entitled "Low-Wage Work in Syracuse: Worker Health in the New Economy," published by the Occupational Health Clinical Centers, Department of Family Medicine, SUNY Upstate Medical University, Syracuse, New York (2014). She was also lead author of an article, "Predictors for Return to Work for those with Occupational Respiratory Disease: Clinical and Structural Factors," published in the *American Journal of Industrial Medicine* (2013).